THINGS THAT MATTER

Special Objects in Our Stories as We Age

Edited by William L. Randall and Matte Robinson

Many of us have particular things in our lives – photographs, paintings, old letters, books, furniture, jewellery, or clothing – that hold special meaning for us. Often, they correspond to pivotal memories and can be central to our sense of self and our life narratives, all the more so as we age. *Things That Matter* sheds important light on the intricate intertwining of mementos with stories – and vice versa – in most people's lives.

The book explores the significance of cherished objects within the life stories of nine participants in a qualitative study of the links between reminiscence and resilience in later life. The researchers who conducted the study represent a variety of fields, including gerontology, social work, ministry, nursing, literature, and education. The book details how life stories can be fraught with a wide range of insights and questions from the memories that get stirred up as people embark on the process of "life review" prompted by the challenges and changes of aging. Shedding light on the complex emotional, psychological, and spiritual findings of the study, *Things That Matter* ultimately reveals the intricacy of personal narrative and the incredible ways in which things and stories are interwoven in our lives over time.

WILLIAM L. RANDALL is a professor emeritus in the Department of Gerontology at St. Thomas University.

MATTE ROBINSON is an associate professor and chair of English at St. Thomas University.

Things That Matter

Special Objects in Our Stories as We Age

EDITED BY WILLIAM L. RANDALL
AND MATTE ROBINSON

UNIVERSITY OF TORONTO PRESS
Toronto Buffalo London

Toronto Buffalo London
utorontopress.com

ISBN 978-1-4875-0665-0 (cloth) ISBN 978-1-4875-3460-8 (EPUB)
ISBN 978-1-4875-2447-0 (paper) ISBN 978-1-4875-3459-2 (PDF)

Library and Archives Canada Cataloguing in Publication

Title: Things that matter : special objects in our stories as we age / edited by William L. Randall and Matte Robinson.
Names: Randall, William Lowell, 1950– editor. | Robinson, Matte, 1976– editor.
Description: Includes bibliographical references and index.
Identifiers: Canadiana (print) 20230495699 | Canadiana (ebook) 20230495737 | ISBN 9781487524470 (paper) | ISBN 9781487506650 (cloth) | ISBN 9781487534592 (PDF) | ISBN 9781487534608 (EPUB)
Subjects: LCSH: Aging. | LCSH: Personal belongings. | LCSH: Narrative inquiry (Research method)
Classification: LCC HQ1061 .T45 2024 | DDC 305.26 – dc23

Cover design: Hannah Gaskamp
Cover image: Cora Woolsey

We wish to acknowledge the land on which the University of Toronto Press operates. This land is the traditional territory of the Wendat, the Anishnaabeg, the Haudenosaunee, the Métis, and the Mississaugas of the Credit First Nation.

University of Toronto Press acknowledges the financial support of the Government of Canada, the Canada Council for the Arts, and the Ontario Arts Council, an agency of the Government of Ontario, for its publishing activities.

Canada Council for the Arts Conseil des Arts du Canada

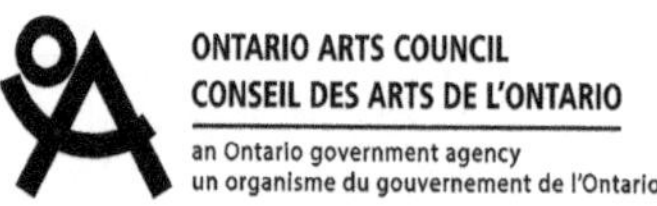

Funded by the Government of Canada | Financé par le gouvernement du Canada | Canada

Contents

Preface

The story of this book is simple enough: we kept talking and talking about *things*. In poring over interview transcripts for the regular meetings of our research team, we kept noticing that the older people who had been interviewed made reference, if only in passing, to particular objects that for one reason or another held particular importance for them, whether or not they themselves had consciously reflected on why this was so. The place of such objects in our participants' lives – or, more accurately, the light that they shed on how they were *storying* their lives – became the focus of our most spirited conversations. It's out of these conversations that this book took shape.

Interestingly enough, the original study on which the book is based wasn't about things at all – as we'll be explaining more in Chapter 1. We didn't explicitly set out to learn what sorts of objects older people "cherish" in their lives, and why (see, e.g., Sherman, 1991b). Instead, as a contribution to thinking in the area known as "narrative gerontology" (Kenyon et al., 2001, 2011), our study was aimed at understanding the nature of resilience in later life, specifically *narrative* resilience. Our guiding hypothesis was that older adults who have what could be called "good strong stories" about their lives (Randall, 2013) will implicitly bring more internal resources to the several challenges of later life, more sense of meaning, purpose, and self-worth. To test this hypothesis and thus get clearer on what qualities might characterize a "strong" story, we put on a series of three one-day workshops one month apart in the winter and spring of 2015 that were designed to assist attendees in expanding and examining their life stories to increasing degrees of depth. Before the series began and after it ended, we interviewed a selection of those who had signed up for it in order to determine what impact, if any, the workshops might have on their self-understanding overall. Our aim, naive though it might seem, was to demonstrate that intentionally exploring our stories can lead to *strengthening* our stories, and thus to enhancing our resilience (Randall, 2020).

During our discussions, however, we increasingly realized that in order to understand how our participants go about storying their lives – and how the workshops themselves broadened, deepened, or even redirected that process – we had to take into consideration the things to which, deliberately or otherwise, they referred. All of this set us on a rather different course. Hence this book. It's still very much a contribution to the field of narrative gerontology, but its exploration of things as portals onto the intricacies of people's storyworlds in later life offers, we believe, a more nuanced sense of the depths and dynamics of those worlds and therefore makes it a uniquely fruitful form of narrative inquiry.

There's another and related reason, though, that this book is unique. It concerns how each of us has looked at the interview "data" through the lens of our own distinct stories, which is inevitable in narrative research of any kind, of course, where some sort of privileged, objective analysis is largely out of the question. That is to say, we found ourselves identifying, often quite intensely, with particular participants, and with the role that the things they singled out appeared to play in their understanding of their lives, whether or not that role was obvious to them themselves. In Part 2 of the book, this led to our engaging in a mode of narrative inquiry that is especially autobiographical – or "autoethnographic" – in nature, insofar as we acknowledged honestly how *our* stories and *their* stories intersect.

We'll be saying more about this intersection near the end of Chapter 1, where we outline the structure of the book as a whole and our respective roles in writing it. In the meantime, it needs admitting that, as a team, we are a rather mixed bag. Though working on this book bound us together like a little family almost, we nonetheless hail from different disciplines, represent different generations, strike different voices on the page, and have differing approaches to thinking about things and stories alike – differences that stand out more clearly in the bios that we've included in Appendix 1. Rather than a weakness, however, we see these differences as a strength of the book, especially given the unique nature of the three huge topics that we're seeking to bring together in it: *ageing, narrative,* and *things.*

First of all, ageing itself is an intrinsically interdisciplinary experience, which means that gerontology has to draw on a wide range of academic fields in order to appreciate the full complexity of its central subject. Put simply, we age not just biologically but biographically as well, not to mention cognitively, emotionally, socially, and spiritually. More to the point, we age in all of these ways at once.

As for narrative, it too is an inherently interdisciplinary topic, as is obvious from the variety of fields into which the so-called narrative turn has increasingly spread. It straddles the border between, on the one hand, literary theory and the humanities in general and, on the other, the social sciences, plus medicine too – witness the advent of "narrative medicine" (Charon, 2006). Rightly or wrongly, narrative itself has become something of a "thing." Even the media bandies the term ever more freely about: "The narrative coming out of the White House this week has been that ..." In this book, of course, we'll be drawing on a narrative perspective in relation primarily to ageing, but it needs noting that scholars have been reflecting on the narrative dimensions of virtually every grand topic there is to reflect on, from time (Ricoeur, 1981), to history (Danto, 1985), to consciousness (Fireman et al., 2003), to emotion (Habermas, 2019), to, well, life (Schiff et al., 2017). That said, there are many different ways of engaging with narrative ideas, let alone different ways of defining "narrative" itself (see, e.g., Reissman & Speedy, 2007, p. 428). Moreover, there are different labels to apply to what it is we're doing on the ground, whether, for instance, it's "narrative research," "narrative analysis," "narrative practice," or "narrative inquiry" – the term that we feel best captures what we're doing in this book and that we'll be saying more about in Chapter 1. This very variety, while it may be frustrating to some, accords well, of course, with the nature of stories themselves. A story is never "about" any one theme alone, be it love, courage, greed, or the like. It is about numerous themes at once, all weaving in and out of one another so seamlessly that it becomes impossible to treat them separately, one theme at a time.

Regarding things ... well, they're everywhere and they're of every kind. Objects, if you will, make great subjects, because everyone has things they want to keep, things they can't forget, things they desire, and things they hold onto for others. And more and more professions revolve directly around them. Scientists study things, inventors invent things, movers move things. Retailers sell people things, and realtors sell people houses big enough to put all their things into. Life transition experts (and we have one on our team!) help people sort through their things, while lawyers deal with the dispersal of things once those people have died. As we'll see in Chapter 3, "thing theorists" theorize about things, while media moguls dream up shows about people who hoard things, or about old things lurking in our attics that might be worth a mint, or weird things buried in the mud behind our houses that could be the clues to unsolved crimes. And so on and so forth. In fact, the fields in which research on things is carried out run the gamut from archeology to architecture, anthropology to sociology, philosophy to linguistics, and marketing to interior design ... the list goes on.

As for what we're doing with things in this book, they serve as our lenses. In other words, it's our participants' stories, or their *storying*, that is our primary focus, and that we're enlisting their things to peer into, not the other way around. This peering, though, has taken us into a bewildering array of topics, most if not all of them hopelessly intertwined. These range from reminiscence to resilience, biographical ageing to autobiographical memory, and legacy to lost possible selves, plus numerous more topics that we'll be touching on in Chapter 2. It's our hope that the three-part structure of the book – from the realm of *theory*, to that of *research* into the meanings of things in our participants' stories, to the world of front-line *practice*, with people, their stories, and their things – will allow readers to reflect from a multiple angles upon the incredible complexity of personal narrative, especially in later life. To repeat, though, *things* is only one lens to look through to appreciate that complexity. Yet it provides a unique means of teasing out the dynamics and enigmas of the narrative self in later life. It's based on this conviction that we offer this book, *Things That Matter*.

Those to whom we offer it include not only researchers and students in gerontology and allied fields, such as health care, counselling, or social work, but anyone who works with older adults in (as we say) a front-line kind of way. By this we mean nurses, doctors, personal support workers, and therapists of various sorts, as well as lawyers, realtors, and retailers too, not to mention life transition professionals (again, we have one on our team), plus spiritual leaders and spiritual carers, whatever the tradition in which they may be rooted. We mean anyone and everyone who interacts with older adults in one fashion or another, who is alert to the subtleties and secrets that can run through their stories, and who seeks to honour those stories in more insightful and, so to speak, *inside-ful* ways. Not only, though, does the book bring together research and practice. By employing a narrative perspective, which as we say is inherently cross-disciplinary in nature, it seeks to bridge the gap between the social sciences and the humanities, all in the service of appreciating the full range of dimensions – including its aesthetic or "poetic" ones – that we believe ageing involves (Randall, 2023).

By way of acknowledgements, *Things That Matter* could not have come into being without the support of numerous colleagues besides those of us who have been involved directly in its writing. Given that the project from which it emerged has been underway since 2011, the list of people we need to note includes several former members of the Centre for Interdisciplinary Research on Narrative, or CIRN, at St. Thomas University, or STU, our home institution. Chief among these would be Dolores Furlong who, before she retired as professor of nursing at the University of New Brunswick, participated in all of our team meetings and often took the lead in presenting our findings at conferences hither and yon. Then there is Elizabeth McKim, professor emerita of English at STU, who has worked closely with Bill over the years in articulating a "poetics of growing old" (Randall & McKim, 2008), who has co-edited with him a journal called *Narrative Works*, and who remained a vital member of CIRN until she, too, retired in 2019.

Included as well are fellow STU professors Sue McKenzie-Mohr, Michelle Lafrance, and Gül Çalişkan, all of whom – Sue especially – immensely enriched our discussions of how our participants go about storying their lives. Christa Blizzard, a student research assistant, conducted all but one of the interviews for Phase 1 of the project (which we'll be explaining in Chapter 1), and so we're profoundly grateful to her. But we're grateful as well to an array of STU undergraduates in both social work and gerontology who helped with our analyses, Shania Arsenault especially, plus a parade of visiting scholars to STU and to CIRN whose presence and expertise we heartily welcomed when puzzling over our interview data. Most notable are Rodrigo Serrat of the University of Barcelona, Bodil Hansen Blix of the University of Trømso, and Charlotte Berendonk of the University of Alberta.

We are deeply grateful, too, to MindCare NB and to the STU Research Office for financial support early on in our research, as well as to the Social Sciences and Humanities Research Council of Canada (SSHRC) for the in-kind support it has provided to CIRN through the tenure of Clive Baldwin, a core member of our team, as Canada Research Chair in Narrative Studies. In a similar vein, we have valued the assistance of Lauren Eagle from STU's Research Office who has been so, so helpful in aiding our research endeavours in a myriad of ways. We are indebted as well, of course, to Meg Patterson, our editor at University of Toronto Press and a supporter of the ideas that we'll be exploring in this book from the time that we first pitched them to her. Last, but hardly least, we are indebted to our participants themselves: the nine women and men whom we'll be discussing in detail in Part 2 of the book. Unbeknownst to them, they inspired us to set forth on this intriguing – and surprising – adventure into the things that matter in the stories of our lives.

One final comment: most of the material that follows was either composed or revised in the middle of a global pandemic, the story of which – at the time that we're writing this preface at least – is still unfolding. And we each have any number of narratives about our experience of living through it. In everyone's story going forward, in other words, there is bound to be a chapter called "COVID-19." But even with vaccines being distributed and communities reopening in ways that seem more or less normal, new variants are on the loose in several corners, and none of us knows quite when or whether the story will end. Our relationships both to the people in our lives and to the things and objects – the *stuff* – around which our lives revolve could be affected forever. Huge questions hang in the air. Are we moving into a world where greed and envy and protectiveness, and the whole mad scramble to amass as much stuff as we possibly can, will intensify all the more? Or perhaps into a chastened, down-sized world where we value one another more than ever before, where we truly appreciate the "little things" in life – a kind word, a sunset, a flower in bloom – and where we cherish whomever and whatever we have? We cherish the friendships and connections we've made during the making of this book, and we gratefully thank all our family members and friends who have supported us. Of those many who are dear to us, we single out Cora Woolsey, a serious thinker about things, who took time out of a busy schedule to produce the painting that graces our book's cover.

PART ONE

Theoretical Meanderings

1 Why Things That Matter? The Context, the Project, and the Book

WILLIAM L. RANDALL

The biography of objects is about their place in the lives of the people who have owned, used, and lived with them. Something of their selves, their personal identity, and their social identity becomes embedded in the object and writing about it begins to bring out their stories – the life of the object becomes a metaphor for those human lives.

– Tim Dant (2001, p. 26)

The Context

To set the stage for this chapter and, in a sense, for the book as a whole, I will begin by sharing a bit about what (at the time of writing) has been happening in my own little life, my own little story.

Six months into my seventieth year, my body has been sending me unsettling messages – a new ache here, a fresh twinge there, a troubling test result or two – that are heightening my awareness of how at long last I am getting *old*, and how I need to make some major life changes ... before it's too late. So it is, then, that I recently sold the house where I had lived for over twenty-three years – literally, the single most consistent "thing" in my life throughout that whole time, and one that's definitely rich in stories! – and moved into an apartment that, hopefully, will see me into my eighties. The past four months have found me pawing through decades of accumulated stuff – papers, books, furniture, clothes, tools, photographs, and just plain junk – and deciding how to strip my world down to what will fit neatly into a two-bedroom flat. It's been a massive exercise in what gerontologists call "socioemotional selectivity" (Carstensen et al., 1999). And all of this has been happening while I'm embarking on the final year of a four-year retirement trajectory out of a faculty position that I've held for twenty years.

On multiple levels, then, I feel myself to be on the verge of what Sarah Lawrence-Lightfoot (2009) labels "the third chapter" of my life-narrative, with whatever adventures, positive or negative, that chapter may turn out to hold. And I'm sensing energies surging inside of me that are pushing me to engage in the very sort of *storywork* that I've been touting in various publications and presentations as essential, not just to *getting* old, but (as I'm fond of saying) to *growing* old in a positive, proactive manner.

This convergence of changes that I'm living through personally could not be more coincidental, even synchronistic, with respect to this book, or at least to my own role in writing it. For while many strands of thinking and theory weave their way through the book, we've been inspired to write it by two intriguing trends – trends that ultimately have to do with practice more than theory and are, so to speak, where the rubber meets the road as far as narrative gerontology is concerned. In a real sense, these constitute the context to which the book speaks, form the backdrop against which we've conceived it, and point to the issues that it seeks to address.

The first trend, which we'll be saying more about in Part 3, is the sprouting up here and there of all sorts of formal and informal groups of older adults who are keen to write the stories of their lives so that they can then share with their offspring and others their unique legacy of experience and wisdom. Along with this is the emergence of books, and even businesses, that guide people in preparing and publishing their memoirs. The "personal history industry" is what it's been called by Anita Hecht and Mary O'Brien Tyrell (2007), who, interestingly, speak of life stories as *heirlooms* – as precious objects in themselves. A second and related trend is the rise of a class of entrepreneurs, like the now-legendary Marie Kondo, who aid older people in "downsizing" and "decluttering" – in deciding what to keep and what to cull – as they prepare to make the transition from a house to an apartment, or a retirement home to a nursing home. Taken together, these two trends reflect complex cognitive processes (like autobiographical reasoning and integrative reminiscence), plus intricate emotional dynamics (like melancholy, nostalgia, and regret), that older people can easily experience, on however subliminal a level. We'll get a more first-hand sense of this complexity in Chapter 15, but in the meantime what both trends have in common is homing in on the things that really matter in older people's lives.

Our aim in this book is to delve deeper into such processes and dynamics by focussing on nine older adults who participated in a series of life-writing workshops as part of a larger project that has been looking into the nature of resilience in later life, one at which we've been labouring for a decade or more. In particular, our aim is to look at the significance of specific things – old photographs, love letters from long ago, items of jewellery, pieces of clothing or furniture, and assorted souvenirs – that these individuals mentioned in the course of the interviews done with them by team member Jennifer Estey (more on her shortly). In other words, we did not set out intentionally to study the place of so-called cherished objects in older people's lives (see, e.g., Sherman, 1991b), which is a worthy endeavour and one I'll be saying more about towards the end of Chapter 2. With no prompting or probing whatever from Jennifer herself, our participants referred to such things entirely on their own, whether or not "cherished" is a word they themselves would have used to describe them. The more we thought about these things, though, whether "cherished" by the participant or simply "important"– important enough for them to mention, at least – the more it seemed to us that they served as symbols of memories, or as metaphors for themes, that were in some way central to that individual's story, that were "identity markers" (Ferraro et al., 2011), entry-points into their distinctive storyworlds. We'll be looking at how their things and their stories are entwined, or more accurately perhaps, how their things can offer pivotal clues as to how they are *storying* their lives (Kenyon et al., 2011).

Throughout these investigations we'll draw on concepts that figure frequently in treatments of the psychology of ageing yet are seldom really linked: concepts such as generativity, autobiographical reasoning, and post-formal thought, all of which, and more, I'll be saying something about in Chapter 2. The perspective from which we're operating here, however, which is primarily a *narrative* one, enables the weaving together of these concepts in ways that present a more intriguing and inviting picture of later life than do prevailing paradigms of ageing. Sadly, the latter implicitly portray it in biomedical terms as, at base, a tragic trajectory towards decrepitude and death, as a "narrative of decline" (Gullette 2004, p. 28). It is in the service of advancing a "counter-story" (Nelson, 2001; Phoenix & Smith, 2011) to this negative narrative of what ageing entails that we embarked on the project from which this book has sprung.

The Project

The road of research often leads to surprises. That's certainly been our experience here. Our intention starting out, in what we refer to now as Phase 1 of our project as a whole, was to investigate the hypothesis that *resilience* – defined as the capacity to cope with adversity and to keep growing through it (or despite it) – is bound up with the sorts of stories that we tell about our lives. Very briefly, our hypothesis has been that human beings are hermeneutical beings. We are makers of meaning

(Reker & Chamberlain, 2000). Moreover, our main means of making it is by composing and communicating stories about the events in our lives, and about our lives as a whole. These stories that we tell (to both others and ourselves) are, in effect, the stories we *are* (Randall, 2014). With advancing age, however, our life stories or narrative identities can, for an array of reasons, be increasingly under threat. They can face a range of serious narrative challenges, among them narrative foreclosure, which I'll say more about in Chapter 2. So then, the stronger the stories people can tell and live, our thinking has gone, then the more "inner resources" they will bring to such challenges, thus the higher their level of resilience (Dubovská et al., 2016).

To test this hypothesis we recruited 110 community-dwelling persons aged sixty-five and over who, in 2011, were living in or around the city of Fredericton, New Brunswick, Canada. Fredericton is the home town of our home base, St. Thomas University (STU) and its Centre for Interdisciplinary Research on Narrative (CIRN), with which all of us are affiliated. All of those recruited into the study, officially entitled "Coping and Adaptation in Later Life," then completed the Connor-Davidson Resilience Scale, or CDRS for short (Connor & Davidson, 2003). The CDRS consists of twenty-five positively worded statements to which participants indicate their degree of agreement on a scale from 0 to 4, for a total possible score, therefore, of 100 out of 100. Sample statements include "I like challenges," "I am able to adapt when changes occur," and "I can deal with whatever comes my way."

The next step was to select fifteen individuals who scored highest on the scale (90–100), fifteen who scored lowest (30–70), and fifteen who scored in the middle (70–90), for a total of forty-five. We then interviewed each of them in a semi-structured manner about their life story in general, their experiences of adversity in particular, and their views concerning the future. All but one of these interviews were conducted by the same interviewer, a female student research assistant. Moreover, all forty-five transcripts were analysed by our multidisciplinary team – representing gerontology, sociology, social work, education, nursing, and English – in terms of the kinds of concepts and criteria that I will be outlining in Chapter 2.

In general, most of our interviewees confirmed our first hypothesis, namely that thick stories correspond to high scores, and thin stories to low ones (Randall et al., 2015). That said, some high scorers told us decidedly thin stories while some low scorers told us remarkably thick ones, where "thick" means, for instance, rich in detail, colourful in dialogue ("I said, she said"), and abundant in stories, long and short, about their lives. This anomaly pushed us to entertain the possibility that the thin stories of the high scorers could be due, in part, to their personal narratives being embedded in larger narrative structures with which they most identify (e.g., those of their family, community, religion, etc.), or by which their identity is subsumed, or in which, between the lines, they find their central source of meaning (Furlong et al., 2015).

To the extent, though, that our hypothesis held – that is, the thicker the story, the greater the resilience – we were emboldened to propose a type of resilience that, to date, has largely been missing from the list of factors most often identified as feeding resilience in later life, such as positive mental health, social engagement and social support, cognitive acuity, financial security, and physical activity. We called it "narrative resilience." In fact, we continue to be convinced of its reality, and of the possibility of fostering it in people's lives through some form or another of what might be called "narrative care" (Kenyon & Randall, 2015).

In Phase 2 of our project, then, we set forth to test the corollary hypothesis, that narrative resilience can be enhanced by assisting people to tell more expanded, more layered, more nuanced, more self-reflective stories about their lives. To that end, we took a group of thirty-eight people, aged fifty-five-plus, through a series of three one-day workshops in the winter and spring of 2015. As Deborah Carr will explain in more detail in Chapter 14, these events were deliberately sequenced to introduce participants to techniques and strategies for exploring the stories of their lives in progressively more extensive and intensive ways from one workshop to the next, with take-home exercises for them to work on in between. Of these thirty-eight individuals, fourteen volunteered to be interviewed at length, before the first workshop and after the last, about their experiences of the workshops themselves and about how, in general, writing their stories affects the way they think and feel about their lives. They also agreed to write out one story in particular that they felt held special meaning for them. Indeed, the second interview began by asking them to comment on the process of *writing* this story in contrast with just telling it in conversation – their response typically being that it took them deeper into the original experience or helped them to see it and interpret it in novel kinds of ways.

Important to note here is that, whereas in Phase 1 we invited participants to tell us the story of their life as a whole, we did not do this with participants in either interview in Phase 2. Rather, we asked them a range of questions concerning their experience of storytelling in general and of writing and reflecting on the stories of their own lives during and after the workshops (see Appendix 2). Yet they still ended up sharing with us the main outlines of their life stories, and possibly lots more that they might not have shared otherwise, given the tenor of the questions and the gently probing manner in which Jennifer asked them. While their stories tended to come out in piecemeal fashion amid their answers, the main turning points, episodes, and chapters were discernible all the same.

It's important to note here as well, though, that participants in Phase 2 also completed four psychometric instruments – pre- and post-, as it were – by way of providing us with some sense not just of their level of resilience (e.g., the CDRS) but also of their sense of meaning in life, their overall well-being, and their degree of "narrative foreclosure" (Bohlmeijer et al., 2011, 2014; Freeman, 2000). Both the workshops and the interviews, we hypothesized, would constitute deepening, thickening experiences that would result in significantly higher scores, certainly in terms of resilience but in terms of the other measures too. Here is where two key surprises emerged.

The first was that we were dealing with what amounted to two types of participants. Our initial assumption in planning the workshops was that those who responded to our advertisement would basically be novices with respect to writing about their lives. However, two of the multiple networks through which we recruited participants were the Writer's Federation of New Brunswick and the New Brunswick Arts Council, one of our funding partners. This meant that roughly half of those who attended are the sort of people who tend to go to writing workshops of *any* kind, in order to pick up more tips and techniques to help them hone their craft. Of the fourteen we interviewed, therefore, six referred to themselves explicitly as "writers" – whether of fiction, non-fiction, poetry, or memoir – while another six were equally insistent that they were *not* writers. The remaining two fell in between. In effect, we had two classes of attendees and interviewees alike. As it became clearer to us just how much their "class," as it were, figured in what people told us about their lives, this factor alone generated considerable discussion among us, about how the two groups differed, to be sure, but also what they had in common.

What they had in common included, first of all, their feeling that there should, indeed, have been two different groups. Non-writers particularly, for example, were likely to speak of feeling "out of place." What they also shared, though, was the view that a key reason for writing about one's life is to share one's story with others (e.g., children, grandchildren), and that "now is the time" to do so. They shared the view, as well, that storytelling generally is a way to appreciate how much our lives are interconnected with those of others.

In terms of the differences, it became apparent as we analysed the interviews that non-writers came to the workshops less familiar overall with the content or material of their lives, almost as if, hitherto, they hadn't really given it much thought. Thus, they found the act of simply getting their stories onto the page a significant task, one for which they were keen to acquire whatever skills they could – the ABCs, as it were, of writing their lives. They were also focussed more on just remembering the events of their life than on reflecting on the meanings those events held for them. If you will, they were more focussed on "the facts, ma'am," not to mention on arranging and narrating those facts in some sort of (usually) chronological order.

The writers, on the other hand, were less interested in such elementary matters, less concerned with the facts than with the meanings behind them. It was as if they saw themselves at a more advanced stage in the whole life-writing endeavour. For one, they were more capable of identifying key themes in their stories and more adept at employing metaphors to reflect upon their lives. Furthermore, when asked questions like "If you could reinvent yourself, what stories would you tell?" they were more able to envision alternative versions of their lives, more in touch with possible selves that they might (or could have) become, or possible lives they might have lived. Overall, they had a more ironic perspective on their lives (Randall, 2013), a more (so to speak) aesthetic detachment from them, plus a more sophisticated capacity for autobiographical reasoning, post-formal thinking, and integrative reminiscence, concepts that I'll say more about in Chapter 2. As far as life-writing in general is concerned, they saw it as a matter of both art and craft, a craft they are ever open to refining, a craft in which editing and rewriting are inescapable components, like learning is too: "autobiographical learning," if you will (Randall, 2010). In other words, they instinctively grasped that writing our life is not simply "to tell our story," to quote memoirist Patricia Hampl (1999), but to "listen to what our stories tell us" (p. 33). On this point, there was a modest but related surprise concerning differences between the two groups. It is not that the numbers of participants involved render our study remotely significant from a statistical standpoint. However, while in three out of six cases non-writers' scores for resilience went up between the first interview and the second (in one instance, by as much as 17.1 per cent), in four out of six cases the scores that writers received went down by as much as 15.7 per cent. This is an apparent anomaly that we'll be returning to briefly in Chapter 2 – although, to be clear, it's ultimately much less statistics than stories by which we're going in this book.

Since the second main surprise is our main focus in this book, we won't elaborate on it here. Suffice it to say that while we asked people a host of questions about their experience of the workshops, about how writing their lives affects how they *story* their lives, and about the place of storytelling in their lives overall (see Appendix 2), we did not deliberately ask them about the place of particular objects in their lives, objects with some sort of symbolic significance. We did not specifically inquire about "the biography of objects," as sociologist Tim Dant (2001, p. 26) puts it in the epigraph at the beginning of this chapter. In fact, only a comparatively few researchers have really done this, among them gerontologist Edmund Sherman (1991b) in his pioneering study of the role of "cherished objects" in personal reminiscence (see also, e.g., Belk, 1988; Csikszentmihalyi & Rochberg-Halton, 1981; Ferraro et al., 2011). Rather, our participants talked about such things entirely of their own volition. As with the differences between writers and non-writers, then, the more we reflected on what they shared about cherished objects, completely voluntarily, the more we were compelled to take notice. And, as Matte will show in Chapter 3, the more we were driven to delve into the complex emotional-existential relationship between the stories people tell about their lives and the things that figure in them: things that, for one reason or another, seem to matter quite a lot.

The Book

An overview is in order here as to how the book is organized and, along with that, of who we each are. Although we're all affiliated with CIRN and therefore, in varying ways, all interested in narrative ideas, all committed to some form of narrative inquiry (however we each understand it), we nevertheless represent a broad range of fields. With that in mind, we've included more extensive sketches of ourselves in Appendix 1, where we talk about what those fields are and outline the nature of our respective interest in stories, in ageing, and in things. By way of a quick introduction, however, here are a few words about each of us in the order that our contributions appear in the book's three parts – which correspond to how material in collections like this is commonly divided, namely theory, research, and practice.

Part 1

I myself am a gerontologist, the only one on the team, in fact. Much of my career has been spent considering how ideas from narrative psychology and related areas can illuminate the complex internal – or biographical – dynamics of later life. It's been devoted to looking into how a *narrative* gerontology can open a space to talk about such elusive yet essential topics as meaning, wisdom, and spirituality; a space where we can talk about the "philosophic homework" of later life (Schachter-Shalomi & Miller, 1995, pp. 124–126) and about the possibility, as I like to say, of not merely *getting* old but of consciously and creatively *growing* old. In this chapter I've offered an overview of the project in which this book is rooted, while in Chapter 2 I'll be introducing various concepts and distinctions that are central to narrative gerontology (or at least my version of it), and that will serve as reference points for our respective reflections in the chapters that constitute Part 2.

Matte Robinson is a professor of English at STU with a keen interest in autobiographical literature, especially the work of Hilda Doolittle, or H.D., and who has tracked with interest – though not contributed to – the emerging field of "thing theory." In Chapter 3 he will draw on such thinking to lay down some theoretical groundwork for our discussions in Part 2 by considering how different writers – philosophers, scientists, social scientists, critics, curators, and poets – write about things, and the implications of their views for the themes that we delve into in this book.

Part 2

Jennifer Estey, or Jenn as she's often called, is a registered social worker. She received her BSW from STU and went on to do a master's degree in interdisciplinary studies. She stands out among us because she is the one person who conducted all of the interviews on our behalf, and in that respect has had the most direct and most personal connection with the interviewees. As for Denise Resmi, she holds a BA from STU in criminology but fell in love with the world of narrative ideas in the course of working as a student research assistant on the resilience project. In Chapter 4, the two of them team up to offer an overview of all nine participants who are our focus in this book before we embark on our respective analyses of the stories – and things – of each one in particular.

In Chapter 5 Matte contemplates the role of sea glass jewellery in the lives and stories of a couple whom we have given the pseudonyms "Mary" and "Bob." In Chapter 6 Jennifer explores the significance of quilting in general, and of one quilt in particular, in the life of "Amelie," while in Chapter 7 I'll ponder the place of a certain ring in the life of "Hermann," whose story, I have realized, resonates uncannily with my own. In Chapter 8 Erin Whitmore, who did her doctorate in nineteenth-century Canadian women's literature and has done extensive work on women's experiences of trauma, writes about the role played in "Harriet's" story by a single page torn from an Italian language textbook, and in the process introduces the concept of "feminist reminiscence." Marcea Ingersoll, who is chair of the School of Education at STU, has been inspired by the work of scholars like Michael Connelly and Jean Clandinin in bringing a narrative perspective to the topics of teaching and learning.

In Chapter 9 she contemplates the role of a packet of love letters in the life story of "Joy."

In Chapter 10 Anthazia Kadir and I explore the significance of a specific beer stein for a participant called "Joan," whom we've nicknamed "Princess." With a background in adult education, Anthazia regularly leads life-writing groups with older adults in which she frequently invites people to write stories around special objects in their lives. She feels particularly called to put on workshops for newcomers to Canada, and indeed played a central role in installing a living exhibit at our regional museum that tells newcomers' stories through the things they chose to place on display. In Chapter 11 Brandi Burtt-Estey, a literary scholar with a strong interest in the boundaries between literature and religion, explores the significance of a collection of frozen red currants in the life of "Susan." In Chapter 12 she and Matte join forces to ponder the personal – and spiritual – significance of a particular table in the life story of "David."

Part 3

This section of the book shifts towards the more applied side of narrative gerontology by looking at the practical implications of the links between stories and things that the chapters in Part 2 have examined. In Chapter 13 I offer an overview of the variables involved in the sorts of life-writing groups in which older adults can express and explore their stories. In Chapter 14 Deborah Carr describes the particular workshops that our participants attended, outlining the kinds of activities, exercises, and strategies that she exposed them to and the sort of storywork she encouraged them to continue doing on their own. A published biographer in her own right and a regular leader of creative writing events for middle-aged and older adults, Deborah was new, at the outset, to the world of narrative theory. However, from her experience of offering such workshops, she soon displayed an instinctive appreciation for the storied complexity of older people's lives, and thus brought a special passion to planning and facilitating these three, intriguing, day-long events. In Chapter 15 Anthazia joins up with Shelley Swift, a certified life transition expert who works with clients, the majority of them older adults, on the pragmatic yet often highly emotional task of deciding which things to keep and which things to cull, which to throw away, give away, or sell. Together, the two of them discuss the ways in which their respective lines of work are in fact closely akin and how, in those lines of work, seemingly so different on the surface, the topics of things and stories are intimately linked.

Finally, in his afterword Clive Baldwin, director of CIRN, professor of social work at STU, and from 2011 to 2021 Canada Research Chair in Narrative Studies, seeks to step back from the book's numerous themes concerning things and stories in later life in order to reflect on the work of cherished objects in shaping our (narrative) identities across the years.

As this outline suggests, an assortment of voices run through the one big conversation that, basically, this book is. These include not just our own voices, but those of the nine individuals who are our focus in Part 2, not to mention those of the scholars whose work we cite in conjunction with the several strands of thought that weave their way throughout that conversation. But while it's a book with many voices, it's also one with many stories. Again, these are not simply the stories of our participants, but of ourselves as well, and the two sets of stories have become enmeshed in ways it's been impossible to avoid, for – as will become clearer in Part 2 – we have inevitably viewed participants' stories through the lenses of our own. Such enmeshment might be seen as a flaw in our methodology, a failure to maintain an unbiased stance towards what our participants shared during Jennifer's interviews with them, what we made of those interviews in our discussions as a research team around what we affectionately dubbed the "sacred CIRN table," and then in the chapters that each of us composed for Part 2. We see things differently, however …

A Word about Narrative Inquiry

Our approach to what our participants spoke about is, admittedly, anything but objective and unbiased. Indeed, the participants on whom each of us chose to write were those for whom we felt an instinctual, often emotional, affinity because of odd sorts of parallels that we sensed between their world and our own, particularly between the things that they revealed to be important to them and comparable things that are important to us, as we explain more fully in Appendix 1. But rather than apologize for this lack of neutrality, we view it as an asset, as a strength almost. This is in keeping with approaches to social science research that are garnering increasing respect and that go by labels like "interpretive ethnography" (Denzin, 1996), "evocative autoethnography" (Bochner & Ellis, 2016), or "relational research" (see, e.g., Chavese et al., 2020). Such approaches come under the still broader label of "narrative inquiry" (Clandinin, 2007).

In narrative inquiry, at least as we're engaged in it here (and each of us has our unique way of doing so), narrative is simultaneously the method with which we study something and the something itself that we're studying, not to mention the overall perspective or paradigm within which the entire enterprise takes place. Narrative inquiry, says one source, views "the story [as] one if not the fundamental unit that accounts for human experience" (Pinnegar & Daynes, 2007, p. 4), and thus the fundamental form assumed by the "data" such inquiry yields. Put simply, Jennifer asked our participants questions and they responded with stories, which we then examined in terms of various concepts and distinctions that narrative scholars have introduced. We're not merely analysing narratives, in other words, but using narrative ideas themselves to guide us in the process, which accords with the distinction that psychologist Donald Polkinghorne has made between "analysis of narratives" and "narrative analysis" (cited in Clandinin, 2007, p. xv).

What is more, narrative inquiry is profoundly relational in nature. In the words of narrative psychologist Ruthellen Josselson (2007), it "consists of obtaining and then reflecting on people's lived experience and, unlike objectifying and aggregating forms of research, is inherently a relational endeavor" (p. 537). As researchers Cheryl Craig and Janice Huber (2007) summarize things in their musings on the "relational reverberations" that narrative inquiry invariably involves, the aim is not to "critique" participants' stories from some privileged, all-knowing stance so much as it is to try and "understand" them (p. 272). The popular English author C.S. Lewis captures the spirit by which such inquiry is informed: "you can't really study people," he once remarked, "you can only get to know them" (Curtis & Eldredge, 1997, p. 114).

A further feature of narrative inquiry that distinguishes it from empirical or quantitative inquiry is its focus on the particular rather than the general. "[N]arrative inquirers," explain Stefinee Pinnegar and Gary Daynes (2007), "embrace the power of the particular for understanding experience" (p. 24). In the case of the particular inquiry that we're reporting on here, our aim has been to get to know – to understand as best we can – how the particular *things* that our participants made mention of are clues to the ways in which they have been, or might be, storying their lives. And in the process, as a kind of by-product – and this stands out for me personally in my reflections on Hermann's story in Chapter 7 – our aim is to understand some of the complexities in our own stories, too.

In a helpful chapter tellingly entitled "Their Story/My Story/Our Story: Including the Researcher's Experience in Interview Research," Carolyn Ellis and Leigh Berger (2002) echo the thinking of many narrative inquirers, "particularly feminists," who "have debunked the myth of value-free scientific inquiry" and "call[ed] for researchers to acknowledge their personal, political, and professional interests" (p. 851).

As their title implies, interviewees' stories and interviewers' stories can't help but intersect. An interview is, effectively, a co-narrated, co-authored creation that would not have come into being had another interviewer conducted it nor had some other person – in this case, each of us – analysed it and interpreted it after the fact. In this respect, narrative inquiry is deeply personal in nature. There are therefore as many types of such inquiry to be done as there are inquirers to do it.

We will get a feeling for all these sorts of intersections in the first chapter of Part 2. There we will see how Jennifer was uniquely touched by, felt perceived by, and developed a distinctive connection with each of her interviewees, as well as how her style of listening may have significantly affected what they shared with her (Randall et al., 2006) and the degree of narrative openness that it invited them to experience. I'll be saying more next chapter about the idea of narrative openness, but in the meantime, this intertwining of stories becomes particularly evident in Jennifer's own chapter on Amelie, where she explores in some detail their mutual passion for quilts. Yet, while in the other chapters in Part 2 the rest of us lacked the direct relationship with the participants that Jennifer enjoyed, there was something in the transcripts of those interviews, there were links that we sensed between the interviewees' stories and our own, that for a range of reasons intrigued us, even charmed us, and that we found ourselves identifying with so intensely that we wanted to crawl inside their worlds. First, though, I'll turn to various concepts and distinctions from the broad field of narrative studies that will accompany us on our crawl.

2 Supporting Things That Matter: Key Concepts and Distinctions

WILLIAM L. RANDALL

If we wish to know about a man [*sic*], we ask "what is his story – his real, inmost story?" – for each of us *is* a biography, a story ... Biologically, physiologically, we are not so different from each other; historically, as narratives – we are each of us unique.

– Oliver Sacks (1987, pp. 110f.)

Biographical Ageing and Narrative Resilience: An Introduction

I will begin by sketching what is, in fact, a critical backdrop to what I'll be doing in this chapter. I mean by this the modest but, thankfully, growing academic interest in what could broadly be called the "inside" of ageing, otherwise referred to as "biographical aging" (Birren et al., 1996; Ruth & Kenyon, 1996). As important as this dimension of ageing would seem to be, however, and certainly as central to our explorations in this book, it has been left largely unacknowledged by mainstream gerontology in that discipline's continuing reliance on a predominantly empirical, biomedical perspective on what ageing is about. According to that perspective, ageing tends to be construed outside-in, so to speak, and in essentially negative terms: not as a perfectly natural stage of the journey of life, not as something to accept, embrace, or at least be open to, but as ultimately a fate to be fought, a condition to be treated, and, in general, a problem – physical, financial, societal – to be solved.

Given this portrayal of ageing as basically a "narrative of decline" (Gullette, 2004), what gets eclipsed, I fear, are equally valid portrayals of ageing as a potentially creative endeavour, as an adventure of development and discovery, and, despite the declines that it certainly entails – perhaps in some ways *because* of them – as a pathway to greater insight and wisdom. To quote Morrie Schwarz, the retired professor dying of ALS who is the central figure in Mitch Albom's (1997) best-selling book *Tuesdays with Morrie*, "aging is not just decay, you know. It's growth" (p. 118). Florida Scott-Maxwell (1968) voices much the same sentiment in her poignant little volume *The Measure of My Days*: "A long life," she says, writing in her eighties, "makes me feel nearer truth, yet it won't go into words … I want to tell people approaching and perhaps fearing age," she continues, "that it is a time of discovery. If they say – 'Of what?', I can only answer, 'we must each find out for ourselves, otherwise it won't be discovery'" (p. 142).

The concepts and distinctions that I'll be flagging in this chapter – and, quite honestly, "flag" is the most that can be managed, for each could take pages to properly explain – provide a language and a framework for the more nuanced, more positive vision of ageing that these kinds of comments imply. In varying ways, they point to the intricate internal dynamics of ageing as it is experienced, subjectively, in the second half of life, dynamics that make ageing every bit as complicated on the biographical front as it is on the biological one. For the most part, they are concepts and distinctions that we can thank fields like narrative gerontology, narrative psychology, and the psychology of ageing for bringing to our attention. Although the connections among them have not yet been made in a systematic manner, this chapter is our way of assembling them together into a rough sort of scaffolding from which we can look into our participants' worlds – which is to say, their *story*worlds – and appreciate whatever sources of resilience sustain them.

As I indicated in Chapter 1, the conviction that motivated our research at the outset is that there is a dimension to resilience in later life that, until quite recently, has not been accorded the attention it deserves. The dimensions that researchers most commonly cite include a person's physical and mental health, cognitive competence, financial situation, social support system, spiritual allegiances and practices, and the like (see Fry & Debats, 2011; Resnick et al., 2011). But the dimension we're most interested in here, while not denying the importance of these others, concerns the nature of our lives as quasi-literary "texts" that we are continually composing and re-composing in memory and imagination. It concerns our "texistence" (Randall & McKim, 2008, p. 5) or our "biographicity" (Alheit, 1995, p. 65). It concerns the "poetics" of our personal development (Randall, 2023). Put most simply, it concerns the "stories" that we tell about our lives, or more accurately perhaps, how we "story" our lives over time, where that word is a verb as much as a noun (see Kenyon et al., 2011). It concerns, therefore, our *narrative* resilience (Randall et al., 2015), the strength that resides, one could say, in our stories themselves.

But this conviction is more than just a random hunch. A growing body of research inspired by the narrative "root metaphor" (Sarbin, 1986) is heightening awareness of a kaleidoscope of variables that make up what has been dubbed "the 'grammar' of resiliency," which is to say "the plots, narrative tones, and degrees of complexity in the stories of ... elders who ... have capacity for resilience" (Ramsey & Bleizner, 2013, p. 8). Indeed, references to such features of stories have threaded their way repeatedly through our discussions as a team, as we've sought to make sense of the mass of material that our interviewees shared.[1] Rightly or wrongly, they have served as the filters through which we've interpreted their words. Though several of them overlap, I've grouped them here for convenience in terms of four broad categories according to which a person's story can conceivably be viewed. They are: content, context, structure, and process – or, if you like, what is *in* the story, what is *behind* the story, how the story is *organized*, and how it is experienced and expressed, which is to say, how it is *told*. As I say, these categories themselves are intertwined, inasmuch as the medium (the telling or the how) and the message (the told or the what) are intimately linked. But they will at least get us started as we situate our thinking here in relation to important thinking that's been done thus far by others.

Content

By "content," I mean essentially what our participants talk about. To start with, this means what they say about basic things like their occupation, their education, their family and relationships, their interests, involvements, and hobbies. But it also means what they do *not* talk about, what they leave for us to guess. It means not just what they reveal but what they conceal; what they foreground and what, intentionally or not, they leave between the lines.

One thing we've been mindful of, for instance, is how they start off: what they come out with when asked – as they were at the outset of the

---

1 To reiterate, in the interviews conducted in Phase 1 of our overall project, we explicitly invited participants to tell us the story of their life as a whole. In fact, that was the interviewer's opening question: "Tell me about your life" – admittedly, a daunting task that few of us are asked to undertake in the course of every day. In contrast, the questions asked in Phase 2 elicited that "whole story" only indirectly. The focus was less on participants' stories per se than on their experience of the workshops, and of writing about their stories as opposed to just talking about them. It was on how *exploring* their story, through the various exercises to which the workshops introduced them, affected their *understanding* of their story. Directly or indirectly, however, both phases elicited a wealth of narrative material. This is why, as I outlined in Chapter 1, the term "narrative inquiry" applies to what we've been doing, for narrative has been, at once, both our method of analysis and the phenomenon that we've been employing it to understand.

interview in Phase 1 of our project – to "tell me about your life." In cases where they give a quick, truncated version of their life – *Well, let's see ... I grew up in Nova Scotia, went to college in Ontario, became a teacher, raised a family, and then retired* – what does such a summary include and what does it omit? What is the "narrative identity card" (Spector-Mersel, 2011, p. 182) with which they lead off? And what can it tell us about their experience, or perception, of their life story as a whole?

At this point, the phrase "life story" itself deserves a stab at definition, for it is hardly a straightforward concept. Psychologist Dan McAdams provides as useful a place as any to get us going. Invoking Erik Erikson's (1968) iconic concept of "identity," McAdams (2001a) equates identity directly with a life story. "*Identity*," he insists, "*is a life story*" (p. 663; emphasis McAdams's), or in other words, "an internalized and evolving personal myth that functions to provide life with unity and purpose" (McAdams, 1996, p. 132). McAdams uses the term "myth," however, not in the sense of an untrue story, one that is make-believe or false. He uses it in the sense of a story that is deep-seated, or "inmost," as Oliver Sacks puts it in the epigraph that leads off this chapter; a story that is below the level of conscious awareness yet foundational to our sense of self.

That this myth is *internalized* is worth noting. It suggests that the stories we tell or write about our lives are externalized expressions of that myth and are to that extent refracted, if not distorted, versions thereof – a difference that I've identified elsewhere (Randall, 2014) in distinguishing between the "inside story" of our lives and the "inside-out story" (pp. 49–56). That it is *evolving* is critical to bear in mind as well. The internalized narrative – the guiding fiction – in terms of which we understand our selves ideally possesses a measure of openness and flexibility. In other words, it is continually changing, subtle and gradual though the changes may be, as we cope with, react to, or accommodate an ever-widening range of experiences and circumstances over the course of our lives. McAdams goes so far as to propose three broad "stages" by which our narrative identity develops across the life span. They are the *pre-mythic* (from infancy to pre-teen years), the *mythic* (from the proverbial "identity crisis" of adolescence into mid-life), and the *post-mythic* (from mid- to later life), which is the stage occupied by the participants in our study here.

Sociolinguist Charlotte Linde (1993) summarizes this ever-changing dimension of a life story in a definition she puts forward in her book *Life Stories: The Quest for Coherence.* "The life story," she writes,

> necessarily changes constantly, by the addition of stories about new events, by the loss of certain old stories, and by the reinterpretation of old stories to express new evaluations. We change our stories at least slightly for each

> new addressee; we change a given story for a given addressee as our relation to that addressee changes; we reshape stories as new events occur and as we acquire new values that change our understanding of past events; and we change our stories as our point of view, our ideology, or our overall understanding changes and reshapes our history. (p. 31)

Still concerning content, it needs stressing that a life story is anything but a monolithic entity. Just as a novel contains multiple episodes, subplots, and chapters, so a life story is really many stories in one ... more or less. We have, for instance, stories about the past but also stories about the future, stories about what might have been and stories about what might still be. We have stories about ourselves alone and, of course, stories about ourselves with others. And we have stories about things, as well! Whatever or whomever our stories are about, they can also, of course, be long or short, big or small, general or specific, fuzzy or precise. And so it goes. As a student of mine once wisely noted in her learning journal, "there's nothing simple about a life story!"

Against the background of this multiplicity of story material, this many-layered side to the stories we *are* (Randall, 2014), we've been especially alert to stories of particular turning points that our participants shared. These can be called "nuclear episodes" (McAdams, 1996, p. 140; McAdams, 1988, pp. 122–175), and they concern particularly critical times in people's lives when they chose *A* over *B*, did *X* rather than *Y*, went here versus there. We've also watched for what might be "self-defining memories" (Baddeley & Singer, 2007) or for "signature stories" (Kenyon & Randall, 1997, pp. 46–49) – or even for what Norwegian gerontologist Oddgeir Synnes (2015) calls "nostalgic stories." In other words, we've watched for stories that may or may not be about turning points per se, but that seem extra polished, as if they were set pieces that the teller trots out on a regular basis, stories that may vary little from one telling to the next in how they are told, what they include, and the "spin" they reflect.

Regarding self-defining memories, Jefferson Singer and Pavel Blagov (2004) identify five core qualities that are characteristic of them, rendering them central to a person's sense of self. These qualities are captured by descriptors such as "vivid," "affectively intense," remembered "repetitively," connected to "other similar memories," and based on an "unresolved conflict of the personality" or some otherwise "enduring concern" (p. 119). Whenever we've detected them at work with particular participants, we've found ourselves wondering what can be inferred from such memories or stories – and as should be evident by now, we view autobiographical memory as *narrative* in nature, as a matter of faction less than fact (see, e.g., Rubin, 1995, p. 2) – about the person's self-understanding as a whole. How pivotal, we've wondered, might these be to their overall "narrative identity" (McLean, 2008), to the evolving, internalized myth that provides their life with unity, purpose, and meaning?

Along similar lines, we've been alert to whether such memories or stories might be for experiences from early rather than recent times in the participant's life, for instance, stories of "firsts" – first kiss, first job, first car, first marriage, and the like, or in other words events that occurred during that period of their development when their narrative identity was in an especially formative phase. Researchers who study the frequency of autobiographical memories across the life course have confirmed a pattern, in fact, whereby we tend to possess disproportionately greater recall for memories from, say, our teen years to late twenties – the beginning in earnest of the "mythic" stage – than we do from those years that fall before and after. How this pattern appears on a graph has become known as the "reminiscence bump" (Neisser & Libby, 2000, p. 318).

As I say, we've also watched for the stories that participants leave *un*told (Randall, 2014, pp. 280–308), the backstories or "shadow stories" (de Medeiros & Rubinstein, 2015) that seem to hover in the background of what they say, the stories behind the story, as it were. This could include stories about their first marriage, for instance, or their years-long battle with cancer, which they hint at in passing but don't elaborate on. When they let it drop briefly that, yes, they are married but then make no further reference to their partner, we naturally asked ourselves "what's the story there?" What could also be involved are stories that are embedded in our bodies themselves, stories hidden in the lines on our face, the slope of our shoulders, the look in our eyes. For the narratives by which we understand ourselves, by which we live, are ultimately embodied. "We are all living history books," claims author Carolyn Myss (1996); "our bodies contain our histories" – to the point, indeed, where "biography becomes biology" (p. 40).

Another lens we've looked through in assessing the material our interviewees shared has to do with the relative thinness or "thickness" of their descriptions of events (see Denzin, 1989, pp. 83–103). When telling stories about particular experiences, do they insert lots of detail and dialogue – *I said, she said*, etc. – or do they speak in vague generalities about their lives? Do they tell lots of stories period, or only a few? Also, do they imply a degree of narrative thickness by alluding to stories that they *could* tell if only there were time, perhaps sprinkling their speech with phrases like "that's a whole other story"? Do there appear to be multiple subplots going on in their lives, and multiple themes running through what they recount, recurring "life themes" (Csikszentimihalyi & Beattie, 1979) perhaps? And are multiple characters mentioned – including the characters, or roles, that they themselves are playing: in other words, the multiple "identity projects" (Staudinger et al., 1995) that they have going (different interests, involvements, commitments), the multiple "sub-Selfs" (Bruner & Kalmar, 1998, p. 320), "possible selves" (Markus & Nurius, 1986), "possible lives" (Brockmeier, 2002), or "unlived lives" (Alheit, 1995, p. 65) that swirl below the lines of what they say: the selves they feel they might have been or might still be? Or do they seem to have few such inner characters, few alternative selves, few other possible lives?

Overall, does what they share reflect a significant degree of "differentiation" (McAdams, 2001a, p. 663) in their personal "storyworld" (Herman, 2008), or does that world seem dominated by one or two subplots at most? Do the words they use and expressions they employ betray a complex, nuanced, multilayered self-awareness, with as much being implied as explicitly stated, or is it a case of what they say being basically what we get? Put differently, how much "narrative complexity" (McAdams, 1988, pp. 105–132) seems at work in the self-storying to which we are privy?

Continuing with content, one topic that is obviously a core focus in this book concerns the role played in our participants' reminiscences by particular objects or things – pictures, letters, items of clothing or furniture, mementos of one sort or other. As Matte will be going into in much more detail in the following chapter, such things have generally been termed "reminiscentia" (Casey, 1987, pp. 110f.; Sherman, 1991b), while those that prompt particularly poignant recollections are referred to as "cherished objects" (Sherman, 1991a, pp. 125f.). In Chapters 5 through 12, we will be attending with particular closeness to participants' self-narrations that revolve around objects of this type, objects that seem fraught somehow with extra meaning, and thus can serve as windows onto the intricate terrain of their inner storyworld.

Context

By the context of our participants' stories, I mean, for starters, the "discursive environment" (Holstein & Gubrium, 2000, p. 228) or the "narrative environment" (Randall & McKim, 2008, pp. 50–57) in which they grew up and by which their "storyworld" (Herman, 2008) has inevitably been shaped. We learned something about this feature of their lives, of course, from their answers to a question that Jennifer asked in the first interview prior to their attending the workshop series: "What role has story telling generally played within your family, both in the past and in the present?" Was the narrative environment of their family of origin, in other words, a comparatively rich one, in which storytelling played a prominent role? If so, then what sorts of stories got told, by whom, and in what ways? Were there certain self-defining stories for the family as a whole? Did certain figures – say, parents or grandparents – stand out as the main story keepers? And how did the stories that they recounted influence the content and structure of participants' own narratives? To quote sociologist Elizabeth Stone (2008) in her book *Black Sheep and Kissing Cousins: How Our Family Stories Shape Us*, how much did such stories get "under their skin" (p. 6) and, for better or worse, inform their narrative identity, stories perhaps that, as First Nations author Thomas King (2003) confesses, "I will be chained to … as long as I live" (p. 9)?

To continue in the same vein, was their household a freewheeling environment in which each member could say whatever they liked, however they wished? Or was it rather rigid, in which content and airtime were tacitly policed and in which children were, as the saying goes, to be seen and not heard? From a young age, were they encouraged to elaborate upon events in their lives in the manner displayed by mothers in the mother-daughter pairs that Robyn Fivush and her colleagues have studied (Fivush, 1994; Fivush et al., 1995)? Or were they coached instead, as such studies indicate boys are more likely to be, not to "go on and on" but rather "stick to the facts" (Nelson & Fivush, 2000)? How in general, we've asked as a team, has the gender of our participants factored into the thickness or thinness of their "storying style" (Randall, 2014, pp. 308–328; O'Neill et al., 2011)? Are women in general, for instance, more apt than men to have thick, layered, differentiated stories about their lives, more inclined than men to be involved in life-writing activities period, to engage explicitly in narrative reflection, to keep themselves narratively open? Are they, overall, more narratively resilient? If so, might this pattern play some part in why they routinely live longer too? Such questions (though perhaps unanswerable) are highly relevant to our study here insofar as only three of the nine participants whom we're discussing in this book are men, and in the three workshops overall the ratio of women attendees to men was two to one.

Beyond the matter of a participant's gender or family of origin, there is the question of what "narrative templates" (Abbott, 2002, p. 7), "narrative resources" (Freeman, 2000, p. 81), or "forms of self-telling" (Bruner, 1987, p. 16) – what life-scripts – appear to have been mediated through the communities or cultures in which participants were shaped by virtue of growing up in, for example, Newfoundland as opposed to New York, or Jamaica instead of Japan. Absorbed by osmosis into their *narrative unconscious* – which is to say "those culturally rooted aspects of one's history that have yet to become an explicit part of one's story" (Freeman, 2010, p. 11) – such templates may continue quietly to guide individuals in fashioning the narratives of self and world through which they understand, and live, their lives.

Another aspect of context is the "narrative positioning" that we sensed our participants were engaged in vis-à-vis their interviewers (see, e.g., Blix et al., 2015; de Medeiros, 2013, pp. 91–101). This is relevant to consider given that the interviewers in both Phase 1 and Phase 2 of the project were female student research assistants. We found ourselves wondering, then, whether female interviewees tended to share story material about their lives, or tended to reminisce, in different ways than males? The point here is that, in the context of an interview, listeners are never simply passive recipients of what is narrated. In a sense, they are co-narrators as well (see Ochs & Capps, 2002), inasmuch as listeners subtly but surely shape what tellers tell (Randall et al., 2006), a point that Jennifer and Denise reflect upon in Chapter 4.

A related consideration in connection with narrative positioning was what was happening in interviewees' lives at the time the interviews took place, or what they anticipated would happen in the future. One woman in Phase 1 of our project, for instance, talked about her life in extremely thick, reflective ways, which suggested to us a great deal of narrative resilience. Yet her score on the CDRS was decidedly low, something that made eminent sense given that she was waiting to undergo open-heart surgery in the weeks immediately ahead. It was as if the shadow story of her (possible) death was hanging over everything else that she shared with the interviewer about her life.

A further matter as regards positioning has to do with the audience the interviewee has in mind. By this I mean not so much the immediate audience they had before them during the interview itself (which Jennifer and Denise will say more about in Chapter 4), but the audience they have in mind for the story – or stories – they say they are hoping to write, or are already engaged in composing. Are they intending that composition for their children and grandchildren primarily, or mainly for themselves?

These sorts of considerations lead to the issue of the "larger stories" (Kenyon & Randall, 1997, pp. 85–95) that, explicitly or otherwise, our participants perceived themselves to live within: stories that may hold as much significance for them, emotionally and existentially, as their own personal narratives, stories in which their individual narratives are "embedded" (Furlong et al., 2015) or by which they are overshadowed: the story of their family, for instance, or of their community, their culture, their religion, the cosmos as a whole. This takes us to the issue of the meta-narratives or, if you will, "master narratives" (Randall & McKim, 2008, pp. 260–267) that they see, and may openly refer to, as infusing their lives with purpose and meaning.

Such master narratives can include, of course, the narrative of decline that has insinuated itself into our society's perception of ageing per se, to the point where, as I say, we tend unwittingly to experience ageing in negative terms, as little more than a downward slide to decrepitude and death. When these master narratives are associated with a particular religion, however, the questions we asked ourselves as a team concerned their influence on the content and structure of the participant's self-storying. Is "God," for example, as much a character in their narrative identity as they are themselves, and if so, a character of what kind – for instance, father or friend, creator or judge? And what themes has their self-storying possibly been seeded with that it wouldn't have been had they identified with the master narrative of some other religion instead, or none at all?

Still on the topic of religion, there is the question not only of what master narrative they referred to but also – in the case of Christianity, for instance – of what version of Christianity. Are they identifying, say, with a fundamentalist form of it, in which all answers to all questions are stridently prescribed and recipes for living life are clearly spelled out, or with a more progressive, more open, less doctrinaire version? That is to say, do they experience their religion as a "rigid, imprisoning structure" or as an "astonishing resource" (Beardslee, 1990, p. 173), or somewhere in between?

Obviously relevant in this regard is the "stage of faith" (Fowler, 1981) participants might be in, at least at the time of Jennifer's interviews with them, whether it be "synthetic-conventional," "individuative-reflective," "conjunctive," and so forth (see also Johnson & Walker, 2016; Walker, 2016, pp. 258f.). However, any opinion regarding this would be pure speculation, for we made no attempt in either Phase 1 or 2 of the project to determine participants' stage of spiritual development, or "ego development" (Loevinger, 1976), or "moral development" (Kohlberg, 1984) – or for that matter, their profile in terms of personality traits, such as the "big five" of neuroticism, extraversion, openness, agreeableness, and conscientiousness (Costa & McRae, 1985). That said, and on this latter point, researchers have found that people who score high on neuroticism tend to tell more negative stories, or more "contaminated sequences" (McAdams, 2006, pp. 213–220), where for instance their life starts out fine but sooner or later falls off the rails. Stories told, however, by people who score high on openness and agreeableness are more "positively toned" (McLean, 2008, p. 1693) and contain proportionately more "redemptive" sequences (McAdams, 2006, pp. 213–220).

Structure

By the structure of participants' self-storying, I mean several things not necessarily obvious from an analysis of content alone. Indeed, gerontologist Edmund Sherman (1991a), widely respected for his research on reminiscence in later life, privileges structure over content when insisting that "it is the form rather than the content that matters most in the study of personal life narratives" (Sherman, 1994, p. 150). Among the features related to form that we've been especially mindful of is the "narrative tone" (McAdams, 1996, p. 136) running through the material that participants shared. For McAdams (1996), narrative tone can range from "blissful optimism" to "biting negativism" (p. 137) or, to invoke the concept of *genre,* from the romantic to the tragic. In a parallel vein, gerontologists Jan-Erik Ruth and Peter Öberg (1996) have singled out six overarching metaphors, or "ways of life" as they call them, that characterized how the elderly Finns whom they interviewed spoke about their personal histories – the bitter life; life as a trapping pit; life as a hurdle race; the devoted, silenced life; life as a job/career; and the sweet life. In his study of the impact of keeping a personal journal on personal development in later life, gerontologist Harry Berman (1994) notes how, in fact, a measure of *re-genre-ation* can occur in our understanding not just of individual (perhaps traumatic) events but of our life as a whole. As our "horizon of self-understanding" shifts over time, or our "landscape of consciousness" (Bruner, 1986) expands, says Berman (1994), "it may become apparent ... that we were not in the middle of the story we thought we were in the middle of" (p. 180). "Perhaps," he says, "we thought our life was a tragedy and all along, unbeknownst to us, it was a romance. Or perhaps we thought our life was almost over, at least in terms of the future holding anything new, and it turned out there was a lot more to it" (p. 180). I'll come back to this possibility later when I look into the concept of *narrative openness.*

Related to differences, and possibly changes, in genre or narrative tone – in storying style – are the various ways in which our participants have characterized themselves in the midst of their life's events, which goes back to the idea of narrative positioning, and also of narrative agency. For instance, do they portray themselves as the protagonist amid the story of their life, a story that they experience as, say, essentially an adventure, in which they possess a healthy measure of narrative agency – or authorship – in how it unfolds and the direction it takes? Or do they talk as if they were little more than a supporting character in their own life-drama, a drama in which someone else possibly – a domineering partner or needy adult child, for instance – plays the lead? Do they speak of themselves as, basically, a hapless victim of circumstances outside their control, or perhaps as an observer, looking on at their lives with an ironic detachment, not as author of their stories so much as reader (see Randall, 2013; Randall, 2014, pp. 314–322)?

Of relevance here is the "locus of control" (Rotter, 1966) that people experience in their lives: whether it is primarily internal or external in nature, whether it resides ultimately within themselves or in conditions and forces outside – the government, for instance, or the omnipresent "They." Relevant as well is the distinction proposed by psychologists Jack Bauer and Sun Park (2010), when discussing late-life resilience, between "growth narratives" and "security narratives" (pp. 66–71). In the former, individuals tend to view their lives as a matter of life-long learning and construe whatever struggles and adversities they face as opportunities for continuing development intellectually, emotionally, and so forth. Someone living and ageing within a security narrative, on the other hand, envisions their main goal as to minimize upheaval and avoid major change; ageing is less about growing and discovering than, as much as possible, settling into – or for – a life of contentment and calm.

Parallel distinctions have also been put forward. Besides Bauer and Park's (2010) own distinction between "eudaimonic well-being" and "hedonic well-being," Bauer and McAdams (2004) speak of "two broad trajectories" that can characterize "adults' stories of life transitions" (p. 573). One is "social-cognitive personality development," which is aimed "toward heightened capacities for mature thinking, complexity of meaning-making" (p. 575) in terms of how we *think* about our lives, and where our overall goal is *maturity*. The other is "social-emotional personality development," where the aim is "toward heightened capacities for psychological health, adjustment, and well-being" (p. 595) in terms of how we *feel* about our lives, and where our overall goal is *happiness*. The difference between the two, we might say, is between ageing on the surface and "aging in depth" (Bianchi, 1991, p. 60).

One obvious way of discussing structure in self-storying has to do with the degree to which the episodes or anecdotes participants recount have a relatively clear beginning, middle, and end – a traditional narrative arc, as it were – as, for instance, a person's "set pieces" (Chandler & Ray, 2002, p. 77) can often possess. Or, in contrast, are they recounted in a higgledy-piggledy style with all manner of digressions, diversions, and self-interruptions that make them difficult to follow and suggest the possibility that the events in question are still in flux in the narrator's own mind, that their details and chronology are not yet sorted out, not yet rendered coherent? If they take any form at all it is that of what sociologist Arthur Frank (2013) would call a "chaos narrative" (pp. 97–114).

Author Margaret Atwood (1996) expresses the essence of such a narrative in her novel *Alias Grace*: "When you are in the middle of the story it isn't a story at all, but only a confusion; a dark roaring, a blindness, a wreckage of shattered glass and splintered wood; like a house in a whirlwind" (p. 298). In short, does there seem to be a unity amid the multiplicity in what we are hearing? Do the many stories that the participant tells seem basically to hang together within some overall narrative frame, or does what we are hearing seem "all over the map"?

This leads to the controversial question of which criteria are appropriate to invoke in evaluating a life story. In an article entitled "Creating a life story: The task of reconciliation," psychologist Peter Coleman (1999) identifies four such criteria: coherence, structure, assimilation, and truth value. McAdams (2001a, p. 663) takes this line of thinking still further with his six "standards" of what he (not uncontroversially) calls "good life-story form": *coherence, openness, credibility, differentiation, reconciliation,* and *generative integration.*

The element of differentiation I have already considered a little in relation to context as well as gender. Openness and generative integration I will be touching on in the next section. Regarding "story coherence," however, researchers Jenna Baddeley and Jefferson Singer (2007, pp. 182f.) have parsed this concept as, itself, entailing different types – for instance, *temporal coherence* (episodes are organized chronologically), *causal coherence* (episodes are sequenced consequentially), and *thematic coherence* (multiple episodes are pulled together under an overarching principle or value, or in light of a particular metaphor). As a criterion for assessing the "goodness" of personal narrative, "coherence" is viewed with some scepticism, however, in many academic corners, surely where cognitive impairment is taken into account (see, e.g., Hydén et al., 2014; Hyvärinen et al., 2010). Or at least it is viewed with the caveat that, as storied beings with multiple "interacting characters" (Hermans, 2001, p. 1) or "sub-Selfs" (Bruner & Kalmar, 1998, p. 320) operating within us on any given day, we are in fact capable of multiple coherences. In the insightful words of autobiography scholar Paul John Eakin (1999), "there are many stories of Self to tell, and many selves to tell them" (p. xi).

In the case of our participants here, however, we can at least ask whether what they shared with us – despite the umms and ahhs and stops and starts that qualitative interviews invariably involve – (a) makes sense and (b) hangs together. Does it correspond to, or is it consistent with, the facts of the person's life, insofar as we are privy to them? Is it, in that sense, credible? Or are there not merely shadow stories lurking between the lines, but glaring gaps in their account overall? Does the story material they divulge in the interviews appear to take into account the good, the bad, and the ugly of their lives – a process that entails a measure of *reconciliation*, and is "one of the most challenging tasks in the making of life stories" (McAdams, 2001a, p. 664)? Or do they gloss over the negative experiences of their lives, experiences that typically "demand more storytelling work" anyway (McAdams, 2008, p. 253; Pals, 2006), and privilege positive experiences instead? If so, they may be said to be opt for happiness over maturity, a preference implied, in fact, by more than one participant whose orientation seemed to go past the so-called positivity effect (Carstensen & Mikels, 2005) that older adults are said to experience anyway and to come under the category of "positive illusion" (Taylor & Brown, 1994). Not that this need be perceived as problematic. Indeed, psychologists Ong and Bergeman (2010) have argued that positivity is itself a factor in late-life resilience, that positive emotions "broaden people's attention and thinking," facilitate a "more holistic processing of information," and "enhance their ability to see the 'big picture'" (p. 245).

Process

The element of process takes us beyond matters of content, context, and even structure – at least as I've been laying them out here – towards still subtler aspects of a person's self-storying, aspects that might not so readily stand out. We can begin, for instance, by citing the concept of "narrative identity processing" that psychologists like Jennifer Pals (2006) have discussed in relation to how an individual makes meaning in the midst of their lives. As "the story species" (Gold, 2002), possessed of "the literary mind" (Turner, 1996), we habitually make sense of events – past, present, and future – by instinctively constructing small stories around them, by conferring on them some sort of narrative shape, and a rudimentary measure of narrative coherence, however unreflective that conferral may be. Often, though, when going through a particularly painful or confusing life event, we can feel the need to process it more consciously with a confidant or counsellor so that we can assign it a greater degree of coherence in our minds and thus, provisionally at least, lay it to one side and get on with our lives. This represents a more sophisticated form of narrative processing known as "autobiographical reasoning" (see Bohn, 2011; Habermas, 2010; Pasupathi & Mansour, 2006; Singer & Bluck, 2001).

Autobiographical reasoning is not just about remembering the past but about reflecting on it too, trying to discern the significance of specific events vis-à-vis our lives, our selves, and our development overall. If you will, it is the difference between an "efferent" reading of a text – in this case, the quasi-literary text of one's own life – and an "aesthetic" reading (Rosenblatt, 1978, pp. 23f.). Simply put, the former entails reading for the events that the story recounts, while the latter is reading for the meaning of these events in relation to the story as a whole (Randall & McKim, 2008, pp. 86f.) – a difference that, as I mentioned in Chapter 1, stood out for us between the writers and the non-writers in our study. Mark Freeman's (2010) phrase for such reasoning is "narrative reflection" (p. 9), or to use the more familiar term, "hindsight." As will become clearer in later chapters, some of our participants seemed to gravitate towards it more naturally and intentionally than others, in some instances – as we will see with Hermann in Part 2 – engaging deliberately in "counterfactual" thinking (Ferguson, 1997) when speculating on how differently their lives might have turned out if they had made different decisions or lived in different times.

Pertinent here is a distinction proposed by narrative psychologist Michael Bamberg (2006) between the narrative activity that we typically engage in when talking with family or friends about what's happening in our daily lives, by telling "small stories," as he calls them, and the more encompassing, more complex mode of narrative activity that we indulge in, usually more rarely, when we step back from the immediacy of the moment and reflect upon our life as a whole. This, in essence, is what we were inviting participants to do in both phases of our project. Bamberg calls the focus of such reflection "big stories." Crudely put, narrative processing corresponds to small story narrative recounting while autobiographical reasoning leans towards "big story narrative reflection" (Spector-Mersel, 2017).

Another interesting distinction to pull in here has been proposed by Susan Bluck and Hsiao-Wen Liao (2013) in their reflections on the intricate relationship between memory and the self: the difference between *chronological self-continuity* and *retrospective self-continuity*. The former is "a continuous, chronological sense of self" that enables us "to organize memory information and exercise daily behaviors" (p. 8) and "is so basic that it is rarely subject to our awareness" (p. 10). At the "higher level" of retrospective self-continuity, however, "individuals not only recognize their basic existence as organisms over chronological time but recall and reflect on their autobiographical history" by engaging in "effortful processes" such as "life review, autobiographical reasoning, integrative reminiscence, and meaning-making" (p. 10). Accordingly, the capacity for retrospective self-continuity "does not simply aid survival, but increases the chances for socio-emotional growth, … for human thriving," by which they mean the ability to "gain self-insight, learn life lessons, and … develop purpose or meaning … to gain a sense of authorship of the life lived; of uniquely *owning* one's life" (p. 10, emphasis theirs).

As with chronological self-continuity, we often take retrospective self-continuity "as a given." However, "we recognize it" – or feel more acutely the need for it – "when it is disrupted." Put differently, "we become aware of [it] most keenly when it is threatened, which may," Bluck and Liao (2013) say, "result in a sense of disorientation and decreased well-being" (p. 10). This trend is extra helpful to bear in mind, therefore, in relation to later life. For, depending on the changes we undergo in our personal circumstances (e.g., illness, relocation, bereavement), entry into old age can be an extremely disruptive experience in itself, a "narrative disruption" (Fireman et al., 2003, pp. 9f.) that challenges our very sense of identity, of self. For this reason, engaging in the kinds of reminiscence activities that life-writing workshops provide can serve the purpose of "narrative repair" (Nelson, 2001), of strengthening or thickening our "inmost" story (Sacks, 1987, p. 105), thus assisting us (inwardly, retrospectively) to *grow* old and not just (automatically, chronologically) *get* old.

This leads us, then, to distinctions that gerontologists have made among the different types of reminiscence in which older adults can engage, and in a sense the "functions" (Webster, 2002) that their reminiscing serves. Although they can be interlaced in the storytelling activity of any given reminiscer on any given occasion, at least six main types of reminiscence have been identified (Wong, 1995). In *narrative* reminiscence we recount past events in a comparatively unreflective, "and then, and then," sort of manner. *Escapist* reminiscence recalls the past in glorified or idealized ways as, so to speak, "the good old days." In *obsessive* reminiscence we return repeatedly to negative events, in line with a particular function of reminiscence labelled "bitterness revival" (see Webster, 2002). With *transmissive* reminiscence, we talk about the past as a means of teaching or informing others in the present. *Instrumental* reminiscence involves, for instance, using memories of how we have coped with past challenges to help us handle present ones. Lastly, *integrative* reminiscence can be thought of as "pulling ourselves together," narratively speaking: the good, the bad, and the ugly in the stories of our lives. As such, it has an especially in-the-moment, dynamic dimension, even a "transformational" one (Kunz & Soltys, 2007): "dynamic reminiscence," a phrase that in fact some researchers have expressly proposed (Chandler & Ray, 2002, pp. 80–92). Scott-Maxwell (1968) captures nicely the gist – and the prize! – of this mode of reminiscence: "when you truly possess all you have been and done, which may take some time, you are fierce with reality" (p. 40). Of these six main types, then, the latter two, instrumental and integrative, are considered particularly "adaptive" (Wong, 1995) inasmuch as they each in their way enhance, if not our fierceness with reality, then at least our sense of retrospective self-continuity. Integrative reminiscence in particular, though, links with the notion of "life review," and thus with the "social-cognitive" trajectory of personal development noted earlier by Bauer and McAdams (2004).

Erik Erikson, along with others since him (see, e.g., Butler, 1963; Haight, 2007), deemed life review to be an innate, naturally occurring psychological process. It is what could be described as a key "developmental task" of later life, and a decidedly *narrative* task at that, insofar as it has to do with making sense of the countless stories, big and small, that we have woven around our lives. Whether spontaneously experienced or prompted from outside, it involves the evaluation and integration of "all one has been and done" and arrives, ideally, at a sense of acceptance, even pride, concerning one's life as a whole, a sense that, all things considered, it has been what it had to be and, "by necessity, permitted of no substitutions" (Erikson, 1963, p. 268). The potential to be gained from engaging in this process, Erikson claimed, is wisdom.

Wisdom is an enormous concept in itself, though despite its assumed association with later life, it is one gerontologists have in general been shy about studying, in part no doubt because of how difficult it is to precisely define. As for Erikson, he defines wisdom somewhat cryptically, if not depressingly, as "detached concern with life itself, in the face of death itself. It maintains and learns to convey the integrity of experience, in spite of bodily decline and mental functions" (Erikson, Erikson, & Kivnick, 1986, pp. 37f.). Such a definition suggests that, whatever exactly wisdom is, an element of paradox and irony, even humour, runs through it (Randall, 2013). Psychologist Jeffrey Webster (2003), who has led the way in attempting to *measure* wisdom, incorporates this element in his "H.E.R.O.E. model" of wisdom, in which key facets of wisdom are having Humour, regulating and accepting the complexity of one's Emotions, Reminiscing/reflecting, being Open to experience, and overcoming and making meaning from a variety of life Experiences (see Bivona et al., 2020).

Another perspective that explicitly incorporates the narrative element that wisdom arguably possesses is particularly pertinent to our inquiries in this book. I refer to a perspective articulated by gerontologist Ruth Ray (2000) in her intriguing book *Beyond Nostalgia: Aging and Life-Story Writing*. The book is a reflection on her experiences of being a researcher-participant in eight different life-writing groups for older adults (the majority of them women) in inner-city and suburban Detroit. As part of her study, she carefully observed the ways that group participants talked and wrote about their stories, as well as how their sharing with one another seemed to contribute to the development of what might be described as a "wisdom environment" (Randall & Kenyon, 2002; Randall & McKim, 2008). In general, this led to her conceiving of wisdom less as a tidy package of lessons learned that an individual can pass along neatly to others than as something more open-ended and dynamic in nature, not to mention more relational, and decidedly more "storied" besides. "A person is truly 'wise,'" writes Ray (2000), "when she is able to see life as an evolving story and to create some distance between self and story by reflecting on it from multiple perspectives. 'Wise' people watch themselves tell life stories, learn from others' stories, and intervene in their own narrative processes to allow for change by admitting new stories and interpretations into their repertoire" (p. 29). We'll return later in the book to this narrative perspective on wisdom. In the meantime, I will return to the topic of life review.

From an Eriksonian perspective, life review is considered not just an innate process but a necessary one as well, above all in the seventh and eighth stages in his model of psychosocial development. As I mentioned already, McAdams (1996) refers to these stages as constituting the "post-mythic" phase of our narrative development (p. 136). During this phase, grappling (however unconsciously) with the issues of "generativity vs stagnation" and "ego integrity vs despair" are, in Erikson's assessment, pivotal developmental tasks that await us – tasks that McAdams combines in his sixth criterion for a good life story, which is "generative integration" (2001a, pp. 664f.). In her chapter in Part 2, Marcea will touch on such concepts in the course of discussing the theme of *legacy* (Kotre, 1999) as it seemed to weave its way through many of our participants' narrations, especially that of Joy. Certainly, a number of participants expressed a keen desire to write their life stories for the benefit of their children and grandchildren. On this point, psychologist John Kotre (1984) insists that a key form of generativity (in addition to the biological, parental, technical, and cultural forms) is "generative transference" (pp. 30f.). Moreover, and in keeping with our focus in this book, he implies that these sorts of written and passed-on stories are themselves "heirlooms" of sorts (see Hecht & Tyrell, 2007). This whole idea of stories themselves as *things* – as cherished objects in their own right – will come up again and again throughout this book.

The question of which modes of reminiscence our participants seemed mainly to engage in surfaced repeatedly in our discussions as a research team. While the probing nature of Jennifer's questions, let alone the activities that Deborah had them do during the workshops themselves, tended to nudge them away from reminiscence of the narrative, obsessive, or escapist type towards more integrative reminiscence instead, we were watchful for whether they responded to this invitation or resisted it. Whether they responded or resisted, possibly opting to focus on the positive over the negative in their lives, we often had the sense that the overall impact of participants' involvement in both the workshops and the interviews was to stir things up. Inviting them, for instance, to entertain "new meanings for old tales" (Chandler & Ray, 2002) conceivably unsettled them to some degree. With a nod to distinctions cited earlier between security narratives and growth narratives, and between social-cognitive and social-emotional development, perhaps it shifted their autobiographical reasoning from being mainly about "self-stability" to being about "self-change" (McLean, 2008, p. 1689).

The latter, claims psychologist Kate McLean, is the opposite of what happens for many as they move into later life, who opt for happiness over maturity and, accordingly, shy away from extensive involvement in life review (see also Bluck 2017; Cappeliez, 2017; Wink & Schiff, 2002). If so, then the combined impact of the workshops and the interviews could be said to have destabilized our participants' customary manner of storying their lives, prompting them to "restory" (Kenyon & Randall, 1997) – or re-genre-ate – to an extent they might not have entertained doing had they not participated in the project. In the process, it could have stirred up a mixture of melancholy and regret as they begin reflecting in some depth on what Arthur Frank (2010) calls their "narrative habitus" (p. 49). By this he means "the collection of stories in which a life is formed and that continue" – for better or worse – "to shape lives" (p. 49): in other words, a person's overall storyworld. In the words of author William Bridges (1980), "each person's life is a story that is telling itself in the living"; accordingly, "each of us resists change because a story is a self-coherent world with its own kind of immune system" (p. 71).

Such an "immune system" may help to explain why our participants' scores on the instruments we had them complete before the first and second interviews – regarding resilience, well-being, and meaning in life – actually went down in many cases rather than up, in direct contradiction to what we expected to see! It was as if we were pressing participants towards big story narrative reflection and thus towards more sophisticated autobiographical reasoning, and with it, restorying, whether they wanted to be pressed in that direction or not – in the process, though, perhaps nudging their storyworld towards greater "narrative openness" (Randall, 2013).

As a concept, narrative openness contrasts with "narrative foreclosure," a condition that Freeman (2010) sees linked to "the conviction that the story of one's life ... has effectively ended ... that the future is a foregone conclusion" (p. 125). In essence, one is living in "epilogue time" (Morson, 1994, p. 193), the post-mythic phase par excellence. Narrative foreclosure is a state of mind and heart to which, for an assortment of reasons, including the sheer power of the narrative of decline, plus the often disruptive effects of the ageing process itself, older adults are especially susceptible (Bohlmeijer et al., 2011). This is why we elected to incorporate the Narrative Foreclosure Scale (Bohlmeijer et al., 2014) into our study. It is one of a number of "narrative challenges" that I've written about elsewhere (see Randall, 2020, p. 448) – such as narrative loss, narrative deprivation, narrative disorientation, and narrative imprisonment – that we can be faced with in later life, challenges to our sense of narrative identity, to our experience of "retrospective self-continuity" (Bluck & Liao, 2013). For that reason it may play no small part in the mild to moderate depression to which many older adults can fall prey, a condition for which, one could argue, the better remedy might be not medication so much as a healthy dose of "narrative care" (Kenyon & Randall, 2015).

Narrative openness, on the other hand, is associated with more positive mental health (see, e.g., Bohlmeijer et al., 2009) and can be signalled by several things. Among these is how receptive our participants have been to the idea of passing on their story, and with it their legacy of knowledge and wisdom, to younger generations – generative transference again (Kotre, 1984). Indeed, as I say, this is an openness that almost all of them implied when asked why they had signed up for the workshops in the first place. It is hinted at, in other words, by how committed they were to "generative narration" (McAdams, 2001a, p. 583).

Narrative openness is also signalled by the range of identity projects and possible selves that figure in our understanding of our lives. It is signalled by the sides of ourselves, possibly long dormant, that we are open to exploring and expressing, especially when asked questions, as in fact Jennifer asked our participants, such as "How, if at all, does writing help generate different perspectives on your life?" and "If you could reinvent yourself, what stories would you tell?" It can be signalled, too, not only by entertaining "multiple fluid narratives" (Bateson, 2007, p. 213) concerning our future, but by being open to different readings of our past, by our ability to appreciate that while past events cannot be changed, our interpretations of them are anything but fixed. Meaning-wise, they are indeterminate. In terms of its interpretative potential, that is to say, autobiographical memory is very much an open text. New meanings can always be gleaned from old tales, and there is no end whatever to what we can discover in the stories of our lives, no end to how much, internally, we can grow. Put in different terms, there is no end to the interest to be earned on our "biographically accrued capital" (Mader, 1996, p. 43). Narrative openness can be signalled as well by the flexibility of the master narratives with which we may identify and the sorts of "counter stories" (Nelson, 2001, pp. 6–9) towards which, however subliminally, we are drawn. Overall, then, narrative openness is, arguably, a critical ingredient in *aging well*, a concept that gerontologist Sherry Chapman (2005) defines in terms of "the on-going co-construction and reconstruction of multiple selves [in] an open-ended process of meaning-making amid later-life events and transitions" (p. 14).

Some of the narrative openness our participants appeared to experience – whether naturally so from the start or enticed to be more so by their involvement in the project itself – may relate to their degree of "narrative literacy" (Baldwin, 2010, pp. 250f.). By narrative literacy is meant their familiarity and comfort with narrative as a metaphor for envisioning their life, for viewing it, for instance, as an ever-evolving *novel* – replete with chapters, characters, subplots, and themes, and which they are situated inside of as author (or co-author), narrator, protagonist, editor, reader, and critic, more or less at once (Randall & Khurshid, 2017).

Certainly, some of our participants, most notably the writers, engaged quite readily in story-talk. One participant, for instance, made repeated references to how in life "we're always editing." Possibly in possession of a more active "narrative imagination" (Andrews, 2014) and a heightened "metaphoric competence" to begin with (Gardner & Winner, 1978), participants like this had little problem applying the story metaphor – or any metaphor, for that matter – to their own lives (Randall, 2011, 2023). It's as if they found it not merely intriguing but empowering, as if it injected them with a new (or renewed) sense of narrative agency, or at the very least afforded them an affectionate, ironic, and conceivably "wise" detachment from the lives that they've lived to date (Randall, 2013). Witness the numerous participants in both phases of the project who came out proudly with statements like "I've had a very, very interesting life" or "I want to write a book someday; it would be a trilogy plus" (see Randall et al., 2015).

They were encouraged to think in storied terms by – besides the exercises that they did during the workshops themselves, plus writing out one of their stories in particular, conceivably a signature story, between the first interview and the second – the very sorts of questions that Jennifer included in the second interview especially. Such questions invited them, for example, to identify any "themes" that ran through their lives and to speculate on what their "next chapter" might be. At the same time, what equips them to entertain a more pointedly narrative perspective on their lives may be the increasing capacity for "postformal thought" that psychologists have claimed comes naturally with later life and is conceivably connected to wisdom in turn (Cohen, 2005, pp. 36–38; see also Csikszentmihalyi & Rathunde, 1990, pp. 30f.).

Post-formal thinking entails the ability to see the forest for the trees and to accept the relativity of all our knowledge, including our knowledge of ourselves. It is the ability to step back and look at our lives as a whole, to accept the ironies and contradictions that run through our nature, and to tolerate, if not celebrate, the uncertainty and ambiguity inherent in our existence, and the variety of interpretations that can be placed on any given event in our life and indeed on our life as a whole. It is the ability, as Ray (2000) would say, "to see life as an evolving story and to create some distance between self and story by reflecting on it from multiple perspectives" (p. 29). And, linked to the development of "a more figurative, symbolic processing style" (Labouvie-Vief, 1990, p. 74) in the autobiographical reasoning in which we engage, it is the ability to appreciate the merits of metaphor and myth as tools for self-understanding – for understanding, and revising, the myth that we make of our own life.

Coincident with the rise of a post-formal style in the cognitive side of our lives are changes on the affective front as well. Gerontologist Gene Cohen (2005), for example, argues that shifts in the structure and functioning of our ageing brains, most importantly improved cooperation between the left hemisphere and the right, equip us generally to manage our emotions better than when we are, say, toddlers or teens. Such shifts, he suggests, also intensify the drive towards "autobiographical expression" (p. 22). Our emotions, in other words, are intimately tied to our memories, and thus – like our memories, like our sense of self – possess a narrative dimension (see, e.g., Habermas, 2019; Ruth & Vilkko, 1996; Singer, 1996). With age, that is, our emotional lives undergo qualitative changes that parallel, and are triggered by, changes in our store of stories as well, whereby that store becomes not just thicker in terms of content (more years, more memories, more stories) but, potentially, more pliable in terms of form. This relates to the process of re-storying, re-interpreting, or re-genre-ating that I've mentioned already and that engaging in a life-writing group, and then being interviewed about what that experience was like, can understandably prompt.

It is for all such reasons, conceivably, that May Sarton (1981) remarks in one of the journals she published late in life how "the past is always changing, is never static, never 'placed' forever like a book on a shelf. As we grow and change," she writes, "we understand things in new ways" (p. 95). In another of her journals, she thus repeats approvingly the observation made by the poet John Hall Wheelock, writing in his nineties, that "as life goes on, it become *more intense* because there are tremendous numbers of associations and so many memories" (cited in Sarton, 1977, p. 231; emphasis mine). And it is such intensity – cognitive and affective alike, in terms of memories and emotions both – that thinking about the things that matter in our stories can intensify all the more, imbuing the past with a poignancy, even beauty, that we were unable to appreciate when the past was our present. "I can only note," writes Virginia Woolf, "that the past is beautiful because one never realizes an emotion at the time. It expands later, and thus we don't have complete emotions about the present, only about the past" (cited in Miller, 2008).

Looking Ahead

This quick and scarcely exhaustive catalogue of terms and distinctions constitutes the rough kind of conceptual scaffolding that I talked about at the start. Introducing them here will provide some sense, I hope, of the peculiar brand of (interdisciplinary) narrative inquiry that we're engaged in within these pages. Obviously, just as each of us gravitated towards one participant over the others, we'll each be leaning on certain of these concepts more than others in our respective analyses, and indeed, in some cases, introduce one or two of our own. With that in mind, I will close with a preview of the directions our respective reflections will take us in Part 2.

Following Chapter 4 and Jennifer and Denise's overview of all our interviewees, in Chapter 5 Matte will explore the importance of sea glass jewellery in the lives of Bob and Mary. Of particular interest, he will elaborate upon how, when we write about special objects, as Mary does, they become transformed into texts and thereby can gather even greater symbolic significance in our lives. In Chapter 6 Jennifer weaves her thoughts concerning Amelie around the concepts of secret stories, turning-point stories, intergenerational narratives, and legacy, which is a theme that, as I say, Marcea zeroes in on in Chapter 9 where she touchingly ponders the story of Joy, in the process identifying a species of personal narrative that she calls "serendipity stories." In Chapter 7 I pick up on such concepts as shadow stories, signature stories, and storying style in my reflections on the parallels between Hermann's story and my own. In Chapter 8 Erin delves deeper into the notion of counter-stories and also of possible selves, specifically "lost possible selves" (King & Mitchell, 2015). In her discussion of Harriet's story, particularly the woman's shadow story of "the violinist who wasn't," she proposes a mode of dynamic reminiscence – and, at the same time, of resistance – that, to my knowledge, few researchers have explicitly named. She calls it *feminist* reminiscence.

In Chapter 10, by Anthazia and me about the beer stein that was cherished by Joan, or Princess as we've dubbed her, we touch on the power of fairy tale motifs as narrative resources in shaping our imagination and inspiring us, possibly, to restory the myth by which we understand who we are, to re-genre-ate it from, for instance, a tragedy to an adventure. We also borrow from Joseph Campbell's vision of "the hero's adventure" or "hero's journey," with its three broad stages of departure, fulfilment, and return (Campbell & Moyers, 1988, pp. 123–163). In Chapter 11, on frozen red currants, Brandi picks up on the notion of texistence, or of our lives themselves as texts we are continually weaving, and ponders the complex interplay between storytelling, memory, and symbol within the world of Susan. Lastly, the place and power of symbol is pivotal to Matte and Brandi's reflections in Chapter 12 on the significance of the mahogany table that has been so central to David and his family across the years.

As a segue to Chapter 3, a few further words are in order regarding the concept of "cherished objects" that is obviously central to what we're exploring in this book and that Clive will be revisiting in the Afterword. As noted already, the gerontologist Edmund Sherman (1991b) has conducted important research into the function of special possessions in older adults' lives – whether photographs, letters, relics, or souvenirs (p. 127) – as "reminiscentia," a term first coined by the philosopher Edward Casey (1987) to refer to "inducers" of reminiscence (p. 127; see also Sherman & Dacher, 2005; Sherman & Newman, 1978). Unlike our project here, however, where mention of such possessions came unbidden from our participants themselves, Sherman (1991b, p. 91) explicitly asked one hundred older adults between age 60 and 102 three key questions: (1) "What kinds of objects or memorabilia ... tend to set you to reminiscing more than others?" (2) "List and describe any personal possession(s) or object(s) that is particularly special to you and that you cherish more than others." And (3) "Why does the object(s) have such special meaning to you?"

Among his findings were that such objects "provide a sense of continuity, security, comfort, and satisfaction" (Sherman, 1991a, p. 125). Accordingly, "those who could identify a most cherished possession generally evidenced higher morale" (p. 125). Moreover, using a cherished object as an aide-memoire enabled individuals "to give much 'thicker' descriptions in their reminiscence," descriptions that "capture the meanings and experiences that have occurred in a rich, dense, detailed manner and create the conditions for interpretation and understanding" (pp. 127f.). In addition, and perhaps equally important, they "serve to reflect meanings related to the past and to integrate former experiences" (p. 125), a finding worth noting, obviously, in connection with *integrative* reminiscence and the concept of retrospective self-continuity.

Since Sherman's initial work, more recent research has corroborated his core findings and explored their practical application in helping older adults accomplish a range of internal developmental tasks that are basically narrative in nature (see Randall, 2020). Besides assisting them to sustain a sense of meaning (Coleman & Wiles, 2020; Phenice & Griffore, 2013; Tobin, 1996) and of identity (Kroger & Adair, 2008; Stevens et al., 2019;), cherished objects can also enable an older adult to carry with them a sense of "home" as they make the often difficult transition to life in an institution – a nursing home, for instance, where they will likely have limited space to bring any possessions at all to remind them of what their life story has been and thus who they *are* (see Green & Ayalon, 2019; Nord, 2013; Rubinstein, 1987; Synnes & Frank, 2020; Van Hoof et al., 2016; Wapner et al., 1990).

All of these are encouraging findings, to be sure. Yet it could be argued that they limit our thinking about things to the utilitarian domain, thus obscuring subtler, more elusive dimensions that special objects can possess, and that this chapter, in its fashion, has been quietly pointing towards, more soulful dimensions, we might even say – dimensions that stand out sharply in the case of David's table. In the simple phrase from Thomas Moore's (1992) book *Care of the Soul*, "things have soul" (p. 269). In the next chapter, then, Matte will move beyond the social sciences to draw upon thinking within the humanities in order to delve deeper into such dimensions, including the distinction between things and objects. He will also look at how writing our stories, which is what we asked our participants to do between the first and second interviews, transforms those stories into texts, and in that respect things, thus rendering the boundary between things and stories all the more deliciously blurred. In the process, he will shed still further light – a much more literary light, if you like – on the emotion-laden, memory-thick, symbol-rich role that things so often play within the stories of our lives.

3 Living in a World of Things: Objects, Tools, and Stories

MATTE ROBINSON

With thanks to Dr. Cora Woolsey

Signatures of all things I am here to read.

– James Joyce, *Ulysses* (1968, p. 42)

As Bill has mentioned already, this book grew out of a larger project, one that I came to late, being relatively new to the study of narrative. I played a role in the conception of this book in part because I am not so new to thinking about things, though I pledge no allegiance to any theory about things: I'm a generalist when it comes to theorizing things. My bits and pieces of expertise – the late work of the poet H.D., the twentieth-century literary occult, and a few other corners of modernist studies – don't directly apply here, which is fine, because for me this book is ultimately for people who have to live and work with things. It is a resource for people who want or need to reflect regularly on their relationship to things and to stories, and so the expertise of any one author is only a way into a broader issue we all share. That said, this chapter does conclude by discussing literary things, because each object discussed in Part 2, over and above what it is for its owner, is presented here as a literary thing, a textual thing.

Bill co-authored a book with one of my mentors, Elizabeth McKim, called *Reading Our Lives: The Poetics of Growing Old* (2008), one of the premises of which is that narrative is hardwired into our brains, and another of which is that a story is only as good as the reading it's given. This chapter weaves *things* into this argument in two ways: by suggesting that things, too, are hardwired into the brain and are intimately tied to language and story, and by distinguishing the literary *thing* – a thing encountered in a story – as a lens through which we can reflect on our own stories in a process that is both integrative and generative. Keeping in mind the distinction between the thing as object of reminiscence and the literary thing it becomes in autobiographical writing, we use things throughout the book, in different ways, to explore the relationship between memory and story.

I can have a thing, write an autobiographical reflection on it, and then I have two things: the thing and the text about the thing. The text may act as a substitute for or supplement to the object written about – I can pass one or both on to my children, for instance – but the story is only as good as the reading it gets. Texts are easily misunderstood when recalled and not revisited: when recalling Robert Frost's famous poem about the two paths in the wood, for instance, many of my students are surprised to find that their memories do not match up with a careful rereading. Most of us first learned that it was a poem about nonconformity, or perhaps about having a strong work ethic, and only later came to realize it was about how we make stories out of random events, imbuing those events with meaning they did not originally possess. The choice of paths appears arbitrary in the speaker's recollection, yet the speaker predicts that ages hence, they will tell the story very differently. I am not sure if I detect a rueful tone to the speaker's prediction, casting a sidelong glance at older people and the way they massage their stories, but turning events into stories seems to be the best way to find some meaning in the choices (guesses) we make as we wend our way along the path of our lives.

Expanding our view to the broader cultural memory of the English language, the original meaning of "thing" in English and related languages is much closer in sense to an event than to a material object. The Old Norse Thing was a forerunner to the British Parliament and is humorously summed up in Rick Riordan's *The Hammer of Thor* (2016): "It's a Thing thing. You wouldn't understand." As best I can tell from the *Oxford English Dictionary*, a "thing" meant an important event – a meeting time and place – for a good long time before it also came to mean the subject of the meeting. Only by extension did it also become an object, some material object imbued with significance and yet, strangely, devoid of it. The significance does not seem to reside in the object but instead in what one does with it.

Things aren't quite the same as material objects, and we should keep that in mind as we discuss cherished objects. Anthropologist Tim Ingold (2011) sees a lot of potential in freeing the concept of the thing from materiality, on the basis of the fact that some things are living things:

> Stripped of the veneer of materiality [living things] are revealed not as quiescent objects but as hives of activity, pulsing with the flows of materials that

> keep them alive … they are, in the first place, organisms, not blobs of solid matter with an added whiff of mentality or agency to liven them up. As such, they are born and grow within the current of materials, and participate from within in their further transformation. (p. 29)

But it is very easy to think of things as discrete lumps of materiality, despite the reality of their being part of the same flow of material and transformation that Ingold describes. The fact that matter resolves itself into lumps of stone and coffee mugs (and, by extension of that fact, into supermassive black holes[1] and neutrinos) at all seems to be a quirk of our senses, ultimately of our brains. In this chapter I explore the way things (much like their sibling, a clever species of ape) flow and transform, in order to highlight the strangeness that occurs when things cross the boundary from the material to the literary.

Literary things are yet another subset of thing, quite distinct from living things, though some literary things take on a life of their own and might then also become mythic things (King Arthur, Lilith, Athena, etc.). The ways literary things are encountered, thought about, felt about, and interacted with are unique. Because this book is about people's stories about their things, I devote the bulk of the chapter to approaching thinking about literary things, such as rabbit holes and halls of mirrors, things many of us have never actually seen, but we know what they are when people say their names.

In this sweeping inventory of things from their place in our brains to their role in a story, I keep two anchor texts by a pair of authors who have done a lot of thinking about things. They are Bill Brown (2001), who invented "thing theory," and Tim Ingold, the eminent anthropologist whose work has already been quoted above (see also Gibson & Ingold, 1994). In his focus on things, humans, and their relationship, Ingold touches on identity as something shared by humans and the things encountered in the world. This chapter in pursuing literary things also chases the elusive occurrence known as the thing as it grew up with the strange critters who first found themselves alongside things in the universe.

---

1 Cosmologist Jana Levin identifies a fissure in the word's various meanings in her *Black Hole Survival Guide* (2020) when she writes that a black hole is "not a thing" because it is empty spacetime, a void. It is not a thing in this sense because it is an absence of any material, and yet as far as most of us are concerned, black holes became things for us some time in the latter half of the twentieth century.

Digging Things Up

> Within what context do we place this social life and history [of things] if not the ever-unfolding world of materials in which the very being of humans, along with that of the non-humans they encounter, is bound up?
>
> – Tim Ingold (2011, p. 31)

Just a few days after I began work on this book, I took the opportunity to do something far removed from the study of literary modernism, my occupation of nearly twenty years: an archaeological excavation. My partner is a bona fide archaeologist, and thanks to her assurances that I was a fast learner, I was allowed to join the excavation team for a week at the site of a 1620s Acadian fortified trading post in southern Nova Scotia. We stayed in a workhouse and spent each day in a pit, carefully excavating with trowel, bucket, dustpan, and brush. It was hell on the hips, and though we were treated like gold (A tent canopy erected over us to block out the sun! Breaks whenever we wanted them!), I confess that I prefer to do my interdisciplinary work around the table at CIRN, which is air-conditioned and has a machine that makes very good coffee. Out on the dig site I would use the trowel to remove layers, looking for artefacts and dumping the loosened dirt into the bucket. When it was near full, I would pass the dirt through a fine-mesh screen to catch any small objects that had escaped my view. There were lots of those.

We were finding plenty of roofing tile, bits of ceramic typical of the culture and the period, rusty clumps that were once nails, amorphous lumps of fire-damaged material, fired lead shot, and other odds and ends that were consistent with what we expected to find because of the stories we knew about the place: there had been a fire, a battle, a settlement, a trading post. But of especial interest was a class of artefact that might provide evidence of interaction between the Acadians and the Mi'kmaq, who had used the site for millennia before the arrival of Europeans. One type of this special category of artefacts was trade beads; the other was the more interesting because it existed only in hypothesis: worked French flint.

It was common practice to fill up ships bound for the Americas with flint, which served as ballast en route and then could be picked over to be worked into flint-and-steel and gunflints. The Mi'kmaq, who had been around much longer, used flint for a vast array of tools – scrapers, blades, projectile points, and probably all sorts of other things besides. All the current theories point to the probability that, in days of early contact, Indigenous people would have noted the abundant ballast material and (re-)worked it into tools from their own toolkit. The Europeans were literally dumping this stuff, and you can find it to this day dotting New Brunswick beaches.

On my second day working I pulled an object out of the ground. I knew right away that it was *something*: it was made of that cloudy-greyish flint, and its shape was oddly regular, round on one side and with two angled planes meeting at a sharp central ridge on the other, like a face-down book. I showed it to my wife; her voice raised half an octave as she shouted out that I'd found a primary flake. I took it to the director. She showed it to a fellow archaeologist; he held it and mimicked striking at it with a rock, imagining the way flakes would break off. He thought it was likely a "strike-a-light," a European thing, but the director was slower to declare what it was. Beginning by noting that she had not seen such a thing yet in this site, she deferred her opinion. A day later, she said she thought that this might be one of the things we were looking for; it seemed deliberately struck with an expert hand in a way that Mi'kmaq people, and not French colonists, would shape stone. But, she cautioned, she was going to finish up her excavation and then spend a year to give herself time to think carefully about it as well as to show it to people she trusted.

Here's what struck me, an outsider who learns fast (I hope): common sense tells me there was a high likelihood of finding one of these things. There's no way shiploads of good, useful flint wouldn't be taken and worked into fine tools, is there? And yet nobody's ever found one. Because nobody's ever found one, archaeologists must consider new finds carefully, ruling out other explanations first. The outsider killing his hips in an admittedly luxurious hole all day wondered what would happen with that thing that came out of the ground, wondered what it was and what it would become.

A Boundary

I interrupt the story about the thing to point out a boundary between the way the social sciences and the humanities map things into the world. This is still me at the archaeological dig, but revisited in the abstract. The humanities, I think, prioritize synthetic knowledge but cannot always agree with the social sciences on how "synthetic knowledge" plays out in the field. I think, in all seriousness, that this disagreement on how to approach a complex set of data marks a (friendly) boundary. It is not *the* boundary, but it is as real as the tape Les Nessman uses to mark out the "walls" of his office in the TV show *WKRP in Cincinnati*.[2] The walls aren't

2 Nessman is miffed that he doesn't have an office, and so there's a running gag about the tape he puts on the floor around his desk. People have to pretend to knock at the door by beating their fist in the air.

there, but their reality is subject to debate, and so the walls are not not-there, as well. It is that kind of boundary that, with our colleagues on the team, Bill and I are exploring in our interdisciplinary approach to narrative, the border zone between what English professor Daniel Albright (1994) speaks of as the "wilderness" of literature and the "garden" of psychology (p. 19). I can most clearly address this boundary in a quick survey of a certain kind of thought about things. I have referred to it as a survey, but it might also be considered a rabbit hole, or a portal discovered in the back of a wardrobe.

A Quick Survey

Someone took that piece of flint and modified it with an abstract form in mind in a process known as poiesis, which means bringing something into being, or simply "making" (you can compare the word to the Latin *facere*, which gives us the word "fact"). By beginning with poiesis, I emphasize the deep connections between making, coming into being, existing, and the poetic, but it is difficult to think of writing a poem in the same way as making a thing. That is because a poem is a kind of thing, and maybe vice versa if you're fancy.

In poeisis the maker, the form, the material, and the telos make up the process of that thing's coming into being (the French word for thing, *chose*, derives from *causa*, cause or reason). Psychologist Donald Polkinghorne (2004) defines "poiesis" as "the art or craft by which natural materials are made into aesthetic or useful objects," an activity that "yields a product or a result that is separate from the person who made it and is available to others for their use and evaluation" (p. 115). So a thing might be understood by the community that produced it as a tool, but some time in the future it will become an artefact: once the thing was found in a hole in the ground, it became, in a way, another thing entirely, available to a new set of others who, while still attuned to the technological processes that brought it into being, were encountering it in a very different sphere of human making. The archaeologist who discovers the thing is attuned to its past use and cultural context but participates in transforming the object into data. The thing has a history, and also a future: as data, though, it exists in the stasis of the archive, without a past or present assigned to it. For Ingold (2011), writing as a form of making is about "*drawing lines*" (p. 179, emphasis his), which evokes both the physical act of writing by hand and the intellectual act of making distinctions that are invisible outside of the act of writing, to be made solid in the imagination as manager Herb Tarlek does with Les Nessman's tape.

The thing I held in my hand is now data,[3] and depending on what is learned about it and its context, it might become, largely, a textual thing, a thing written about, a means by which the story of the place and people of a certain era can be read and interpreted. Archaeologists are only some of the scholars who deal with material objects in this way. The philosopher Bruno Latour (2005) focusses on metal weights attached to European room keys to illustrate the ways in which objects are imbued with force, power, and significance equiprimordial to the "sign" of the semioticians (pp. 106f.). There seems little to add to a theory that sees objects and humans as co-agents in a networked world, but there does remain, outside the job of data analysis, the problem of the thing, whose mystery is not quite plumbed. The networked world in which the thing is found in its original context and the classificatory archive-world in which it will be deposited in a plastic baggie also intersect with a literary world that destabilizes these relations, a world haunted by the noumenal otherness of the quasi-immortal thing and its materiality, or by its very mortal "owner." It will be helpful, going forward, to conceive of humans as something other than *owners* of things, since the things outlast their humans – maybe something like "caretaker," or "steward," but there are probably better words.

Protean Things

As the piece of worked flint makes its way into the text of local archaeology, the artefact will transform from the mysterious object it is only once the archaeological community has decided what it is. Its physical presence will remain in environmentally controlled storage somewhere, strictly held in stasis. Meanwhile, many people will encounter it for the first time not as this thing at all, but as the text-thing it has become. Free now to signify in this new context, the artefact-as-literary-entity will still bump up against strong resistance to becoming something other than what it is: the scientific method, peer review, competing theories, further excavations will all attempt to limit the play of the thing's identity past the transformations it has so far undergone. The thing is now fixed – not owned, but identified and catalogued in the controlled surroundings of the archive. Thought of in this way, its nearest neighbour will be a key with a heavy fob, not an ornate basket of porcupine quills.

3 Just as the stories of the things and their caretakers collected in this volume are first encountered by us as data.

That is so, anyway, until someone, perhaps a writer of Mi'kmaq heritage, encounters it – say the actual artefact is repatriated – and writes about it in far different contexts, perhaps as an effort to resituate it within the cultural, historical, and spiritual terms that it has been removed from, or as inspiration or symbol from which new poetic meanings can be wrought, written into a poem, song, or story. It could become an image (a sketch, perhaps, or an image that resonates somehow) used by a new generation who claim its signifying power. The image could be reproduced in much more than textbooks and articles, posts and memes. What happens to that thing once its image has become a symbol? Then its thingness really cannot be controlled; its identity is destabilized as it becomes a literary object of a different sort: available to any reader, present or future, it can take on any of a myriad of new meanings while still being somehow tethered to that thing first encountered (by me anyway) in a hole in the ground. The kind of generativity things have is their promise of enduring. I pass on my things to be cherished, sold, broken, or lost; I do not have a future, but the thing does, and it will have many caretakers or stewards before it, too, perishes. It will almost certainly reveal itself to be protean, to be very different things at different times and places, while somehow remaining itself. Things, having this quality, add something to our stories and to our readings of those stories; seeing people's stories through the lens of things adds a dimension beyond the personal, the family, the community: others, complete strangers, might have a stake in any given thing's past and future.

This Thing Is an Object, but Is It Cherished?

Even the literary object retains some connection to the thing itself, brief as a flash though that encounter may be. And it is this sense of the thing, as fetishized and so pushing against the boundaries that tell it what it really is, that has concerned those of us sitting around the CIRN table discussing the objects we encountered in the interview transcripts and stories of our participants. That's what I saw, anyway, but then I'm new. Not an outsider, but like I was at the dig: just new. People trained in English are drawn to ambiguity like slugs are drawn to the one plant in the yard you care about for its volatile compounds. That was known before I took on this project, and so it is no surprise that this is not a straightforward book about "cherished objects": Bill and I instead came up with a different book, about *things that matter.*

To cherish is to hold something beloved, which to be sure tells something about the subject-object relationship, but nothing about the thing itself. The artefact discussed above, as a cherished thing, is currently in the stasis of the archive, a catalogue number: it is not cherished by anyone, so instruments designed to detect "cherished-ness" will not detect it. We don't know what it is because we don't know who worked it. Perhaps it will become a cherished object for reasons the system that recovered it has begun to address but has not fully considered.

There are many points to be considered by those who administer that system:

- Objects of reminiscence need not be cherished nor even kept to trigger reminiscence; the story or even mention of the object is an adequate substitute.
- Not all the objects treated in this book are cherished, but all of them are important.
- Though some objects begin as "reminiscentia," their primary function can be understood to be the generation of new thinking, new narrative threads.
- When the object is passed on, it opens itself up to further generativity, and when it is lost and recovered, to further still.
- Objects can "speak" to the investigators in different ways than they do to the participants, having become data.

The purpose of this list is not to diminish the notion of cherished objects but to expand the discussion to other types of objects significant to narrative, in order to prepare the ground for some of the things discussed in this book.

The boundaries between the humanities and social sciences are crossed all the time at universities, often in obvious ways – you can read a novel about ageing in gerontology class or take a survey course on literature about archaeology – but each field will emphasize different things, and will emphasize things differently. In the spirit of Randall and McKim's (2008) survey of insights into narrative and the brain, I turn to things, language, story, and the brain en route to looking at that subset of things I call the literary thing.

Things, Tools, Narrative

Thinking about things has, over the past century, been closely tied in with the most fundamental ontological questions that can be asked: What is being? Why is there being rather than nothing? René Descartes seemed to banish things, as objects, to some anti-realm set over against the subject, the ego, the self. The subject-object boundary became, for a time, the front in a battle between idealists and materialists. In the twentieth century, phenomenologists evaded the mind-matter distinction altogether by focussing on the points of encounter between humans and things. In an oft-written-about section of Martin Heidegger's *Being and Time* about the way everyday things are encountered, tools are observed to be ready-to-hand: when I am at work with my hammer in my workshop, the hammer becomes in a sense invisible to me, just as my heartbeat or my little toe is. The entire workshop, in fact, with its screwdrivers, chisels, and drills hanging ready for when I need them, is invisible by extension. It is not even correct to say that they are an extension of myself, because my own body, my own sense of myself as a separate ego, is part of that invisibility, the world as it manifests to me in working, or to put it another way, it is easier to think about being wrapped up in a world of things without positing a mind-body distinction in the first place.

Heidegger contrasts this state with the present-at-hand, which changes the essential relationship with the object: in various ways, if the hammer breaks or a chisel is missing from its hook, or a thumb rather than a nail is hit, the thing stands apart from this world as a deficiency. You've hit your thumb when you wanted to hit the nail on the head. There you stand, clearly *very* separate from the broken hammer, and consider it, or maybe you distract yourself by staring at the chalk outline on the pegboard considering the chisel in its absence, or maybe you just swear loudly, sucking your thumb. These are radically separate ways of being in the world, and it seems to me that only a sense based on deficiency can function as the point of departure for Cartesian enquiry. Rather than begin with the thinking self, it is possible to begin an enquiry into being with beings and things united in their world of poiesis.

Deficiency or Excess?

Bill Brown, whose 2001 special edition of *Critical Enquiry* introduced "thing theory" to a wider scholarly audience, uses the definition of "thing" that arises from Heidegger's and other works as his own point of departure for considering things in literature and culture. An object, when removed from its ready-to-hand state, becomes a thing, which can now be considered in various attitudes involving critical distance, such as study, scientific enquiry, or art. Say any word ten times and it will become an abstraction; hold a thing in front of you and call it something over and over, you'll stop thinking about it. You'll already know what it is, so you'll think about it that way. Objects are abstractions, but things are real.

For Brown, the object as deficiency, removed from its usual sphere and considered, like a fish out of water, in a calculating, classifying manner, is not what a thing is. Heidegger will turn his attention to things in his enquiry into being, which will lead him to works of art and poetry. Brown, who begins with fiction and poetry, uses the concept of things as "excess" (rather than deficiency) of objects to open up avenues of enquiry about things' role in literature, culture, politics, economics, academics, and other areas of life. The sense of things as an object's excess, "as what exceeds their mere materialization as objects or their mere utilization as objects – their force as sensuous presence or as a metaphysical presence, the magic by which objects become values, fetishes, idols, and totems" (Brown, 2001, p. 5), is what guides his enquiry.

Thing theory is not an attempt to escape the social or the political but rather an attempt to bring things in, as it were for the first time, to the discussion of the world by turning to them and seeing what they can tell us. Things. This is not a way of granting agency to a thing because of a postulated methodological exigency, but rather to attend to the "thingness" of things in order to help speak to some original constitution of what it might be to be human ("Thing" is also the name for an animated severed hand in *The Addams Family* and *Good Eats*). Many of the fruitful discussions that can arise from such thinking take place in English departments (really!), but another, parallel discussion arises from the hard sciences.

Things only really exist on the human scale, unlike objects. Zoom in far enough and objects dance along the borderline between matter and energy, expressing themselves as waves or particles. What they might be, beyond waves or particles, is not accessible to human experience. The floor, the table, our bodies are all mostly empty space, held together not by the continuity of stuff but by fundamental forces, yet on the human scale these bonds configure themselves into stuff, which on a less coarse scale resolves into objects. Some of those objects also become things for us, as presumably they all once were things. If "thingness" is the excess of objects, it is also a way that stuff configures itself for and through the human world, and this fact of "thingness" is the ground for the narrative mind. The fact that we are storytelling beings, beings who make sense of time in the first place through narrativizing life, is also the fact that we are with things,[4] and not just objects, and that things generate stories.

Siblings

In episode 2 of *The History of the World in 100 Objects*, British museum curator Neil MacGregor (2010) considers a stone chopping tool from

4 I have read about young chimpanzees who keep and care for special sticks, almost as though they were dolls, so I hasten to add that "thingness" might not be an exclusively human experience.

the Olduvai Gorge, from the lower Palaeolithic, made by an early hominin nearly two million years ago. It belongs to the so-called Oldowan tradition, the first tools known to be made by hominins. Identifying the species that began making these tools has proved difficult, but it was likely an australopithecine or an early member of the genus *homo.* MacGregor's podcast tells the story of history through things, and he believes that tools are the first things, as I have been using the term here: "unlike [animals], we make tools before we need them. And once we have used them, we keep them to use again." This process, according to MacGregor, implicates tools in the evolution of the human brain. Unlike other apes' symmetrical brains, our asymmetrical brains have evolved in tandem with an ever-expanding toolbox: we make and adopt a tool, the brain evolves for its use, and from that knowledge base we make other, more complex tools, all in a chain that results in a mutually developing relationship between things and neural structure. David Attenborough, appearing on the podcast, notes a kind of excess in the Oldowan chopper and things like it: they are well made, more than is necessary to do the job of scraping. The chopper represents for McGregor and Attenborough a capacity not only for making the tool, but also for imagining how it might be better made.

In his book based on the podcast, MacGregor (2011) makes his point clearer: "from the point where our ancestors started making tools like this, people have been unable to survive without the things they make; in this sense, it is making things that makes us human" (p. 11). And surely becoming a thing and not a mere object is tied in with technology: I cannot do without the device I couldn't have conceived of when I became an adult, nor would I enjoy life without working lights, heaters, toilets, and taps. The Olduvai tool, according to MacGregor, "represents the moment at which we became distinctly smarter, with an impulse not just to make things but to imagine how we could make things 'better'" (p. 11). MacGregor and Brown appear to be talking about the same thing: a kind of excess in things that seems to arise from the creation, or poiesis, of the things themselves: I whittle a bird or write a blues song with a sense of all the other whittled birds and written blues songs, and also with a sense of how some day I might be able to make better ones. Given a certain level of skill, improvements in my ability as whittler or blues writer become invisible to a general audience and only noticeable to experts. Literary things – both the things depicted in stories and the stories themselves – are distinguished by level of skill: some writers are well trained, and some are writers' writers. But literary things also demand training of their readers: stories are only as good as their readers, and all of us, after a certain time, can become experts in our own stories through a process of narrative reflection and enquiry.

The idea that the language-using mind evolved as a result of and alongside of toolmaking is not new (see Hewes, 1995; Stout & Chaminade, 2012) and has seen many variations over the centuries. Supporting MacGregor's assertions about brain change and Oldowan technology, some studies suggest that Oldowan tools trace a boundary between the human brain and those of other known primates. At two million years ago, the advent of Oldowan tools marks the farthest boundary for the development of language, and evidence is mounting that these tools helped pave the way for modern, language-using, narrating human beings with senses of self. The long-lived Oldowan technology seemed to facilitate the development of language, whereas a relatively sophisticated language is believed to be essential to making the Acheulian technology that replaced it.[5] Storytelling is a little inconvenient without language, language and making co-evolved, so things and stories can be thought of as siblings. Poets still, by and large, focus on things, and those of us who study poets are trained to note the way poets work the encounter with things.

Language was almost certainly not being used by the early *Homo hominins* who were flaking cores to make Oldowan tools such as the scraper in the British Museum, but language had likely developed by the time Acheulian bifaces were being produced. Other evidence, such as morphological changes in early hominins that coincide with Oldowan technology, suggests as well that something happened to our common ancestors once they started making tools, a something that also led to language.

A more recent study (Morgan et al., 2015) further investigates the Oldowan-Acheulian shift, noting that the former tradition stayed relatively the same for approximately seven hundred thousand years, indicating a cultural stasis inconsistent with what one would expect to be found

5 The evidence gathered by FDG-PET and fMRI scans of participants learning Oldowan toolmaking skills, combined with research on human and non-human brains and clues from the fossil record, supports theories that "selection acting on Oldowan toolmaking capacities could have favoured the elaboration of a praxic system that was subsequently co-opted to support the enhanced articulatory control required for speech" (Morgan et al., sec. 3a). The significantly more complex late Acheulian toolmaking technology, which arose much later, "provides a second behaviourally and chronologically grounded functional/anatomical link between technological and linguistic capacities, further extending the plausible context for co-evolutionary interactions (e.g., behavioural, developmental and/or evolutionary co-option)" (sec. 3b).

in a community with complex language. Tests on transmission methods of these two tool traditions "support a gene-culture co-evolutionary account of human evolution in which reliance on Oldowan tools would have generated selection favouring teaching and, ultimately, language" ("Introduction"). The human capacity for language seems to have developed during those hundreds of thousands of years alongside the toolmaking (poiesis), which "generated selection favouring increasingly complex teaching and language" ("Discussion"). Speech has been shown to be the most effective, time-saving way to pass on the skills necessary to produce these tools, but also the use and manufacture of the tools makes more use of the same neural systems that are associated with language. An even more recent study by Lombao et al. (2017) concludes that by the time the very complex Acheulian tools were being made, language would almost certainly have to play into the ways those technologies are passed on to future generations. Language, according to this theory, first emerges as a means of better passing on knowledge and skills, originally tied to making things. Autobiographical narratives are not so far from this early development.

Randall and McKim's *Reading Our Lives* builds upon the foundation of the "narrative mind," a model of mind supported by an interdisciplinary group of thinkers including psychologists Jerome Bruner, Mark Freeman, and Dan McAdams. Antonio Damasio's "core self" is posited as the milestone in the developing self that first allows for a sense of selfhood through the nascent twin awareness of narrative and metaphor (Randall & McKim, 2008), but it is important to note that the core self itself "is born as a result of our encounters with objects" (p. 24). Supplemented by the observations of phenomenologists and neuroscientists, this observation places things in the role of midwife to the self, or perhaps better in line with the studies detailed above, the thing is the (narrative, narrating) self's older sibling. Brown in his way addresses the same concerns, in contemplating things, as the researchers studying chipped stone dug out of the ground: that humans are wrapped up in things; that both self and thing grew up together as part and parcel of the same world; that narrative, thingness, and complex, abstract modes of thought all are inseparable from what it is to be a human being. Things, like humans, are mortal, though their lifespans are often longer than any individual human's: when the last person dies, the last things of the human world will revert to objects, unless they are some day appropriated by another narrating species.

For some of our participants this is no simple thought experiment. You are ageing and you must downsize, that large thing has to go, and your kids can't take it. You go to the writing workshop where you're supposed to learn how to write about yourself. Instead you write about the thing. You're losing the thing – or are you?

Things as Literary Images

The last goal of this chapter is to consider what happens to a thing as it makes the transition to narrative, taking on literary duties. This is the point where some of my expertise in modernist writing kicks in. Modernist writers and artists, as well as theorists of modernism, have been most keenly attentive to this question, from French painter Marcel Duchamp's interrogation of manufactured objects (the famous urinal-cum-fountain; see Franklin, 2000) to the literary imagists and their successors, the objectivists, for whom there are "no ideas but in things." In attempting to strip poetry of its artifice and return to the essential, gestural beginnings of poetry, imagism – the intersection of things, humans, and the media that represented them – paved a new way to understand the symbolic value of things in literature. Rather than as contrived metonyms, symbols – grounded in the image – took on new agency as ambiguous figures that were on the one hand bounded and hard edged and on the other gravity wells for metaphor, without being metaphors themselves. In the chapters in Part 2, we aim for the things themselves in the stories and interview transcripts from our various participants, letting particular things engender the stories of the individuals connected to them. In doing so, sometimes the stories that emerge cast a different light on the stories the participants are striving to tell.

Poetry

When a group of young poets sought, around the time of the First World War, to revolutionize poetry in English, they did so by cutting out the excess. All the unnecessary ornament, artifice, convention, and habit that had accrued – including rhyme and regular metre, and also to a great extent including figurative language including metaphor and symbol – was eliminated in a process of reduction that, they hoped, would result in poetry that was stripped to its essence. The poems that emerged were short, concise, and centred on images, which poet Ezra Pound (1954) defined as "that which presents an intellectual and emotional complex in an instant of time" (p. 4).

Most of these images were crisp depictions of things. Like the gestural line that suggested an elaborate shape or movement, the image was the living pulse of the imagist poem. The sculptor Constantin Brancusi's "Bird in Space," a lithe line of metal, could be considered sculpture's response to the imagist poem, with its seeming striving for the essence both of the metal itself and of the bird in flight.

Imagism was originally styled with a final "e" to evoke an earlier movement, "symbolisme," which it sought to replace. Ezra Pound, imagism's most strident spokesperson, complained that for symbolists, symbolist symbols had a "fixed value" and were not really symbols but metonyms. I think that most of his colleagues agreed with him on this point. The school of symbolism would clearly influence Freud, who saw "symbols" found in dreams to be metonyms or metaphors whose corresponding vehicles were hidden or repressed. While imagist symbols had abstract value, they were grounded in clear, economical descriptions of real things. The things do not vanish into the symbol, and no one-to-one relationship exists between the symbol and something else. The image of imagism invites a new kind of symbol that does not point, but gathers. Tim Ingold (2011) also prefers to understand writing as "a species of gathering" (p. 179), which for him combines the skill of the maker (*tekne*) with the act of weaving (*texere*) that informs our ideas of text and of making in general.[6]

The modernist reformulation of the idea of the symbol, based on concrete things but having abstract value, would come to dominate literary definitions of the symbol. The *Oxford Dictionary of Literary Terms* (Baldick, 2008, s.v. "symbol") concludes that "it is ... usually too simple to say that a literary symbol 'stands for' some idea as if it were just a convenient substitute for a fixed meaning; it is usually a substantial image in its own right, around which further significances may gather according to differing interpretations." In the 1916 collection *Sea Garden* by H.D., for example, various flowers are the subject of short, ode-like poems that work to complicate the conventional symbolism associated with roses, lilies, and other flowers, while also steadfastly refusing to rob them of their thingness by subsuming them into larger signifying codes. Modernist scholar Burton Hatlen (1995), who prefers the term "image" to "symbol," notes that "in these poems, meanings develop that transcend the individual images. Nevertheless, these images retain their integral unity" in "new, distinctly post-symbolist methods of making meaning" (p. 124). Rather than understand these objects as symbols in the traditional sense, Hatlen emphasizes that any given poem from the collection "does not say a single word about the observer or her longings: instead

6 Jennifer and Brandi, in Chapters 6 and 11 respectively, dig into the idea of weaving, textiles, and identity, and in Chapter 12 on the table, Brandi and I explore its owner's exploration of things, symbols, and gathering.

the poem focuses on a dynamic process that is happening 'out there,' in the world of objects." This represents "a distinctively Imagist poetics, one that opened up powerful new possibilities for all poets, women and men" (p. 127). What I think is most characteristic of the symbol in this modernist literary sense is that the object is characterized by a hard-edged clarity with "clearly demarcated boundaries" (p. 114) and yet it generates post-formal thought that knows no closure except, somehow, within the horizon of the thing in its world.

In other words, for Hatlen H.D. is making things in her poetry, not symbols. The things are as real as Les Nessman's tape walls, and they require our knowledge of seasides and of plants to come into play. But once you can imagine a particular beach on the coast and you can picture a flower you can imagine growing there, stunted and slashed by wind, salt, and sand – once you come face-to-face with the thing she's writing about – you start to see it as a symbol because it's a poem after all, and a text is a kind of thing as well, as Marcea will explore in Chapter 9.

Back to Thing Theory, and Virginia Woolf

Not far from the imagist poetry of H.D. is the modernist fiction of Virginia Woolf (1985), whose story "Solid Objects" serves as Bill Brown's (1999) point of departure for his early work on thing theory, "The secret life of things." I now quote at length from each, one after the other, in order to highlight the way that Woolf's fiction is born out of the foam of things' excess:

> As he was choosing which of these things to make it, still working his fingers in the water, they curled round something hard – a full drop of solid matter – and gradually dislodged a large irregular lump, and brought it to the surface. When the sand coating was wiped off, a green tint appeared. It was a lump of glass, so thick as to be almost opaque; the smoothing of the sea had completely worn off any edge or shape, so that it was impossible to say whether it had been bottle, tumbler or window-pane; it was nothing but glass; it was almost a precious stone. You had only to enclose it in a rim of gold, or pierce it with a wire, and it became a jewel; part of a necklace, or a dull, green light upon a finger. Perhaps after all it was really a gem; something worn by a dark Princess trailing her finger in the water as she sat in the stern of the boat and listened to the slaves singing as they rowed her across the Bay. Or the oak sides of a sunk Elizabethan treasure-chest had split apart, and, rolled over and over, over and over, its emeralds had come at last to shore. John turned it in his hands; he held it to the light; he held it so that its irregular mass blotted out the body and extended right arm of

> his friend. The green thinned and thickened slightly as it was held against the sky or against the body. It pleased him; it puzzled him; it was so hard, so concentrated, so definite an object compared with the vague sea and the hazy shore. (Woolf, 1985, p. 55)

For Brown, Woolf has hit upon the ways in which things spill over the boundaries between worlds, revealing the human world. Woolf's prose is attentive to the way the

> thing becomes manifest between multiple objectifications. Within the shimmering splinters of glass, glass can become something else. Or, to offer another narrative example (of what can be exemplified only syntactically, only in time): in the process of using a knife as a screwdriver, of dislocating it from one routinized objectification and deploying it otherwise, we have the chance (if just a chance) to sense its presence (its thinness ... its sharpness and flatness ... the peculiarity of its scalloped handle, slightly loose ... its knifeness and what exceeds that knifeness) as though for the first time. For the first time, perhaps, we thus also sense the norms by which we customarily deploy both knife and screwdriver. My concern, then, is not to unveil the meaning of things in their proper thingness, nor to describe the fate of pure objects abstracted from their use, and neither is it to privilege the thing (*das Ding*) over things (*die Sachen*). For the life of things made manifest in the time of misuse is, should we look, a secret in plain sight – not a life behind or beneath the object but a life that is its fluctuating shape and substance and surface, a life that the subject must catalyze but cannot contain. (Brown, 1999, p. 3)

What I get out of this, both Woolf and Brown, is that things can act as a lens through which everything familiar can be seen in a new way. The impulse always seems to be to skip over the things, to leap instinctively to their use, or their social value, or their personal significance. Holding fast to the thing as something not subsumed in these intellectual schemes forces us to reflect on stories that we thought we already understood. It is that lens, subtle as invisible boundaries, that this book offers to a narrative enquiry into the complexity of older adults' inner storyworlds.

Looking Things Up

One of the roots of the word "thing" is the Germanic *þengas*, "a time to gather" (*OED*). This phrase comes close to the subtitle of the story, really a meditation, written by the final participant we discuss in Part 2: "Mahogany Table: Bringing Things Together" (see Chapter 12). In meditating quite explicitly on his family's table's symbolic value as a tool not only for reminiscence but for gathering or meeting, the participant – David – has touched another earlier definition of the word "thing," straight out of the Old Norse that gave it to us: a meeting or gathering. The thing in question in David's meditation, the table, becomes the site of all human interaction, the original gathering place.

The sense of thing as "gathering" is important here: it's one of a few connotations of the word that help the thinker approach the question of the thingness of things. David uses the word "gathering" in multiple ways to suggest the way the table is a place of gathering along several horizons, from family gatherings all the way to the gathering of those things that make community and, ultimately, humanity possible by virtue of its being there. We gather to share food and stories. The table as symbol partakes of this gathering, that freeing of things in and for their thingness. They are not objects set against subjects, nor are they mere reminiscentia or fetishized objects. Rather, they maintain their mystery while gathering unto themselves metaphorical associations that cross the boundaries of what any owner or author could intend.

Putting "Ekphrasis" in the Wrong Syllabus

The existing order is complete before the new work arrives; for order to persist after the supervention of novelty, the *whole* existing order must be, if ever so slightly, altered; and so the relations, proportions, values of each work of art toward the whole are readjusted; and this is conformity between the old and the new.

– T.S. Eliot (2005, p. 153)

Asking "What's that?" while indicating a thing that has been brought up in a narrative can open new ways, supported by the narrative, of thinking about that thing. The family couch is a thing, but isn't the spot on the left side equally a thing? With its two skewed springs and stains on the arm, which the spouse, children, and one of the cats fight over because it has the best view of the television? So maybe it's only that spot on the couch that is meaningful, cherished. Should that spot be cut out and made into a memento?

Or could the narratives and other symbols associated with that spot be explored by other means, say in writing about them? As for defining "thing," the etymology is clouded, and the set of possible objects it includes is comically buried. A massive black hole holds our galaxy together, but it only became a thing in the twentieth century, first called "dark star" or "gravitationally collapsed object" until some wisecracker thought of the

Black Hole of Calcutta (which is now Kolkata; "Calcutta" is only a thing now in things named after it, such as the black hole and the gambling scheme). It became all the more a thing when it was first imaged in 2019. Yet when I look up "black hole" the definition I get is the opposite of what I think of as a "thing." I am assured, nonetheless, that a black hole is a thing, and I am equally assured, by those in the know, that it isn't.

There is nothing more alien from the ordinary world of things – a world of human manufacture full of coffee cups and glowing screens and right angles – than this monstrous but equally real and observable thing, which belongs to the world of human making now that it has been appropriated by a team of scientists working with a global array of networked telescopes. It is narrative resilience, the narrating subject's ability to be ductile, that moves over and lets a black hole into the human world. Cup of coffee in hand, sitting in a favourite spot on the couch, humanity calls the family around to look at the new image on a screen.[7] The known laws of nature are updated and narrativized in order to find the place this new thing occupies: "Gravity won't break, but all space and time has to fold in when there's a black hole, and if you get close to it you will stay young while those you left behind will age before you can return, though to you it would only have been a few hours" (Levin 2020). The black hole has been there all along, invisibly holding the galaxy together, but only in its appropriation to the human world has it become a thing, and it's forced us to reconsider what a "thing" is. Either way, it fits into the categories "real" and "improbable," and things are all over that.

The interviews with our participants were full of narrative, and in nearly all of them a thing helped to anchor that narrative. The attitudes to things, however, varied. After Jennifer and Denise offer brief introductions of all nine participants in Chapter 4, our next chapter focusses on a couple who have no trouble leaving things behind so long as there are copies, while our last chapter, Chapter 12, examines the lengthy piece written by David about a particular family heirloom (the table) that can, in a sense, substitute for the physical presence of the heirloom itself. Between these two strategies are several other potential attitudes we can have to things in the narratives of our lives, and the ability to have ductile narratives, or narrative resilience (Randall, et al, 2015), may well have a salutary effect on our resilience in general.

Literary scholar Northrop Frye (1990) remarks that "what is true for us is what we have made ... a creation in which we have participated, whether we

7 I think that the image depicts all the stuff that accrues around the black hole and not the black hole itself, and so strictly speaking it is an image of the things that point to the black hole, which is not a thing by some definitions but is nevertheless there.

have been in on the making of it or the responding to it" (p. 82). For Frye, it is a given that everything real is "in contrast to our dreams … a human creation, and whatever human beings have made human beings can remake" (p. 82). We cannot forget "the reality which is real because it is a created fiction, and recognized to be as such" (p. 82). The power of literature to remake the thing – as Victor Hugo's novel remade Notre Dame Cathedral – and the power of Les Nessman to create walls out of lines on the floor is not a special case of the thing, but a fundamental condition of thingness.

Poiesis is the making that produces the human world, and poetry is, to some extent or another, the contemplation of things in the human world, through the human speaker. Sometimes the speaker is Martian or divine, but the poem is written in lines by a human hand, gathering, weaving lines; sometimes the world is distorted or strange, but this is simply the way in which poetry highlights some systems while downplaying others, just as an x-ray is no good for what an ultrasound can do. The human-thing relationship is intimate; the human's mortality is bound to the thing's mortality, and the thing teaches that death is a gradual process of decomposition in which only meaningful things hold any distinction. The Grecian urn is torn from its original context, to which it cannot be restored because only museums exist now of its civilization,[8] and yet the youth and vitality of the figures adorning it, frozen in time, are the object of a poem that ends "Beauty is truth, truth beauty, – that is all / Ye know on earth, and all ye need to know." What remains strong in things – and in people – is their place in the human world. Ekphrasis or "speaking out," from the verb meaning "to proclaim or call an inanimate object by name," is the kind of asking that attends to things in narrative; ekphrastic writing, or the asking of questions inviting an ekphrastic response to things, produces thoughtful reflection on why this particular thing has a name (a story, an occurrence), a meaning that is important for the narrative, and so might go some distance towards answering the question "What are we to do with things?"

Sure, it's a stretch to call what we're doing in this book ekphrasis. We are not writing poetry responding to art or craft: we are writing academic work responding to data. But some of our data *is* writing about art and craft, and so our book responds to those responses. It attends to things that are real enough, but our readers will never see them. To someone somewhere, some are cherished, which we all should remember, because to you and me, they're textual things encountered by us as though for the first time.

---

8 Anyway, Keats had made the image out of several urns he'd seen, not one.

PART TWO

Research Adventures

4 Things and Stories: Our Participants' Worlds at a Glance

JENNIFER ESTEY AND DENISE RESMI

Every person's life is worth a novel.

– Erving Polster (1987)

Our goal in this chapter is to offer sketches of nine of the older adults who attended the three workshops that Deborah Carr facilitated as part of our project looking into the nature of narrative resilience in later life. (See Chapter 14 for her description of these events.) Of the thirty-five who attended in total and, in turn, the fourteen who agreed to be interviewed before the first workshop and after the third, these nine individuals, entirely without prompting, and either during the interviews or in the pieces of writing they did in between, highlighted certain objects that seemed particularly significant for them. Since these objects themselves take centre stage in this part of the book, our aim here is to outline the lives of the "storytellers" (Mishler, 1991, p. 119) behind them. Before we get to that, though, a few words are in order about Jennifer's experience as an interviewer, since of all of us she enjoyed the most personal relationship with these individuals, and about Denise's experience as a research assistant.

In both interviews, Jennifer saw herself playing the role of storylistener as much as, if not more than, interviewer. Using scripted questions prepared beforehand (see Appendix 2), as well as prompts such as "mm-hm" or, at times, just a smile or nod, she encouraged the storyteller to give, as much as possible, long, rich, and detailed responses. At the same time, she remained attentive and refrained from interrupting, for ultimately it was the storytellers themselves who chose how they responded, sharing as much or as little as they wished. That said, many of them obviously felt comfortable enough with her to share funny, sad, harrowing, and sometimes long-hidden aspects of their stories. Conducting these interviews was thus deeply humbling for her, a trained social worker, and triggered a great deal of introspection about what it means to relate to and with other people.

She found herself wondering, for instance, how she had influenced the content of the interview, being very much aware that in qualitative research generally, and definitely in narrative inquiry, listeners invariably shape what tellers tell (Randall et al., 2006). And she wondered what aspects of her approach had invited her interviewees to trust her sufficiently to reveal so much detail about themselves. Is it that they perceived her to be not just kind and a good listener, but also non-judgmental? A white woman with blue eyes and dark brown hair, worn almost always in a tight ponytail, she tended to dress casually in jeans, loose fitting T-shirts, and running shoes, and without makeup – an outfit more suitable for visiting friends perhaps than for conducting interviews. Yet this simple style itself, she felt, might have contributed to the positive rapport she developed with them. She wondered too, though, whether their openness with her was related to the fact that they knew the interactions between the two of them would be short-lived and thus that there were little or no long-term consequences to what they would say. While numerous other questions are still unanswered, she believes overall that the opportunity of gaining intimate insight into these people's lives was very much a privilege.

What is more, her interviews with them changed how she views storytelling itself. They revealed to her how vulnerable a storyteller can be, and how that very vulnerability creates a certain level of intimacy. While storytelling can be a surface-level activity, for the purpose of entertainment, of sharing information, or of teaching, she realized that it can be profoundly personal as well. And it can be profoundly physical too, in the sense that the stories people tell are on some level the stories they *are*, and as such are embodied. The looks and lines on their faces, and their gestures and postures, attest to untold stories and shadow stories that may hover in the wings. Although Jennifer can't, of course, speak to the feelings that the participants themselves had about the interviews, she found herself concerned at times that their sharing of such intimate stories might be unsettling for them, stirring up still deeper stories that were troubling to recall. Many such concerns, of course, were mitigated by the positive feedback she received from them, not to mention the encouraging comments she got from members of the research team.

In contrast to Jennifer, Denise never met the participants face to face. Brought into the project as a research assistant during the analysis phase, she nonetheless came to know them quite intimately from all of the transcripts and recordings that the interviews produced and that she carefully reviewed. Filtered through pages and pages of paper and the speakers of her computer, the participants' unique personalities thus gradually revealed themselves to her, and she found herself deeply moved by the things they chose to hold onto in the course of their lives.

There is, first of all, the tangible, the objects themselves: items that survived multiple moves, or were painstakingly crafted, or were unexpectedly uncovered in abandoned lots. But there is also the intangible: the memories, the hurts, and the possible selves (Markus & Nurius, 1986) that the participants carried with them and held close to their hearts. While some participants engage with these objects regularly, for others, empowered by Deborah's workshops and Jenn's gentle probing, it was their first time to do so in their sixty- or seventy-odd years. In the whole intriguing matter of what memories resurface, in what ways, in a person's latter years, Denise has found a certain poignancy and mystery. And if nothing else, it has left her with a profound curiosity for her own story too. Though the future carries an obvious allure, with its unknowns and its possibilities, she has come to realize that our past, while seemingly less exciting, possesses an abundance of material from which to extract meaning and to springboard our way to greater growth.

Our Interviewees and Their Objects

Our main aim in this chapter is to outline the lives of each of our nine central storytellers, as Jennifer got to know them in the course of the interviews she did with them and as Denise became acquainted with them while poring through the pages of what they said. It might be helpful first to summarize briefly the objects they have each made reference to, since that's what they have in common and it's what we'll be zeroing in on in Part 2.

Known in our study as LS20 and LS21 (LS stands for "life story"), "Mary" and "Bob," as Matte refers to them, are a married couple whose principal hobby has been creating jewellery out of sea glass. Indeed, members of their family have contributed to their expansive collection of glass by combing the beaches for pieces that they can work with. But this hasn't just been a pastime for them; it's been a source of income too, not to mention an inspiration for their writing. While the two have actively collected objects, by contrast the life of LS18, whom Brandi calls "Susan," revolves in many ways around story. The activities she participates in, in other words, are specifically chosen to acquire material for her writing. For instance, she has been using decades-old frozen red currants picked by her now-deceased mother to dye yarn so that she can write a story about the process of doing so. As for LS06, whom Jennifer calls "Amelie," she threads together the past, the present, and the future through the various quilts that she creates.

Both LS27, whom Bill and Anthazia refer to as "Joan," and also as "Princess," and LS08, whom Erin calls "Harriet," divulged what were actually quite difficult stories. Joan had journeyed across the sea to England in search of her past, and returned with her grandfather's beer stein, an object that represented an inaccessible legacy yet was monumental in terms of helping her to understand important pieces about her identity that had previously remained in doubt. As for Harriet, her story demonstrates how a page torn from a textbook can point to a path not taken, and to the possible selves she might otherwise have lived.

The labyrinth ring worn by LS19, or "Hermann," as Bill calls him, serves as a symbol for his life as a journey through a maze with many different turning points, which he proceeds through with curiosity and a sense of adventure, uncertain where it will lead. On the other hand, LS29, or "Joy," as Marcea refers to her, says that her life has come "full circle," a statement inspired by rereading a series of letters written to her years ago by a much older male friend. Reflecting on this relationship, one of unrequited love on his part that spanned more than two decades and that reading the letters brought back to mind for her, has given her a fresh perspective on it. Lastly, LS16 – or "David," as Matte and Brandi have christened him – takes us on a journey from the cosmos to his kitchen table, an object for which he holds a deep and abiding affection as a place of gathering.

Our Interviewees' Stories

Bob and Mary

The interviews with Bob and Mary take place in the living room of their two-storey suburban home. After coming in the entryway, Jenn finds a neat, orderly, open-concept space whose walls display beach-themed art. Mary offers her a hot cup of loose-leaf tea, which she gratefully accepts and places on the shadow box coffee table whose contents – sand, shells, and sea glass – are also reminiscent of the beach. A fireplace provides a warm, comforting ambiance. Jennifer sits in a chair and Bob or Mary each sit in one as well, or else on the sofa, where they can make eye contact with her throughout the interviews. Though the two of them are both at home during both sets of interviews, neither interrupts the other's interview. We'll begin with Mary's story.

Now seventy-four, and a self-described writer (2-II), Mary reflects on growing up in New Brunswick. From a young age, she knew that she would leave her small town because she was self-confident and, in her words, "directed" (9-II). Two incidents in particular shaped her life early on and appeared to be especially self-defining for her.

The first took place when she was twelve. One day she went down to the river with several of her cousins. One of the older boys, Jack, had brought along a camera and asked her to pose with his sister at the water's edge. He kept telling them to back up, his goal being for them to fall into the water, not knowing that neither girl swam well at all. His plan worked perfectly and both girls tumbled in. When he saw them struggling to surface, however, he jumped in and pulled his sister from the water. Mary, though, was caught in the current and quickly dragged below the surface. Close to drowning, she lost consciousness and recalls having an out-of-body experience. After Jack dragged her, too, from the water and performed CPR on her, she finally came to. The incident left her with a lifelong fear of water.

The second occurred when she was fifteen and had been told by her male classmates that girls were less capable and less intelligent than boys. To prove them wrong, she spent the summer peeling pulpwood with her father, working twelve-hour shifts a day, beginning at 6 a.m. While she didn't exactly enjoy the work, since it was difficult, back-breaking, and dirty, the sense of accomplishment she derived was well worth it, and the whole experience revealed her strengths to her. As she put it, "it was one of the most important things that happened in my life" (62-II).

Bob's work as an RCMP officer required them to relocate frequently, seven moves in total, Mary recalls. They also travelled widely, having vacationed in numerous countries, including South Africa, Tunisia, and Hong Kong, and visited almost every state in the United States. For thirty-two years, she sent annual letters to family members in which she recounted the events of the preceding year, including their travels, as well as those moments that gave her "goosebumps" (3-I) or, as she said, could not "be contained" within herself (7-I). For instance, as she sat one time in the ruins of an ancient coliseum, she thought, "This is where St. Paul addressed the Ephesians" (7-I). It was, she said, an "out of this world moment" (7-I). These letters to friends and family proved invaluable to her writing as they contained a wealth of material, offering long-forgotten details of special past events.

Mary also wrote about her involvement in community yard sales. For several years she not only attended them but played a key role in organizing them, and held fond memories of the community coming together around them. She also became fascinated with how objects themselves travel and then cycle back into the sales. For example, she once sold a tablecloth that she had purchased in Europe, and ten years later, she tried to buy it back, forgetting it had once been hers!

When Bob walks into the room for his first interview, he starts right in sharing stories, speaking for a good ten minutes before Jennifer asks if she can turn on the recorder, to which, of course, he immediately agrees. The chair he sits in is at an awkward angle to her, though, so eye contact between them is difficult at times. During the interview he eats grapes, which he offers to Jennifer but, due to dietary restrictions, she declines. Over the grapes, he settled in to telling her about his life.

Now seventy-five, Bob grew up in Atlantic Canada within a close-knit family. He and his brother were always devising ways to make money, including splitting wood, tearing batteries apart, and collecting worms to sell as bait for fish. He recalled paper routes where each newspaper sold for five cents. He was grateful, though, that his parents taught him and his siblings to be independent and accountable for their actions. In addition, his mother kept them busy by teaching them how to prepare dinner, something that left him with a lifelong love of cooking. As an adult, he often experiments with different dishes, and together he and Mary have hosted several large dinner parties.

At eighteen years old he applied to become an RCMP officer. Once accepted, he boarded the train for the police academy in Saskatchewan, thus beginning a career that lasted thirty-six years. He took great pride in his work and was pleased that his grandson wanted to follow in his footsteps. When Bob discussed his work, he became animated and excitement poured out of him, leading him at times to jump out of his chair. This excitement flowed through the many stories that he tells Jenn about some of the highlights in his career, including his involvement in large drug busts, high-speed car chases, and working security for celebrities and world leaders. These, he feels strongly, would make captivating stories for the next generation.

Outside of his work, he pursued various hobbies, including hunting, fishing, snowshoeing, and skiing. As he has aged, however, and many of these activities have become too difficult for him, he has started painting, writing, playing cards, and making sea glass jewellery.

Sea glass jewellery – which they have sold at craft fairs for as much as $150 per piece – has been a significant part of the couple's life for the previous six years. Sea glass is glass that has been weathered in sand and salt water over time, and been polished by it into a smooth surface. With the help of their grandchildren, who became involved in collecting it from the beach near their son's seaside cottage, they have accumulated over twenty thousand pieces that they have carefully catalogued and stored in their basement. While Bob has taken the lead in making the jewellery, Mary has researched and written about the origins of the glass itself.

As the sea glass chapter has wound down in their story as a couple, their principal "we-story," as it were (Singer & Skerrett, 2014), the two of them have become more focussed on writing, and it's their aim to co-author a booklet for their grandchildren. Though this sort of endeavour has been entirely new to Bob, he's delighted by the memories the writing has triggered. As the self-identified writer in the partnership, Mary feels more experienced, though, and is the one who edits their work. Feeling very much that he is *not* a writer, Bob prefers to stick to the facts and keep embellishments to a minimum, in the hope that readers will get a realistic sense of who he was. For him, the biggest challenge is sequencing the events that he writes about, not coming up with content per se. There is no danger of his lacking that, he explains, for he feels he could write volumes about his childhood, his interests, and certainly his career.

Susan

Like Bob and Mary, Susan, aged sixty-one, engages in numerous hobbies and activities. Set in a rural location, her home itself makes it clear that she is engaged in a variety of creative endeavours and that she very much, as she says, "lives in" her space. A collector of items that energize and inspire her, she definitely has eclectic tastes.

Jennifer walks in the front door and up a set of stairs into an open-concept living room. She sits in a chair to the right, with Susan across from her on the couch. As she scans her surroundings, Jennifer observes an overwhelming assortment of things. To her left, the office door is ajar, permitting her to see four walls with bookcases, and lots of boxes sprawled across the floor, some stacked in teetering piles, their lids protruding from overfill. Straight ahead is the dining room where a variety of plants are hanging from the ceiling, sitting on the table, or perched upon shelves. Knick-knacks with no apparent theme linking them together are scattered across shelves, side tables, and stands. The walls hold several types of paintings, many of them Susan's own work. During one of the two interviews, she shows Jennifer an incomplete work that's been inspired by a large, cylindrical glass potpourri jar and the yellow curtains that hang in the dining room window. Her inspiration, it is clear, stems from the things that surround her.

During the first interview, Susan alludes to the death of her parents, but explains to Jennifer that this is a story she feels is untellable: "I really haven't written about their deaths," she says. "I've written about them and lots of stories about them, but I haven't really written about their deaths and they were kind of horrendous. They were accidental deaths" (14-I). Yet by the second interview, she tells Jennifer this "untellable" story, explaining that having a non-judgmental audience helps her to share more, a comment that Jennifer still thinks about. "How come she felt able to tell me?" Jennifer asks herself. "What was it about my demeanour or my attitude that helped her feel able to share that? Was she the villain in her story? Was she feeling responsible or guilty for their deaths? Did she think I would mirror these feelings? Based on what she shared, did I feel sympathy, empathy, or sorrow for her loss rather than scepticism? Or contempt? What changed for her through the process of the workshops or the interviews themselves?"

Susan identifies herself clearly as a writer. From an early age, she was a voracious reader and her parents were both storytellers, instilling in her a lasting love of narrative. Her mother in particular would entertain her and her siblings by telling them stories about growing up during the Great Depression and World War Two. Her father, in contrast, told fewer stories; that is, until he revisited his childhood home, at which point, Susan says, "a switch turned on" (27-I). It's as if the homestead itself triggered all manner of memories for him, and so lots of stories and anecdotes began to emerge.

Loving the natural world, Susan refers to "a major part of the fabric of my family life" being cabins or camps (1-II). She recalls helping her father build one when she was a small child. It's where she penned her first poem and where, later, she retreated during her graduate studies. She wrote her master's thesis in biology surrounded by her subject matter, nature. Wanting her son to have similar experiences with nature, she and her husband began building another camp when he was three. Once completed, it became the backdrop for countless family gatherings, late nights playing Yahtzee, and summer days spent relaxing. In time, however, the couple found it too difficult to visit the secluded location, and with heavy hearts they sold it and bought a new, more accessible camp.

Susan's mother died under difficult circumstances, and her father passed away soon after. Both parents' deaths were traumatic and therefore difficult for her to address directly. In an indirect way, however, she has found a means of writing about her parents and, in particular, revisiting her mother's memory. Before her death, the woman had picked currants and asked Susan to freeze them. Having kept them for over a decade, Susan has recently decided to use them as dye. In their transformed state, both the currants and the yarn that she has dyed from them have therefore become something new that she intends to write about.

The plant dye project is significant because it represents a key theme running through Susan's sense of narrative identity: that of the scientist-turned-artist. Having recently retired from a thirty-three-year government career composing dry, technical reports, she suddenly has more time to engage in a range of projects, among them blogging, journaling, painting, quilting, and family genealogy. In each of them, she has been highly productive. Her blog has had over 650 posts, her paintings are auctioned at local establishments, and she has become her family's repository of genealogical information. At the heart of it all for her, however, has been writing. Dedicating almost sixty hours a week to it and her other creative activities, she has written five collections of poetry and two books; she frequently attends writing workshops, such as the three that were part of this project; and she is a member of two writing groups. Throughout the interviews, she makes numerous allusions to her "writing life."

Her husband is an active supporter of her several endeavours, running the household errands so as to give her more free time and often serving as her first audience. At various times during the interviews, she emphasizes how much fun they have together. The contrast in their personalities, she believes, creates a balance between them. "I see the whole world through glory glasses," she explains to Jennifer; "everything is the way I want to see it, not the way it actually is. But my husband sees ... black and white. He's able to kind of give me a bit of truth" (10-II).

Susan speaks of being inspired at times to write about something from her life, whether it be a childhood memory or a walk through the woods with her husband. And sometimes, in fact, she sets out to experience things with the express purpose of writing about them. Even seemingly insignificant things, like a rug, can launch a new project for her, and thus form the basis of a story. She tells Jennifer, for instance, about how when her son was a teen they would play Dungeons and Dragons together and how, through the medium of fantasy storytelling, they could resolve real-life issues between them. Almost every facet of her life, it appears, is susceptible to being storied.

Susan is eager to publish more of her work. Before the workshops, she focussed on fiction, but the workshops have invited her to do more memoir work instead. In writing about her mother's life, which she considered putting into poetry, she has realized, though, how much of what makes it into her fiction comes from her own life. Often when she reads a piece to her husband, for example, he will remark upon the similarities between the two – between her fiction and her life.

Amelie

Amelie, aged sixty-five, lives in a two-storey house located in a subdivision just outside of Fredericton. Her husband, a diehard do-it-yourself-er, does home maintenance and has given their dwelling some unique design characteristics, such as built-in bookshelves that span the length of the living room wall, plus stairs he has hand-painted with a fake brick-and-mortar look. The house is orderly and well-kept, although the "brick" at the top of the stairs has been worn off by their dog, who often sleeps there.

Amelie comes from a family rich in stories. In many of them her grandfather was a larger-than-life character, having left Europe at the age of eleven, worked on a boat, travelled the world, and learned seven languages. Amelie wants to transcribe the tapes of him recounting such stories in order to preserve their historical value.

She grew up in northern New Brunswick, but she felt like she never really "fit in" when she was younger (23-II). She had one close friend, however. The two were born just four days apart, with their mothers in adjacent hospital beds. By fourth grade, their friendship was well established. Their biggest adventure together was in 1968 when they turned eighteen and hitchhiked across New Brunswick and Prince Edward Island.

After leaving notes for their families, they sneaked out in the dead of night with less than twenty dollars between them. For sleeping arrangements along the way, they went sometimes to the local police station and, with varying success, would ask for a jail cell in which to spend the night. Amelie still has the two maps that detail the routes that they followed. The first one is of the Atlantic provinces with the planned itinerary drawn carefully in pen. Whenever they deviated from it, however, the original line was crossed out and redrawn to where they ended up travelling instead. On the second, a map of New Brunswick alone, they wrote one-line descriptions of each of the people who picked them up. Amelie rarely shares her hitchhiking story, however, feeling that it could be a bad influence on her children and grandchildren. Yet this short trip continues to stand out for her because it was one of the few times in her life when she was carefree and without responsibility. In contrast, the years to come proved rather challenging.

At nineteen, Amelie married a former classmate, "Frank." Despite her desire to become a medical doctor, she became a teacher instead, as was expected of many young women at the time. As much as she loved the work, it was difficult to sustain her growing family – at one point, all three children were under the age of three – on a teacher's meagre salary. So, she and Frank lived from pay cheque to pay cheque, struggling under the weight of their combined student debt. To help supplement their income, she worked for a time as a bartender. She would teach during the day, start her shift at the bar at 8 p.m., finish at 2 a.m., and then return to school just a few hours later. She had very little time off. Even maternity leave, as was customary at the time, was only one week long. Frank, also a teacher, joined her in bartending, bringing the total number of jobs that they held down between them to four. Any extra money they made was carefully saved, however, until their hard work and frugality allowed them to get ahead enough to begin investing in real estate. It was determination, she told Jennifer, that was the key to her success, and she is proud that her children possess similarly hard-working spirits.

While the hitchhiking trip was the beginning of her travels, that sort of adventure has remained a common theme throughout her life. For example, she spent a summer one time working in Africa and, more recently, she has visited China, where she and her sister walked along the Great Wall, literally following in the footsteps of her grandfather. She also travelled across Canada in a motorhome. Between travelling, working, and managing a family, Amelie feels that she has been busy enough to fill four lifetimes rather than merely one.

Twenty years ago, Amelie was diagnosed with multiple sclerosis. At first, the symptoms were so severe that she could barely walk. Her memory and vision were impaired as well, forcing her to leave her career of twenty-five years. Though she claimed that she remained a "teacher at heart" (49-II), these changes were devastating for someone who defined herself by her work ethic and her self-sufficiency.

Notwithstanding these challenges, she has retained her sense of determination and, with treatment, managed her condition well. She translates articles in English for French publications, knits for farmers' markets, and has volunteered for five years at the local hospice. She is also an avid quilter, combining writing and quilting by recording the histories of many of the quilts she creates. Some of these stories are light hearted, focussing on details such as the origins of the fabrics, while others are more troubling. She was working on a quilt, for instance, the day that she heard about 9/11. In total, she has written over eighty such stories, which she stores in binders and shares with others in her quilting circle.

For Amelie, it is crucial to be adaptable. Her personal philosophy is that if circumstances prevent you from doing what you want, then you must do something else. She does not want to take a break, in other words, because there is always still more to do.

Before attending the workshops, Amelie dabbled in writing out of a wish to pass on her love of stories to her granddaughter. To accomplish this goal, she wrote short stories specifically tailored to the young girl's interests, each one ending with a message or moral, making it possible for her to transmit wisdom to the next generation, a good example of transmissive reminiscence, or of generative transference. Inspired by her grandfather's stories, though, Amelie now wants to capture the facts, as well as the historical context, of her own story. Through her writing, not unlike her quilting, she seeks to weave together the threads of the past, the present, and the future. That said, she avoids emotional writing, for she finds it difficult to reflect on tough times. In keeping with a trend that gerontologists have identified (Carstensen & Mikels, 2005), she prefers to stay positive instead.

Joan

Joan, aged seventy, is interviewed at her cozy single-storey row house in the city, where she lives alone. With a strong nod to her heritage, she calls it "my English cottage" (34-I, 15-II). Jennifer sits on the couch in full view of the kitchenette, living area, and bedroom. To the right is a bookshelf where many of Joan's possessions are on display, including family photographs, her grandchildren's paintings, and her grandfather's beer stein.

Born in England, she moved to Canada with her mother when Joan was just an infant. She never met her father and, outside of her mother and half-siblings, had few close family relationships. When she was two years old, her mother was incarcerated and Joan was left to the foster care system. At first she was placed with her half-siblings, but ultimately they were separated. She recalls five different placements and living in three different homes between the ages of fourteen and sixteen.

Joan describes herself as a survivor, for when she was in foster care she was frequently mistreated. Having had, basically, to fend for herself from the age of nine, she felt isolated, and as a result struggled in high school, ultimately dropping out. While her peers used drugs and alcohol, however, she felt it was important for her to stay sober and in control. Also unlike her counterparts, she actively sought employment. One of the first of her many jobs was babysitting two little girls. Whenever possible throughout this period, she would write to her mother in prison, as well as her grandfather back home in England.

Her unusual upbringing affected her relationships. For example, she became engaged but once her fiancé's family learned of her lineage he called things off. Soon after, still relatively young, she married someone else, but her mother-in-law harboured reservations about her, saying things like "you just don't know where this girl came from" (30-II). She had two daughters with the man before the marriage ended in divorce.

When Joan was twenty-six she wanted to complete her high school diploma. As she was waiting to register, however, she was told that she could apply to university as a mature student. A self-declared "lifelong learner," she went on to get her bachelor's degree in psychology (10-I). At the time, of course, it was uncommon for women to go to university at all, but she was determined to provide a better life for her children. A single mother, she worked at a restaurant while attending university in order to make ends meet. In one of the courses she took, she recounted her life story to her classmates, who were all surprised at how well adjusted she was, considering everything she had experienced.

One thing that has always bothered Joan is the sense of having no roots. This has left her wondering for much of her life about her true identity. In the late 1980s her grandfather's second wife passed away and left her a small sum of money, so she decided to use it to take her daughters with her back to England to visit her grandfather's estate, where she hoped she would find some answers.

The manor house itself was gone, however, and three new houses had been built on the ground where it once stood. She asked the locals what happened; one neighbour told her it had been demolished quite suddenly in the middle of the night. Walking across the newly empty lot the next morning, he had discovered a beer stein sticking out of the debris. To her delight, he presented Joan with it and said to her, "we knew you existed; we just didn't know where you were" (1-II). This simple, bare acknowledgment of her identity was nothing short of monumental for her. As she later expressed it in the story she had written, "those were the most powerful words anyone could ever have said to me." After so many years of upheaval and uncertainty, it confirmed that she in fact belonged somewhere. The beer stein now sits proudly on her living room shelf.

All throughout her life, being told that she couldn't do something has motivated Joan to do just that. So not only did she get her BA but, eventually, she earned her master's in counselling and psychology. With pride, she describes herself to Jennifer as "a high school dropout with a Masters" (10-I, 56-I).

Many of Joan's friends have urged her to write about her life because it seems to them such a compelling story, but she has felt too busy living life to stop and write about it – until recently, that is. Although the process of writing is new to her, she hopes to use it to help her explore in greater depth themes such as love and forgiveness and, above all, her relationship with her mother.

Harriet

Prior to the first interview getting underway, Harriet, aged seventy-eight, takes Jennifer for a walk along the managed trails of her multi-acre property in rural New Brunswick. Jennifer finds the landscape stunning, its natural beauty enhanced by multiple feeders that attract all manner of birds and squirrels, its vast silence broken only by their chirps and cheeps. Inside Harriet's house a large picture window provides a view of this expansive outside world. Welcoming Jennifer in, Harriet gives her a tour of the well-maintained two-storey structure, its freshly painted walls modern in tone while its furniture is elegant and classically styled.

During the interviews, the two sit across from one another and exchange eye contact easily. While many of Harriet's stories appear rather polished, as if they were set pieces that she's told several times before, the one that seems to Jennifer most central is not – the story about the violin. Harriet had always wanted to become a violinist, she tells Jennifer, but it had not been possible. When asked why she doesn't take it up now, she seems perplexed, and explains that to be a good violinist one must begin as a child.

Jennifer perceives Harriet to be a woman who has lived a life full of meaning and purpose, who could have recounted any number of polished stories – about being a fierce opponent of war, a caring woman of faith, the founder of a retreat centre, and so forth. Instead, she chooses to talk about something that she has rarely, if ever, talked about before with anyone. Jennifer still gets goosebumps when she thinks how meaningful this story was and how grateful she is that Harriet elected to share it with her. The reason behind her decision remains unclear, however, for following the interviews she expresses to Jennifer her uncertainty as to why she shared it at all, having assumed that she had long since buried it in the past.

Harriet was born in England, two years before the Second World War. During the war, as was the case with many children at the time, she was evacuated from the city to a home in the country where a family took her in. She remembers feeding horses sugar cubes, playing with a Scottish terrier, and enjoying the tranquility of the countryside. Her five-year-old brother, however, was sent to work on a farm where the conditions were gruelling and many children died of malnutrition – an experience that left him with a life-long refusal to talk about his childhood. After six years, she reluctantly returned to the city, very sad to have to go back home. In fact, she barely recognized her mother, who spent little time rebuilding the bond between them. The aftermath of the war, she found, was shocking, and she tells Jennifer that she became a nervous and detached young girl.

The relationship between Harriet and her brother was complicated. Her mother favoured him over her, which Harriet speculated was due to the woman's guilt for sending him to the farms, or possibly due to their Italian culture, where traditionally boys are favoured over girls. In any event, despite having tried for many years, the two siblings were never able to develop a positive relationship. The war-time separation, austere life conditions in general, and then, later, their mother's death all contributed to the distance between them.

Unhappy, Harriet fell behind in school, yet her mother seemed not to care, so long as the girl would eventually marry. She was pulled out of her depressed, dispassionate state, however, when the school introduced music lessons, for she was given the violin to learn. She fell in love with it at once. She remembers playing a hymn, and in the story she wrote she describes the notes as "sweet beyond any imaginings." Music gave her comfort in the midst of so much uncertainty, and she yearned to become a violinist herself. In her excitement, she brought the violin home one day to practice. At the time, her brother was learning Italian. Reciting lines from his textbook, he read out loud the words "God protect you from a bad neighbour and a student learning the violin." Not realizing that he was reciting a line from a textbook, their mother took this to mean that the violin was distracting him from his studies, and so, without any discussion of the matter, she forbade Harriet to play again.

It was not until four decades later that she learned the real reason for the violin ban. By chance, she stumbled across a university-level textbook for beginner's Italian, the same book that her brother had used so many years before. She found the page containing that fateful line, and finally realizing what had happened, copied it and kept it. At Jennifer's request, Harriet gave her a copy to show to our CIRN research team.

Her inability to practice the violin, she believes, contributed to her lack of self-confidence throughout adolescence. Whenever she listens to an orchestra, her eyes tear up as she thinks of the life she could have had as a professional violinist, the unlived life she might have known. During the interview, therefore, she finds the subject very difficult to discuss. Upon reflection, though, she has reassured herself that the turn her life took, despite not being what she had envisioned, has been satisfying all the same.

Hermann

Aged fifty-seven and the youngest participant in the workshops, Hermann asks to be interviewed on campus, so he and Jennifer meet at CIRN, a spacious room with large windows and several tables arranged in a circle – the same room where the research team meets. The two of them sit across from one another with lots of eye contact between them as the interviews unfold, Hermann moving his hands frequently as he speaks.

Born in Germany, he was raised Roman Catholic and, in keeping with family tradition, became an altar boy. He vividly remembers his aunts praying with their rosary beads. At age six, he saw two figures standing in the garden outside of the living room window. Certain that they were angels, he ran to the next room to tell his mother. "The way you behave," she said to him dismissively, "I don't think angels would come to you" (13-I). For a long time, he says, her words deeply affected him. However, he tells Jennifer that he's recently discussed the incident with her and the two of them have had a good laugh about it all.

In his early teens, Hermann's family moved to Southeast Asia, where aside from the familiar Christian churches he was exposed to a melting pot of Buddhism, Hinduism, and other religions. His visits to various holy sites proved, he says, to be a "journey of discovery" (16-II) in which he realized it was possible to part with his inherited Catholic tradition. Despite this exposure to a wider world of the spirit, though, he went on to study theology, the only thing keeping him from entering the priesthood being the fact that he was married. Eventually, however, he and his wife divorced, and he still recalls how the church's disapproval of divorce caused tension in his parish.

His second wife being a Lutheran, he was happy to switch to her denomination. In 2002 the couple moved from Germany to a remote village in British Columbia. He vividly recalls flying over Whistler Mountain and being astounded by the landscape. There was a sense of "coming home," he says, even though the two of them had never visited Canada before (18-I). Since the village where they lived was so isolated, the only church was a Presbyterian one, but as it was attended by people of many different denominations, they felt very welcome.

When real estate costs skyrocketed, it became too expensive for them to remain there, so having been offered a teaching position back east, he and his wife relocated to New Brunswick, where eventually they found a church with a pastor whose liberal views suited their own. Their fellow parishioners seemed similarly minded – until they expressed intolerance towards a homosexual couple in the congregation. This bothered Hermann and his wife greatly so, once more, the two of them felt the need to find a new church.

At some point, Hermann acquired a ring designed by an Indigenous artist in the form of a labyrinth. He wears the ring nearly every day, and identifies strongly with the figure depicted in the midst of it: a wanderer through life's many twists and turns. When asked by Deborah during the last workshop to sketch the storyline of his life, he drew a combination of a labyrinth and a maze.

One of the turning points in his life's own labyrinth was in 2008 when he travelled to Asia and was again exposed to Buddhism. He found himself particularly moved by all the prayer flags that figured in people's practice of it and began questioning his own spirituality and his ambivalence towards Christianity. So, upon his return to Canada he transitioned to atheism. That said, he was unused to thinking of himself in this way. How would this change his lifestyle? he wondered. Might the way he has ended up somehow change his past? In order to understand his journey better, he started writing about it. In 2011 he began journaling on a daily basis. Indeed, he regrets not starting sooner because writing, which he describes as "a different kind of thinking" (2-II), helps him to process his thoughts, he says, and to "relive the day" (3-I). Having learned about so many different religious views, Hermann also began recognizing how a great many of the world's stories that are used for teaching lessons, despite coming from different cultural contexts, help to maintain the essence of human togetherness. They serve, that is, to unify people.

Hermann is interested, too, in writing about the history of National Socialism. In fact, he often speculates on what his life would have looked like if he had been born before the Second World War. Raised in Germany himself, he has observed how much this dark period is still embedded in people's daily lives (see Marks, 2011) and is a larger story they continue to be shaped by. Indulging in "counterfactual" speculation (Ferguson, 1997, p. 2), he also asks himself how he would have behaved if he had encountered the situations that his parents and grandparents did, whether he would have abided by the changes that the Third Reich imposed or have resisted them. If so, he wondered, what might have happened and how would the context of his life have shifted?

Joy

The two interviews with Joy, aged seventy-four, take place in her mini-home, an extremely welcoming environment beautifully laid out with oversized leather furniture. Classical music plays softly in the background. During the first interview, she sits on the sofa and Jennifer is seated across from her in a large, comfortable chair, with Joy's dog sprawled across her lap. When they are done, the woman gives her a tour of her home. As they walk along, Joy picks up different photographs and talks about each of them. One is of her mother who, in her seventies, looked like she was in her thirties and could have graced the cover of any beauty magazine.

Joy was an only child, and not having siblings left her frequently feeling lonely and bored. To entertain herself, as well as to record her thoughts, she began early on keeping a journal. Her journals, she tells Jennifer, "saw her grow up," for they documented her transition from adolescence to adulthood (3-I). As much as she loved to read and write, though, the process inevitably grew tiring, and she concluded that if she was bored then she must have become boring. So, as a way to get out of the house and do something constructive, she started volunteering.

Her earliest commitment, at age fifteen, was as a friendly visitor in a nursing home. Even as a teenager she related to older adults remarkably well. She tells Jennifer of growing especially close to a patient who was nearly one hundred. Speaking to her and other older adults, she says, was like "opening a pirate's chest full of jewels" (3-I). All throughout her life, she has loved writing to the many senior pen pals whom she acquired from such visits. These exchanges have had a "richness" to them that she cherishes to this day, and indeed she alludes frequently to how her life has been influenced by and "interwoven" with the lives of these elder mentors (3-I).

These sorts of positive experiences encouraged her to broaden her horizons. An article in *Reader's Digest* written in the 1950s or 1960s proved especially inspiring in this regard, so much so that she has kept a copy of it as a reminder to herself to seize opportunities and remain open-minded. It was entitled "Try Everything Once" (20-II). At the time, however, Joy was anxious about what life would look like if she failed to venture outside of her hometown after high school. There was a real possibility, she was convinced, that she would stagnate while others moved on. Though unsure if she wanted to marry, she certainly didn't want to risk a reputation as a "spinster" (39-II). She yearned to travel and continue studying. Her mother, however, was opposed to the idea and became quite distressed at the prospect of her daughter moving away. Her father was more sympathetic even if, for her mother's sake, he asked Joy to wait a few years. While she resented this restriction at the time, she now recognizes that she was far too naive to move to a big city alone.

Her first solo vacation was a trip by train to a neighbouring province. Sitting across from her in the railway car was a seventy-four-year-old man named "Scott" whom she noticed was meticulously dressed and had a refined manner of speaking. (She later learned he was an engineer from Canada's west coast.) The two of them talked about the weather and other trivial topics until they began bonding over their mutual love of poetry. They enjoyed their conversation so much that, upon reaching their destination, they exchanged contact information and a correspondence began between them that lasted nearly twenty years. Initially, she thought of him as just another of her senior pen pals, but as the letters that he wrote to her accumulated, she began to suspect that he harboured deep feelings for her, even if the fifty-plus-year age difference prevented them from ever becoming romantically involved.

Two years after that fateful train ride, by then in her twenties, Joy moved to Montreal to begin life on her own, though the move proved rather challenging. Having grown up accustomed to her family providing her with the necessities of life, she struggled to manage her finances. When she was first approved for a credit card, she spent nearly two thousand dollars on new clothing. As a consequence of her inexperience in budgeting, she lived from pay cheque to pay cheque for the first few months, getting by on a diet of jam sandwiches and little more.

There was also an incident with her landlord. After receiving complaints about excessive noise, he summoned her to his apartment, believing her to be the culprit. He circled her wielding a knife, demanding that she move out immediately. She had nowhere else to go, however, and her parents' hostility to her move in the first place made calling them out of the question. The next day, the landlord discovered that it was the tenants across the hall from her who had been responsible for the complaint; he apologized profusely and told her that she was like a daughter to him. To cope with the hardships brought on by such bizarre situations, Joy turned again to her journals. Where once writing had been boring, she now found it to be therapeutic.

Joy wrote to Scott regularly, and they in fact saw each other once a year. Either he flew to her or he paid for a ticket for her to visit him. Eventually, though, she met someone closer to her own age and became engaged. Once she told Scott, their visits ceased altogether and the tone of his letters grew steadily more platonic. Nevertheless, they continued their correspondence right up until his death.

Scott published a collection of poetry in which his love for her is the subject of many of the works included in it. Joy calls the book a piece of "his immortality" (15-II). Just as she describes her life as being interwoven with her senior mentors, so she weaves Scott's words carefully into her own, placing excerpts of his writing into the dialogues she composed for the story she wrote between the first interview and the second. She's been surprised, in fact, at how much the process of writing has challenged her and at the emotions it has unearthed. "I thought it would be easy," she tells Jennifer. "I didn't realize the emotion that it would bring to the fore and I'm now looking at it, at the whole experience, from the view of a different, an older woman. I had a different perspective than I did as a, a twenty-year old, of course" (2-II).

At the time of the interviews, Joy was the same age that Scott had been when the two first met, a coincidence that has led her to reminisce about him often. When he died, he left her his mother's wedding ring and jewellery box, both of which she has carefully kept, along with all of the letters he wrote to her across the years. For such reasons, she tells Jennifer, she feels her life has come "full circle" (1-I).

One further thing … Joy is fascinated by genealogy, and given this interest in the past, wants to pass down something to her children. She hopes they will be able to pull out funny anecdotes from her writing and, in this way, get a sense of what her life was like. Certainly, these were the sorts of stories that she loved hearing most from her own mother and grandmother. Having already drafted her obituary to capture her sense of who she was and who she cared about, it's as if she knows already how she wants to be remembered.

David

David asked if he could be interviewed on campus, so he and Jennifer meet in a small office at the university that is sparsely furnished with two chairs and a small round table. Such a stark setting doesn't appear to faze him, however, for he tells her his story with great enthusiasm. As he sits back in his chair, he appears extremely relaxed, gesturing energetically with his hands to enhance what he is saying.

A retired lawyer in his late sixties, David was born in Jamaica but did his law studies in the United Kingdom, which is where he met his wife. Together, they moved back to the Caribbean, where he practised for twelve years, during which time they had four children. Jamaica was also the birthplace of their dining room table, which David himself had designed in collaboration with a local woodworker and storyteller. Three types of African mahogany were chosen to create the five-foot-long structure, plus benches to match. Both the materials and the design were intimately connected to David's belief system and his experience of spirituality. To reflect a monastic aesthetic, for instance, benches were built instead of chairs.

David is a practising Christian who enjoys spending his early mornings in prayer and meditation. Though his ancestry is Jewish, he reckons that his family converted to Christianity during his grandfather's generation. In the past, he has made various pilgrimages to Europe, and plans to do so again in the future. He regularly contemplates humanity's interconnectedness and our relationship to the Earth, and he admires

Indigenous spirituality in particular because of its rituals and its care for the land. So intimately is spirituality bound up with identity for him that, as Jennifer notes in listening to him talk, he can switch from the sacred to the mundane and back again in a single breath.

In 1976, David and his wife relocated the family to Canada in the face of escalating conflict and violence at home in Jamaica. In order to transport the table, however, it had to be taken apart and then reassembled by him and his son at its new destination. He recalls how difficult it was to move it, and at the same time how uncertain was its future.

In his legal career, David needed to do extensive research in preparing for his cases. When he spoke before a courtroom, it was crucial to be unbiased; opinions were to be avoided. This training, while helpful to being a lawyer, was detrimental, he feels, to being a writer. As a result, it's been a challenge for him to inject his personality into his writing. To make it more personal, he has considered writing his life story in the form of a letter addressed to his children, although even in this format, he admits, the researcher in him can't resist inserting the proper footnotes and citations.

It's the urging of his son that has led to him writing his story. As for his own father, the man had intended to put his life down on paper but died before he could do so. Having been highly attuned to Jamaica and its politics, he would have had much insight into the situation that drove David and his family to leave the place. Unable to ask his father, David has been determined to learn "what makes it tick" (11-II) because he believes he and his children are, in many ways, "products of the trauma" (5-II) that they witnessed there. Jamaica remains for him a larger story that has shaped their lives profoundly and haunts him still. Ironically, though the children themselves have visited the island since moving to Canada, he hasn't yet been able to bring himself to return.

David doesn't want to deprive his children of his story but, except for having done sporadic journaling, he is relatively new to the practice of writing about his life, which is why he signed up for the workshops in the first place. In his final interview with Jennifer, though, he tells her that they have already helped him to examine his life and his values in different and meaningful ways.

Final Words

Each of these participants, with no prompting whatever from Jennifer, wove mention of certain objects into what they chose to share with her about their lives. In many respects, these objects serve as conduits for conveying a fuller understanding of their internal storyworlds. In this chapter, we have provided more details concerning the broader context of each such world. In the chapters that follow, we will be pondering more deeply the complex relationship that each participant has with the things they singled out as holding a unique significance within it.

5 Sea Glass Jewellery: New Chapters for Old Things

MATTE ROBINSON

Any object, intensely regarded, may be a gate of access to the incorruptible eon of the gods.

–James Joyce, *Ulysses* (1968, p. 413)

A piece of sea glass in Virginia Woolf's story that I quoted from in Chapter 3 comes to embody the mutability of life, the ability of things to transform and simultaneously be transformed. Before I look at the place of sea glass in the lives of Bob and Mary, it's interesting how Bill Brown (1999), in "The Secret Life of Things," uses Woolf's glass as the master metaphor in a critical reorientation or call to return to the strangeness of things:

> Familiar materials – glass, china, iron – are debanalized, appearing all but magical: "it was impossible to say whether it had been bottle, tumbler, or window-pane; it was nothing but glass; it was almost a precious stone" … Not objects, but materials – "nothing but glass" – have been released from any readiness-to-hand. Free from their incorporation into the familiar object world, they seem to assume lives of their own as John grants them a kind of agency. (pp. 6f.)

The "agency" Brown refers to is different from Bruno Latour's envisioning of objects' agency (see Chapter 3). While actor-network theorists would find agency in patterns of human-object interaction, Brown's approach is attentive to the ways things reveal or conceal themselves in particular moments, in particular circumstances. So attention to an object's place within a system – economic, semiotic, or otherwise – will never arrive at its thingness: "producing a thing – effecting thingness – depends … on a fetishistic overvaluation or misappropriation, on an irregular if not unreasonable reobjectification of the object that dislodges it from the circuits through which it is what it typically is" (Brown, 1999, pp. 2f.). In attending to the "excess" of things, rather than their deficiency – or better yet, in reframing deficiency as only one kind of excess – the thing is now understood as that part of the object that interacts with the human world. Thing theory as I appropriate it here does not dispute the existence of non-interactive matter, which in its absence can only elicit a being-toward rather than a being-with; I conjure it because I hope that in recognizing the thing's capacity to surprise, to shock, to overflow the boundaries of the systems woven to contain it, thing theory might provide a complementary lens for approaching the various objects that we're discussing in Part 2.

Though there might be no way to write a poem about a rose without conjuring up many traditions' worth of codes dictating what a rose means in a literary work (modified by its colour, its provenance, its thorniness, etc.), modernist poetry attended to ways a rose might, in an instant of time shaken loose of those traditional associations, come to structure and offer possibilities within the work itself. Traditional literary forms and devices were subverted or jettisoned altogether to allow each work to prod the strangeness of the thing, and perhaps even to let that strangeness take on an agentic role in the shaping of its narrative. With its new attention to things, literary modernism is attuned to things' involvement in particular environments at particular times with particular people (the Circe episode in *Ulysses*, with the room full of objects interjecting and modifying the narrative, is an extreme example of this impulse). Without this thingly turn, it is difficult to conceive of the current *Oxford Dictionary of Literary Terms*' assessment of the literary symbol as "a substantial image in its own right, around which further significances may gather according to differing interpretations" (Baldick, 2008, s.v. "symbol").

Bob and Mary, the married couple who have taken up sea glass jewellery-making, do not reflect to any great extent upon the role of sea glass (the thousands of objects catalogued in their basement) or the craft objects they fashion from it. The transcript of the interviews with Bob, for instance, plus the piece of writing that he did, are thick with the names of objects, building materials, lists and terse descriptions of the types of things found all around him, even when he has not been in contact with these things for decades. Consider this example from the story that he wrote between the first interview and the second: "In all, there were approximately 25 or so Quonset single story homes set on wooden pilings, about 2.5 ft. clear of the ground, the outside was covered with green grit tar paper approximately 2 feet wide and nailed from top to bottom every 4 inches or so with large headed tar nails. The inside walls and divisions were made of donna conna wall board, with all walls open at the top." The world he lives in, as he describes it, is a world of things, but usually these things are subject to systems for which they are of use, either as tools or as a mode that might reveal a forest, for instance, as so many cords of firewood and board feet of lumber. Techne rather than poiesis guides this form of revealing, for the most part. The things available to him in the story that he wrote between the two interviews are there to be noted as material or, better, to be exploited by young, hard-working entrepreneurs: "We could dig and uncover the old iron ore nuggets from days of yore and sell them at the junk yard for a penny a pound. The owner would occasionally hire us to break old batteries apart for the lead and we did that a few times until the acid burned holes in a pair of pants, mother ended that" (p. 1).

The sea glass for him has a similar quality, collected and catalogued in his basement, in reserve for his hobby: "I've got over twenty thousand pieces of sea glass in the basement that we work with and putter around with" (6-I). This hobby is unique for him, though, in that it gathers the whole family together, unlike such solitary "puttering" as fly-tying or oil painting: "the kids know all that, the grandkids know a lot about it and they're into picking it" (6-I). His wife's interviews, which I'll be looking at shortly, express many fears about families' potential to fracture, including her own. The picture he paints in his, of the family together at the beach by his son's cottage, each pursuing a suitable activity organized around sea glass jewellery-making, offers an image that stands guard against potential fracture. Mary, the kids, and the grandkids are the "pickers" while he, with a workbench set up right at the beach, can "be busy"; the new set-up is "great" because it offers an alternative to the more active outdoor activities which he used to pursue before arthritis set in. The individual bits of sea glass remain substantial things in their own right, but further significances gather around them, strengthening the thing named "family" and the thing named "marriage," becoming woven into the narrative of their lives.

Mary has more interest in the things themselves, but never in terms of the immediate and unmediated encounter with things that Brown describes (who does?). Rather, the pieces of sea glass that they collect inspire readings in archaeology and history so that she can better place the objects and her relationship to them: "I have five books on sea glass that does classification, it tells the story of sea glass, it tells the story of the person who's picking the sea glass. It tells of people who leave their vocation and they go and they study, uh, the art of fine jewellery and then use sea glass" (32-II). She is also interested in the potential of the finished jewellery to produce new stories – each piece is unique and sometimes can trigger memories in people who encounter them. The opportunity for such encounters, and for the couple to do something together, comes at an annual craft festival to which they travel to show and sell their work.

One memorable encounter is with a woman who, eyeing their display, picked up a piece that also included sea-polished ceramic shards that had been gathered at the beach. These were fragments of dishes, and the stranger recognized the patterns as identical to those on her grandmother's dishes, which she remembered from childhood visits to her house. These new connections made of stray, transformed things are electrifying. "[I]t was ... a goose bump moment," she says, "and I thought I should have taken the picture of her with that because that was, that's what it's all about is finding how that story connects to your life or how you would like it to connect to your life. So again, just a fascinating thing about life that just comes along and, and you're lucky to find it" (19-I). In refashioning fragments plucked from the shore into art objects on display, the couple has created a piece of reminiscentia for a stranger in an exchange far more complex than that of mere buying and selling.

When they were younger, Bob and Mary used to organize highly popular garage sales for their neighbourhood each year (the tradition continues with different organizers) that found new homes for often high-end household objects. Mary expresses an unsentimental attitude towards things as cherished objects: "you can't just keep storing things in the hope that maybe your grandchildren would see it differently and I'm sure down the road a grandchild or grandchild's, or great grandchild would say, 'Oh my God, they had a spinning wheel that, that you could use, you know, I would have loved to have had that.' But that's gone in a garage sale" (13-I). The couple's new activity reproduces the movement and exchange of potentially cherished objects, and though the things themselves have been sold to strangers, they remain important to the couple's narrative, to their "we-story," as it were (Singer & Skerrett, 2014). She remembers the teak dining set and china cabinet that she sold at the first garage sale, and she plans to compose a piece on the garage sale tradition once she has more time to write. The couple is preparing to retire from sea glass jewellery-making, just as they did from the garage sales, and she is making lists of writing projects she will be able to undertake once that space has been freed up by the sea glass's absence.

Were you to read the stories these two present, they would point in definite directions, would tell of the kind of lessons and warnings they want to leave for posterity. The objects in his story are all things marshalled by enterprising poor young men to turn a profit. Her one-page story, which ends with the line "it was one of life's best lessons," tells of a young woman standing up to a powerful and well-connected man who had her fired unjustly. The anxiety about their children's generation is not at all disguised, especially in her interviews, which warn of being comfortable in a privileged lifestyle when hordes of more enterprising people in less fortunate circumstances are arriving with their sights set on the kind of successes each member of the couple sought so resolutely in the wilder past.

These "lessons" are fine and useful, but the sea glass lets a more vulnerable, and equally valuable, story be told, not the least because it opens up, alongside the family roles he calls "vegetating" (reclining on the beach, reading about the history of sea glass), "keeping busy" (setting up kit and workbench at the beach), and "picking" (the grandchildren's role), an aesthetic mode. In collaborating on the production of craft objects, the couple must work at new ways of seeing things. For example, though the neurological theory supporting its exercises may today be inadequate, the perennially popular manual *Drawing on the Right Side of the Brain* teaches art newcomers how to see things in a way suitable for drawing by introducing tricks aimed at bypassing the usual habits of seeing. These can be as simple as turning something upside down and drawing it, an act that Bill Brown characterizes as "reobjectification that is a kind of misuse" (1999, p. 7).

Sea glass as thing encountered on the beach glimmers with a film of such misuses through its protean transformations, allowing it to reorient and restructure the given narrative in the way that a modernist image grounds the poem in its poiesis. What are first encountered as fragments like gems are wrought into things, each of which has a kind of narrative generativity. In fact, now that the couple is downsizing and must abandon its large collection of sea glass, the craft-things are to be converted to text-things, which have even more potential to gather new meaning, to have their own agency. Now in their seventies, Bob and Mary still look on the sea glass as something new, even though the activity will be coming to an end after this year. As Mary says to Jennifer, "I am going to write about this new hobby that my husband and I have discovered, uh, sea glass picking and making sea glass jewellery" (32-II). For the next chapter of her life, writing will be the new activity to focus on. In part this is out of necessity, because of the downsizing, but it is also another way of engaging with things, even as the things themselves are lost: the things are converted into symbols or images.

Something interesting happens when Mary's words are interpreted through the lens of things. In preparing stories, she appears to want to lend the narratives themselves a thingly quality, polishing them into nearly impersonal fables or "lessons" that can be passed down and exist independently of her own subjective existence.[1] But the things in such narratives have other ideas, disrupting the subject-object relations upon which these plans are built. In order to clarify this claim, I must spend some time fleshing out Mary's narrative as she presents it in the interviews and in her submitted story.

Mary's Official Narratives, Exoteric and Esoteric

Mary is a well-travelled, successful person who stands up for herself, keeps her own counsel, and has much to say about many matters. But her focus seems to return to a sense of the self as a moral entity, with a role to play in the greater community, who must for duty's sake tamp down any undue sense of entitlement or self-importance. At the same time, she takes pride in being part of a community of strong women, resilient elders, and dutiful citizens. She has taught children (she liked them, she says, but did not love them), helped the less fortunate (by buying them livestock in her children's name), started a tradition (garage sales), taken up a satisfying retirement hobby (making and selling sea glass jewellery), worked many jobs (she could work as she chose because her husband was in a secure and lucrative career in the RCMP), and travelled the world (at times making travelling her job as well).

There are also, in the interviews, a few things that she wants to talk about but that take a long while to come out, requiring foreshadowing through oblique mentions here and there immediately followed by tangents. The second interview seems about to end at a few points, but it does not, and as it goes on she deviates more and more from the questions, commenting on how she is losing track. There must be a reason for this delay to the ending of such a long interview, and it seems that she might be trying to find a way to address these things that she has been hinting at all along but could not find the opportunity to discuss. Eventually, she tells Jennifer about them, more or less. One is a situation in her life, with her family. The other is a story that she thinks is foundational, one of her three "big stories." Both take dozens and dozens of pages to emerge.

The first is maybe better divided in two. Something in recent years, involving the estate of a relative, has shaken her faith in people, particularly family. It has taken her some time to recover from the experience, and she clearly is still working through what she wants to take from it. She

1 Cf. the last stanza of Robert Frost's "The Road Not Taken" vis-à-vis the rest of the poem.

does not give many details, only enough to let us know that she is shocked and disturbed at the revelation that there are "self-entitled" (67-II) people in her life, in particular one "close relative" who she judges is "on some level mentally ill" (67-II). This person has introduced, in this late chapter of her narrative and her family's, "lies," "deceit," and "so much that has never touched my life before" (67-II). Neither peeling pulp for the summer as a youth (to show the men that she can play their game) nor fighting powerful doctors as the administrator of a medical centre (for similar reasons) has prepared her for this challenge from within, this woman close to her who says, defiantly, "no one tells me what to do" (68-II). There is a ready answer to this defiance: "law, ... government, ... church, ... your school, ... your boss" all get to tell you what to do (68-II), but the answer does not seem to penetrate enough to remove the wounding thorn. In confronting someone who does not recognize these authorities, this structure, this moral code, she has had to resort to an unfeeling state, to "nothing" (68-II). The details she provides are still not enough for a reader to flesh out the details of the situation or to express them in terms of plot, character, or crisis. They are there, behind the words, but inaccessible. This is an untellable story, a shadow narrative.

Whatever the situation is, it seems to have affected the way that she thinks about her own children; though she does not call them "entitled," there is the familiar generational disagreement about how kids should be raised that comes up again and again. Implied is a kind of selfishness, that these new parents feel "it's their time and their, their generation's time and they don't see a lot beyond that" (11-II), and that they are paying too much attention to their kids, spending time with them whenever they want, worrying about their needs and desires too much, something her generation would never do. This has left her feeling alienated. While she is welcome to go to ringette and hockey games, it appears that she would rather engage with her grandchildren on her own terms, but the parents pay so much attention to their kids that there is not much of a role left for the grandparents to play. There is an additional dark undertone to this particular story, signalled by her prediction that in a few years "it's all going to explode" (13-II).

What might be at stake, to her mind, is a failure to pass on a certain moral quality, certain values about charity and helping the needy. She used to donate animals to needy South American families (she's not entirely sure if they're South American, but she thinks so) in her children's name, hoping that her children would then pick up the habit, take up the torch, and continue to buy chickens and goats for less fortunate families. The fact that the children show no interest speaks to the insularity she fears in their generation, at least in their region and economic class. What of "the personal values that kids don't always follow through with" (37-II)? A clue to the identity of the deeper threat is found in *Silent Spring* (38-II), Rachel Carson's (1962) landmark in environmental writing, a text that helped form Mary's sense of her own generation: "It's been longer coming than I think she thought it would be," she explains to Jennifer, but it is being brought by migrants who have known a different world from the one in which her children were raised, who require only a part in that same world. "They" are coming "in boatloads" and saying "the time's here" (38-II). The message? "If you don't share, there are more of them than there are of you and they're just going to take over anyway and you might not live through this" (38-II). By enjoying privilege and not sharing, by hoarding and walling yourself off from the rest of the world, you are a fool to "not expect something to explode" (38-II).

The words "it" and "them" and "us," possible to understand in some immediate sense but impossible to pin to an exact person or group, stand in stark contrast to the objects in her basement, fragments of past times and lives turned to jewels by the tides. In touching one she can treat it as an archaeological artefact, listing its era, the watercourse it was found by, and details of its manufacture. When she turns it into jewellery, it will be able to produce new stories, on display to the public. But this "it" she speaks of is intensely private and stubbornly immaterial. It can only be described in metaphorical language, such as the "explosion."

There are two kinds of "explosion" she expects will happen soon: one, a disaster arising from intersecting environmental and socio-economic crises and the other, a social values explosion coming from – or at least indicated by – a generation's short-sighted if well-intentioned childrearing that produces hopelessly selfish children. The message that is not getting across?: "You, as a child are not the most important child in this world" (38-II). She hopes that the grandchildren, anyway, will figure it out. There doesn't seem to be time anymore for the children to learn.

There is a distinct theme, in the interviews, of loss of faith in family. Family you don't choose, whereas you choose your friends and, to some extent, your mentors. In the case of families, she "only know[s] one family" that has not broken down (25-II), a group of strong women, "three girls" (25-II). It is implied that her family has already exploded (the untellable story), but there is some hope that something unifying skips a generation. The grandchildren collect small, naturally polished particles of glass they find along the beach and keep it for their grandparents; she, meanwhile, has turned to writing workshops so that she can polish her prose into useful, discrete lessons that her grandchildren can read.

Maybe closest to the bone on the family issue is her being part of what she frequently calls the first "sandwich generation." Repeatedly she asserts that she does not want to outlive her usefulness, to become an object of pity. She is dealing with having children with whom she is less close than she'd maybe expected, but also she has frequent contact with a difficult mother, one who is never satisfied. Her mother is ninety-five and has macular degeneration that has done away with her ability to see the world around her. But instead of an absence of vision, she lives among vivid and often frightful images, like a waking dream. There are grave-faced children who stare at her silently, there is an old man at the base of the bed, there is a "drop-off" just to the bed's side. It is implied, but not stated, that being caught in an inescapable world of hallucination is for Mary a terrifying prospect, brought far too close to home in the figure of her ageing mother.

The mother wants constant attention and limits, by virtue of her condition, the movements of her daughters. "She's just lived too long" (75-II) is the assessment. Before he died, her father said, "you can never satisfy that woman" (75-II). This predicament reminds her of the Prince song "When Doves Cry" (1984), though she can't remember the title and can only remember a line about the singer being like their mother, who is "never satisfied." She tries twice to remember and twice cannot recall what the song says about the father. She tries to reconstruct her memory of the song, though, imagining that the father is never "living up to their standard or something like that" (75-II). She is searching for the words "too bold."

There is a sharp distinction between "never living up to their standard" and being "too bold," especially considering the bold, fearless character that bears her identity in her narratives. Her tale of having defied the men closest to her, and indeed the patriarchy, by spending a summer doing men's work peeling pulp, is kept to the length of a fable, easy to read, easy to interpret as both a life lesson and an origin story for a resilient person. Her second "big story," of standing up to a powerful doctor, is so polished as to be considered a "life lesson." Clearly, what has drawn her to the workshops is practical help in converting some formative events of her life into well-wrought stories, things which can be passed on to a further generation. Like many such stories they may be seen to act like parables, with a literal and esoteric meaning, the latter having to do with "them," "us," and "it," while the former teaches such conventional lessons as standing up to injustice, strengthening the community of women in families, being honest, having integrity, and showing competence.

The third "big story" is a different sort altogether. When she is twelve, she goes out with cousins, one of whom "likes" her even though he's several years older. He wants to take her picture in her bathing suit, and though she is unwilling she eventually submits to standing by the water next to his sister. He tells them to back up so that they can get in the picture, and they fall down an embankment into deep water. Neither of them can swim, and in struggling to get air they prevent one another from getting a firm hold on a small ledge. The people on land have witnessed a practical joke and, not knowing that the girls cannot swim, think they are horsing around and make no attempt to help. The photographer, suddenly remembering that his sister cannot swim, dives in and drags her out, but Mary is left behind to float towards the rapids. Once she is in them, it all moves too fast for anyone to help.

She almost drowns, thanks to a combination of ignorance and incompetence on the part of the people who put her in this situation. What results is what she calls an "out-of-body experience" (she's read a book on the subject) but might also be called a "near-death experience": she hears a hum and realizes that she's "flying" by a "hydro line" (63-II) with "ten or twelve" "black birds." Below her she can see the little waterfall where they will find her "body" – she says "they find my body," underscoring the fact that at that moment, she is not in it. Her vision fades to nothing and there is only the hum, then gradually she begins to see again. She is still hovering above her body, but it is now laid to rest "in [her] casket" (64-II). At the coffin-side are two figures, her mother and a boy, not the photographer, but someone *she* likes. Then she wakes up, vomiting water (64-II).

There are clear parallels between this formative experience and her discomfort in thinking about her mother, who plays a coffin-side cameo in the dream. The "out-of-body" near-death experience takes place in a non-world in which things appear as symbols of some sort (black birds) but are not actually what they appear: they are constructed out of some dream-fabric of significance without a physical counterpart. Though the waterfall is where her body will end up, in her vision it is some sort of waterfall-double, living in the same world that has a casket with her body in it. Even the guy is not the guy she is physically with, but an absent object of desire. He is not who he seems to be. It is a world of hallucination, not of things.

She wishes she could have learned from this experience that death is a gentle thing, but this story does not lend itself to polishing into a "lesson." There is something about it that eludes her, some significance she has not grasped, and so it cannot be passed down safely – who knows what's in it? Instead of a compact narrative lesson about resilience, she acquires a lifelong fear of swimming from the "trauma" (64-II), one that mars her attempt to get her son swimming lessons. The way she tells it, then, unlike the other two stories, she did not get anything from this experience, did not grow, did not become the character that she wants to be. What could be the value of such a story?

It is a brush with the supernatural, and though she is silent on its significance, she is thinking about it. Why didn't it help her deal with the idea of death? What is its significance? What connection does it have to the strange daily visions that her mother now has? Mary is a woman who loves to organize. She wants everything to be in its place. She gains some satisfaction in knowing that her granddaughter has inherited from her this organizing trait. But where do you put an experience like this? How does it fit in? What does it do to character development? What does it tell about the world around you? What if, in the middle of a live feed, there were an alien visitation, but the feed just kept rolling on through the years, without commenting?

For "years" (64-II) the visions would haunt her, and she can put that down to trauma. But her mother's strange visions? Her children's myopia about the coming "explosions"? Both involve a kind of forgetting, each kind peculiar to its generation. In families, between generations, forgetting happens, and things that are passed on must have their own agency or they, too, will be forgotten. Her stories are mere details of a subjective, half-understood life unless they are polished into "lessons," which then acquire thingness and can be distributed as heirlooms. Other stories will die with her, and these are the stories that resist object-ness and yet also, somehow, trace the limits of what a life is – something bordering on death. The explosions will come because of a failure to pass on; the hallucinations come because of a deferment of passing on.

In the end she must abandon family, since after all you die on your own and you're responsible for your own happiness and sadness (21-II). You can't blame people or circumstances. She has a plan for when her husband dies, and her mother has already lived too long. Her children have their own lives. She has worked to become a "world person" (65-II), something greater than the single ego that makes its way through the world. She has touched on a prediction about an upcoming explosion and a vision that took her out of her body as important ways that her identity is changed by that quest.

But there is this "new" hobby to consider, which is soon to end its existence as a real activity but will be the subject of her next piece of writing. Something about it seems to counteract the foregrounded narrative, with its heavy sense of fracture, forgetfulness, loss, and breaking away. It springs from things that were fractured, lost, forgotten, and divorced from their context. These sea glass fragments, and the jewellery she will fashion out of them with her husband, have united the three generations, have strengthened the marital bond now that the older rituals have been exhausted, and are generative in that they add new twists and wrinkles to their lives, thanks to the sale and display of the jewellery. And they promise a new kind of story, yet to be written, that does not merely, on the one hand, amount to a generalized law or, on the other, promise insight valuable only to the private life of a mortal individual. This is a story about the family, written in the present tense or something very near it, that involves surprising transformations and the recovery of beauty from a broken past.

Things Found Along the Strand

Edmund Sherman (1991b) identifies three general types of reminiscentia in his article "Reminiscentia: Cherished Objects as Memorabilia in Late Life Reminiscence": those used to remember specific events or persons or even "whole eras," those that are "special or cherished," and those that can "stimulate recollection of the past *in general* rather than any specifics within it" (p. 194). This third category comes closer to the modernist symbol (see Chapter 3 and above) because of its more abstract value: Proust's narrator bites into a madeleine and is flooded in memories that generate, through what Edward Casey (1987) calls a sequence of "internal horizons" (p. 207), the enormous text of *A la recherche du temps perdu*. It is significant, though, that in the case of Proust's narrator, he does not know that the object, a simple pastry, will generate these memories. It is neither cherished nor special, nor is it selected or kept for the sake of remembering. Instead, it generates the memory spontaneously.

What of the sea glass? There are over twenty thousand pieces in Bob and Mary's basement, none of which is cherished as memorabilia. Even the crafts made of them are from recent times and could not be considered as reminiscentia. They are, at most, *potential* reminiscentia. A necklace, say, made of red glass collected by one of the grandchildren, might in seventy years' time be a true cherished object, passed on with its accompanying stories to a new generation. But if the sea glass is not really cherished in itself, not used to regenerate narrative associated with memory, it nevertheless is remarkable, especially in its transition from thing to literary image or symbol.

These and related objects, once made part of a text, begin to gather meaning to themselves and thereby enrich the reading of the text, without their having necessarily been placed there to do so, as literary devices are usually thought to function. These symbols, in the sense that I've sketched above, can even be characterized as *inverted* reminiscentia. Instead of objects that recall memories that can be formed into a narrative, these are objects first "found" within the text, and they can generate new narratives, or modify existing ones, out of the very thinginess that only reveals itself through the text. They were included in someone's life story along with other objects being described (the nails in the wall studs, the broken batteries), as one of them, but reveal themselves in the text to be literary objects of a different sort. Their value as symbols may not be fully seen until the text is read, in order to be shared, edited, reworked, and so on. They can enrich – thicken – the narrative as it is crafted, edited, or simply reread, and thereby have a profound effect upon the way the world is experienced through that narrative. They belong to the sphere of the narrative as literary text, and may be used alongside other modes of analysis, such as thematic lines, plots, genre, and the like (see Dubovska et al., 2016). They work by means of "metaphorical association" (Randall, 2011, p. 24). Indeed, they can be understood as dense nodes that act as gravity wells for strands of metaphorical thought.

Bob and Mary certainly have each thought about sea glass jewellery, but not necessarily its symbolic value in the story of their lives, both separate and together. When each set of interviews is taken separately, the sea glass jewellery does not stand out. Mary's second interview alone is almost one hundred pages long, covering numerous topics, and her written story does not mention the jewellery at all. Bob's interviews and written story, while not particularly reflective, are nonetheless rich in objects, of which the jewellery is only one example. It is mentioned briefly in both interviews, but not in his story. However, when considered as a window into these intersecting lives, the sea glass, transformed into artwork and then commodified as items to be sold in another province, becomes a powerful emblem of narrative openness and, indeed, resilience.

The crafts are products of an activity taken up at a period in their lives when some old, familiar activities are no longer available. Though the children are grown and have left the family home, they too are involved in this activity and can remain connected to it throughout the year, collecting sea glass no matter where they are in the world and bringing it back to the parents. The grandchildren, too, pick it for their grandparents. The displaying and selling of the crafts at the festival allow them to continue their family hobby of commercial ventures, like the garage sales, but in the context of a relaxed vacation on a resort island, organized by someone else instead of themselves. The activity brings the couple together, but also fosters separate hobbies. Bob enjoys the organizing and fashioning of the jewellery, and he keeps thousands of pieces catalogued in the basement, along with the records that he kept during his career with the police. Mary has delved into the history and archaeology of these artefacts – each colour and style of sea glass, some adorned with stamps or writing, tells a story and can point to a particular time, nationality, and vessel, leading to learning about the historical periods and people who would have used them. The transformation of these artefacts, fragments from others' pasts, into new, crafted artefacts, and their subsequent commodification, make each one a new potential cherished object, for themselves as well as for those who are given or buy them, who thus become part of the story.

The shared activity "has opened up a whole new world," according to Mary, but like the garage sales before it, the sea glass hobby is winding down:

> Seven years this new discovery of sea glass has become a very focal point. A shared hobby that has been wonderful. We have learned, uh, we have worked, we have shared with other people. It's been … a sheer joy. So now … we're coming sort of to the end of that, now writing is becoming the major point of what we're doing as a couple and that we feel, you know, really involved in. (86-II)

Writing represents another step in the transformation of sea glass. Glass on a ship is shattered and over many years is tumbled into a sea jewel, which is picked up, catalogued, fashioned into crafts, given away or sold, and now will become both symbol and subject of a narrative. Indeed, Mary tells Jennifer in the second interview that the sea glass will be the subject of her next piece of writing. Taken as a symbol, the sea glass and things like it thus have a transformational quality. A keepsake or memento, say an old coin, becomes something else when it is fashioned into a necklace or a pin. It remains a cherished object but is also now an art object made from the raw material of the keepsake. Once written or spoken about in a story, it can take on a symbolic quality in the literary sense, opening itself up to accumulation of meaning and association. Mary intends to write about the sea glass, but the story she chose for her interviews is about her childhood. Bob mentions the sea glass as well, listing it among other things in his basement and mentioning their shared hobby. The richness of its symbolic value may come out once Mary writes her narrative about it; it certainly has come out in the interviews.

The symbol as I've been discussing it here opens up possibilities for narrative resilience not only as a form of reminiscentia, or a transformed cherished object, but as something that disrupts and deepens – even creates – the time of a narrative. The genealogy of materials and artefacts that make up the sea glass jewellery, as well as the family table that Brandi and I will discuss in Chapter 12, points in far-off directions across space and time, over and above the artefacts' immediate value as reminiscentia. Once those artefacts are woven into a text – whether or not they are being deliberately used as symbols – they also expand along the lines of Casey's "internal horizons," not in the deeply personal world of space-memory that Proust's prose occupies, but to the cosmic, primordial, mythical, supernatural, and divine. The literary object-as-symbol gathers the world and lets the world appear.

As I say, the last chapter in this part of the book will consider a table, which in a lengthy written piece submitted by its owner, David, gathers together the family that has sat around it, the artisan who created it, the wood from which it was made, and the place where the trees that provided it grow. And eventually it gathers storytelling itself, both the acts of storytelling told around the table and the temporal world that emerges from the narrativizing of experience. In *Rewriting the Self*, Mark Freeman (1993, pp. 50–80) uses Helen Keller's autobiography to illustrate how, in a very real sense, time and storytelling emerge at the same moment, out of a process that also produces the sense of self. Likewise, and as we shall see in Chapter 12, David sees the very origin of humanity in the gathering from which the table emerges and which it, as thing, stands in for and preserves, even if the object itself is no longer present and only its narrative stand-in remains. The sea glass, fragmented and spread out in thousands of discrete bits, does not have this table's mass, but it is more closely related to the table than to mementos or to Sherman's three types of reminiscentia.

As generative narrative objects, "covert symbols" such as the sea glass serve as reminiscentia in reverse. They open up or inspire new narrative directions or dimensions, fending off narrative foreclosure by thickening and enriching life narratives, lending complexity, ambiguity, ductility, and irony to the mixtures of pleasure and pain, regret and nostalgia, hope and fear that life narratives invariably reflect. Overt symbols can do so too, of course, but in the hidden or covert symbols one may seek new, undiscovered narrative threads that lead to the kind of richness our team believes is linked to inner resilience (Randall et al., 2015).

Mary has real fears arising from watching her children become parents, her family members revealing their selfishness and amorality, her mother "living too long," her nagging memory of a near death experience. But she is remarkably proactive about finding ways to be resilient, letting go of things – not just furniture, but hobbies and occupations – and moving on to the next new thing. Her plans for the next chapter in her life story include writing on several topics (she keeps a running list of subjects she wishes to write about). Some of that writing will involve reminiscence, some will require her to use various writers' tricks, like those that Deborah introduced in the workshops (see Chapter 14), to polish her stories into digestible lessons that can be passed on to others. The things she writes about, such as the sea glass, may well afford her an openness to the activity peculiar to writing autobiographical narrative: sea glass and other potential symbols in her writing offer her the opportunity to reframe and deepen her own story, offering new plot and character points that need to be developed in its next chapters.

The "next chapter" is the challenge of narrative: the sense of impending closure suggests a natural end to a chapter, and if there have been many chapters, it is natural to ask, if only for a moment, "will there *be* a next chapter?" After all, "no new chapters" need not mean death: it may mean settling into a place, a role, and playing that part (the parent of a young child, the homeowner wrestling with a mortgage, the worker who has tired of a job, the new resident of a nursing home). A better way to describe an autobiography's narrative is "the last chapter for a while," which means that though it may have been the best years of one's life, there are no stories associated with it (perhaps not a coincidence). It could be that stories are life affirming only at times when circumstances are not at their best. Both Bob and Mary have kept records and catalogues, but they have been nearly merciless in disposing of (potentially cherished) things … nearly. They have maintained connections to a few things: he to the aesthetic product of his "keeping busy," like an oil painting or a fishing fly, she to the well-crafted story that also teaches a lesson. Stories, though, are for the times in life when you have less energy to kayak, run, spearhead, get into vehicle chases, fight the powers that be. Storytime is separate, set off from the rest of life. A quiet time, maybe a bedtime, maybe a time in a classroom, but always a time for gathering thoughts.

Narrative itself may write its own chapter into this couple's lives. Her education in creative writing might cause her to consider ways of telling stories beyond the well-polished lesson or fable. The bravery that shows through in her willingness to talk to Jennifer, a stranger (not to mention the strangers who would go on to analyse her interviews), about such profound and troubling experiences in her life – to share such a gift with our research team – speaks to our suspicion that the ability to tell a thicker, richer story about one's life is linked in some important way to resilience. She might then explore her near-death experience, for example, in fiction. His oil painting may take on a more central role now that he can no longer draw from his stash of sea glass. We know that he is content and that she has a plan for when he dies, but contentment and settling into a new phase do not mean the end of autobiography, or death. The (temporary) end of story is sometimes the beginning of poetry.

6 Apple Quilt: Repositories and Legacies

JENNIFER ESTEY

Memories can cut both ways – they can depress us or elevate our spirit; they can bind us or set us free.

– Paul Wong (1995, p. 35)

As Denise and I suggested in Chapter 4, cherished objects can act as conduits for the passing down of memories from one generation to another. This kind of generational continuity is something I have experienced personally, as my grandparents have passed down to me hand-sewn quilts that were made by my great-grandmothers. One of these, sewn by my grandmother's mother, stands out in particular.

Along with a teacup and saucer, it is the only object I own that once belonged to her. It has two solid pieces of fabric tacked together with white yarn that secures a solid piece of cotton batting, its top patterned with randomly scattered fall-coloured leaves. Someday, I will pass it on to the next generation. I will share stories about my grandmother, to be sure, for I know her very well, but also about my great-grandmother, whom I never knew because she died before my birth. However, I have heard lots of stories about her from others in my family, stories that convey her kindness, patience, and calm, her self-sacrifice and her loving demeanour: qualities I like to think she passed on to me.

This cherished possession in my life draws on the collective memory – on the stories – of all those who knew her to form an image in my mind of her identity, of who she was (Bakhurst, 2001). Although their stories about her are, technically speaking, unrelated to the quilt itself, whenever I see it I think about and in some ways "remember" her.

For such reasons, I have chosen in this chapter to focus on Amelie, for she was, among other things, an avid quilter. When she showed me what she calls her "apple quilt," which I'll be discussing in more detail later on, I felt an especially deep connection to her and her stories. During our two interviews, though, she discussed not only quilting but, directly or otherwise, history, generativity, legacy, and the matter of continuity between the generations of her family, all of them subjects to which I could very much relate. In what follows, I'd like to explore the role of quilts as repositories of stories and, as such, as legacies in their own right.

Self, Identity, and Secrets

As an interview participant, Amelie was bursting with stories and had a range of experiences she wanted to share, from hobbies to health, relationships to friendships, and employment to education. In this way, the data from her interviews reflected "a conversation of narrators" in which, rather than a "single, linear narrative voice" (Raggatt, 2006), multiple "personifications" emerged, such as quilter, mother, teacher, and volunteer, each one revealing a separate facet of identity in her polyphonic story.

Every story has different threads or topics that the teller can explore. During my interviews with Amelie, it seemed that some topics were more difficult than others to disclose, and some were not to be shared at all, were "secret stories" (Kenyon & Randall, 1997, p. 49). "Just because it happened," she explained to me, "just because it was true, it doesn't mean that you have to share it ... They say secrets are statements that you give to one person at a time ... I don't have any burning desire to reveal secrets" (41-II). This hesitancy to reveal aspects about her life could be taken to illustrate a dialogical view of the self that draws upon the thinking of Mikhail Bakhtin. Psychologist Hubert Hermans (2001) explains what that view entails:

> [We] conceptualize the self in terms of a dynamic multiplicity of relatively autonomous I-positions. In this conception, the I has the possibility to move from one spatial position to another in accordance with changes in situation and time. The I fluctuates among different and even opposed positions, and has the capacity imaginatively to endow each position with a voice so that dialogical relations between voices can be established ... Each of them has a story to tell about his or her own experience, from his or her own stance ... resulting in a complex narratively structured self. (p. 248)[1]

1 *Editors' note*: Dialogic entities are things in their own right, while monologic entities are mere objects. To be dialogic is not to assume that things (fungi, the world, stars) are conscious, but neither is it to conceive of them as objects that cannot have consciousness. Amelie's own story here is conceived as a quilt, a collection of things with stories.

One story that Amelie chose not to share with her children and grandchildren, particularly in her role as mother and grandmother respectively, characterizes her as a hitchhiker. She and her childhood friend, Sarah, had decided early on that they very much wanted to travel. However, her mother's reaction to the idea was terrifying: "If you leave the house before you're eighteen, I'm sending the police after you" (16-I). So, they watched the calendar carefully, and in 1968, when Amelie turned eighteen, the two of them began planning their trip in earnest. The evening before they set out, they bummed a dollar from each of their friends for the grand total of twelve dollars between them. "We didn't have very many friends," she chuckled (16-I). Leaving notes for each of their families, they sneaked out of their houses in the dead of the night.

Amelie had heard somewhere that if you went to a jail and asked for a place to stay, the police were obliged to offer protection and provide you a bed for the night. The two of them soon found out this wasn't true, so they ended up staying in a variety of places – including lighthouses, hotels, and (only when there was space) jail cells. With the aid of two maps that she has held on to all these years, she outlined to me the route they had originally planned to take, along with the one they actually followed. In total, they were gone for over two weeks, a tremendous adventure overall, one of her signature stories, for sure. Still, Amelie was insistent: "I can't tell anybody about my hitchhiking trip … I can't ever tell!" (16-I). If her children and grandchildren were to find out about her escapades, she felt that they would have something to hold over her head.[2] Quoting an adage that her mother had passed down to her, she said, "Not all truths are to be told" (40-II).

Quilting

"I'm a quilter," Amelie announced to me in no uncertain terms. "That's my passion" (47-I). With this in mind, I'd like to touch on the development of quilting down through history, for in many ways it demonstrates how the features of quilt-making that Amelie so keenly values, such as building a social network, have been prevalent for a long time.

The word "quilt," which derives from the Latin *culcita*, literally means "stuffed sack" (Betterton, 2015). The process of creating a quilt combines two types of needlework. The first is patchwork, which entails piecing together scraps of fabric of various shapes and sizes to create a

2 *Editors' note*: The paradox here is worth noting: she has told, and yet she has not – indeed, "can't ever tell."

unified whole that will serve as either the top or bottom layer. The kinds of fabric that quilters have used depends, obviously, on availability and reflected the era in question. For instance, silk was commonly used in the seventeenth and eighteenth centuries, while in the nineteenth century it was more likely to be cotton and wool (Webster, 2008). Second, the two layers are fastened together, with loose material, such as cotton batting, distributed uniformly between them. The final product varies based on the chosen materials. The top could be a single piece of fabric, multiple scraps of fabric, appliqué, or a combination of them all (Betterton, 2015).[3]

Though quilting has existed for centuries, it has changed over time, based upon the surrounding cultural and political environment. In the seventeenth century, for example, life on the American frontier was difficult due to the scarcity of resources, thus requiring hard work, discipline, and frugality to ensure survival – something that the Protestant work ethic keenly promoted (Cheek & Piercy, 2004). At the same time as quilting provided women with opportunities to socialize, it also satisfied the expectation of producing items that were useful, not frivolous, items that served a host of practical purposes, from providing warmth to raising money to wrapping the dead (Cheek & Piercy, 2004; Ettinger & Hoffman, 1990; Webster, 2008).

In the latter half of the nineteenth century, the trend towards industrialization resulted in an increasing division between the public sphere, outside the household, and the private sphere, inside it (Ettinger & Hoffman, 1990), a division that was, of course, decidedly gendered. Whereas men worked in factories, in the public sphere, women stayed home and engaged in activities like quilting, tasks that embodied the prevailing social values of patience, precision, and skill. Moreover, and in contrast to the corresponding viewpoint that linked idleness with evil, the quilts that such dutiful women created could be donated to those less fortunate than themselves (Ettinger & Hoffman, 1990).

Traditionally, women were in many ways voiceless, both publicly and politically. Their quilts, however, served as a means of communicating their social worth. During the nineteenth century in the United States, for example, the ability of a young woman to engage in needlework demonstrated her worth as a wife. A young woman who could quilt not only

3 *Editors' note*: These materials make up the thing, the quilt, but might not Amelie's life itself be viewed through the lens of things called quilts? A quilt can display images with stories – some known, some not.

fulfilled societal expectations but was more marketable to male suitors (Ettinger & Hoffman, 1990), whereas young women who could not were considered unprepared for marriage.

In the last quarter of the nineteenth century, amid the Victorian era, patchwork quilts made of various materials, including ribbon, silk, velvet, and brocades pieced together, were highly decorative pieces that showed off how skilfully and elaborately they had been sewn (Betterton, 2015).[4] Such quilts were designed to be aesthetically pleasing (Senft, 1995) and to be displayed on furniture, in stark contrast to those designed in the seventeenth century. In the nineteenth century, that is to say, a shift was evident from quilting as utility to quilting as leisure or hobby, indeed as art.

Apart from this shift, one characteristic of quilting that has persevered over the centuries is its collaborative nature. As a child, for example, Amelie had few friends who shared her interests in reading and writing. But in adulthood, as she became involved in quilting and teaching quilting classes, she describes having "dozens and dozens of friends" whose interests she shares (22-II).

NAMES Quilt

Quilt designs and styles tend to reflect different regions, time periods, and countries of origin. Moreover, many have been designed to tell stories – there's the close link, again, between stories and things – that represent broader social-cultural contexts, which can be mythical, biblical, historical, or political in nature (Wilson, 2009). For instance, the "NAMES Project AIDS Memorial Quilt," conceived originally by Cleve Jones, has helped to transform cultural and political responses to the AIDS pandemic in the United States (Morris, 2011). The largest ongoing community art project in the world, it has served as a symbol to raise awareness, promote education, reduce stigma and fear, foster connectedness, and mourn and memorialize those who succumbed to the disease (AIDS Memorial Quilt, n.d.).

Each panel of the quilt measures three by six feet, the approximate size of a coffin, and the panels are sewn together into twelve-by-twelve-foot squares (Morris, 2011). In 1987, at the time it was first displayed

4 *Editors' note*: One can therefore easily forget a story attached to an image displayed on the quilt: it hides in plain sight. For the quilt is busy signifying skill, marketability, or as-yet-undreamt possibilities. People look through it to something else, ignoring that square with a map.

in conjunction with the national march on Washington for gay and lesbian rights at the National Mall, it contained over 1,920 panels, each one signifying a deceased person. Today, there are more than 50,000 panels commemorating the lives of over 105,000 people, and the quilt as a whole continues to grow. Praised as "a beautiful tribute to those lost to the devastation of HIV/AIDS," it is a reminder to "us all of our responsibility to tell the personal stories lovingly stitched into every panel" (AIDS Memorial Quilt, n.d.). It inspires us to remember the past, to engage with issues in the present, and to seek to change the future in order to end the AIDS pandemic altogether. It is a memorial that will exist for generations to come.

Just as quilts can be used to memorialize the dead, so, too, can they celebrate a birth, mark the recovery from illness, and process difficult emotions associated with the dissolution of a marriage (Cheek & Yaure, 2017). In fact, Amelie has integrated several of these things into her own experience of quilting. For example, when a fellow member of the quilting community dies, their relatives will often bring her the deceased's unfinished quilts for her to date and store and at times even to complete, and then to incorporate into her own collection. Completing the unfinished quilts is a way for her to connect the present with history, something she values deeply, she says, since it "relates to the development of the world as we know it" (58-II).

As an example of this kind of connection, Amelie told me how, each summer, she typically moves the wooden frame that holds the pieces of her quilts in place out into the sunroom. In the fall, when it gets too cold to continue, she moves it back inside. On the morning of 11 September 2001, while she was doing precisely that, her neighbour phoned her and told her to turn on the television. When she did, she learned that at 7:45 a.m., New York time, a jet filled with passengers had flown into one of the two towers of the World Trade Center (Hillstrom, 2012). After the initial crash, she thought that maybe it was an accident, but as she continued watching, she learned it was but the first in a series of attacks that, without question, significantly affected the course of recent history. In honour of this significance, and not only to mark this personal "flashbulb memory" (Schacter, 1996, pp. 195–201) but to preserve a piece of history for future generations, Amelie named the quilt on which she was then working "Stars over Manhattan" (22-II).

Generativity

Erikson (1963) has defined "generativity" as, essentially, concern for guiding or for contributing in some constructive way to the next generation, a concern that he believed was at the forefront of our lives in stage 7 of his model of psychosocial development, or roughly from age forty to sixty-five. During this time, we tend to have developed our own unique sense of identity and are involved in some way in caring for and about the next generation, and in seeking ways to pass on to it our unique legacy. Generativity can occur on a small scale, from parents to children within the same household, or on a larger scale – in churches, schools, neighbourhoods, and communities (McAdams & Logan, 2004). By the same token, it can be manifested not solely in mid-life but will "ebb and flow at different times in the life cycle" (p. 18).

Generative actions include teaching, mentoring, volunteering, participating in church activities, and participating in politics (McAdams & Logan, 2004). On all such fronts, Amelie is a highly generative individual. She has volunteered for the local hospice, delivered Meals on Wheels, visited friends in nursing homes, taught school for twenty-five years, and as a parent, taught her own children and grandchildren too. She has also participated in quilting guilds, where she has passed on her knowledge, experience, and skills to others who share her interest in the craft. As she explained to me, "it's very valuable to be able to, to leave something behind and I'd like to do that" (8-I).

If a life is understood as in some way a *story*, then one could say that it has a beginning, middle, and end. As people age – as they age biographically, that is – they become more aware of the eventual ending of their stories, more aware that there are fewer years ahead for them in the future than behind them in the past. Biography, writes Bakhurst (2001), is "one of innumerable ways we sustain an image of our past. Through the written word, photograph, film, audio and video recording, ritual and memorial, and so on, the past is constantly made present. This is no small fact, but a defining feature of the human condition as it now is" (p. 185). Amelie would agree. In her words, "it's really important for people to leave their experiences ... All my life I have preferred to read non-fiction and I've read a lot of biographies ... I've learned from those people," she says (8-I), alluding to what could be called *biographical* generativity. But quilting itself can also be a form of generativity.

Cheek and Yaure (2017) describe the act of passing quilts on to others as elevating them from mere objects to "symbol[s] of caring and shared experience[s]" (p. 40). Over time, Amelie has amassed an impressive collection of quilts, to the point where the provincial museum has expressed great interest in it and she has agreed to donate it. Doing so, she feels, will be a means of passing on her own unique legacy and, at the same time, affording the general public access to their distinct historical value.

But it is more than just the quilts themselves that, in her mind, figure in this legacy. So, too, does writing about them.

Writing offers her an opportunity to reminisce about the story of each individual quilt, and indeed she has written over eighty quilting stories, which she has had published in the magazine *Burda Style*. The process of writing provides her a way of reflecting upon the motivation behind creating the quilt, and the mental and emotional labour that went into designing it. It can also serve as an outlet for resolving past issues (Cheek & Yaure, 2017). The argument has been put forward, in fact, that quilting and writing are similar endeavours (Rogerson, 1998), both possessing a generative dimension: a quilter sews random pieces of fabric to create a quilt and a writer connects an assortment of ideas to produce a text. As for Amelie, she not only uses both of these media but – in her quilting stories – she integrates them as well.

When I asked her what writing means for her, she explained that it prompts her to ask "Is that what happened?" (9-I). It pushes her to step out and see what other people are seeing. For her, the writer can see the story not as it was experienced, but as an objective observer looking on from the outside – a process that has helped her to cope with personal experiences that are particularly charged in nature. In the moment, she says, she is an emotional writer, but when she later reads what she has composed, she will often rip it up – or as the case may be, burn her journals – because such writing, she says, leads her to feel depressed. Once a crisis is over, so she explained to me, people need to move on. Accordingly, she does not dwell on negative events and does not want to pass on negativity to others. She would rather focus on the positive, and leave the next generations with the lessons she has learned.

Overall, quilts can be meaningful gifts to give or to receive. Gifting a quilt is itself a highly generative activity insofar as it provides an opportunity for preserving traditions, and memories, that others can cherish in turn (Cheek & Yaure, 2017). It can provide them with a greater sense of stability and continuity, and help them live more fulfilling and meaningful lives (Baumeister & Vohs, 2002).

The Quilting Language

While in Amelie's home, I noticed a bag of quilts by the front door, quilts hanging on the wall, quilts folded neatly on the couch, and quilts draped over the backs of chairs. I found myself wondering what the presence of so many quilts suggested, what it – what they – were saying.

In an intriguing article entitled "Quilt Language," Mara Witzling (2009) makes the observation that "quilts speak through their formal qualities, their use of fabric, and their social context" (p. 219). They speak, for example, through their design, whether it be a commonly used pattern or one peculiar to an individual quilter. A number of familiar ones have been used down through the years, including Ohio Sunflower, Double Irish Chain, Tree of Life, and The Log Cabin. If you like, these patterns are a means for quilters to communicate their experiences without providing a literal description of them but rather through the quilt's distinctive visual qualities (Witzling, 2009).

As I noted already, it is a common practice to give the finished quilt a name (Webster, 2008). Indeed, many designs have well-known names that have been used repeatedly by generations of women. The Five-Pointed Star, for example, is patterned so that the centre of each block of the quilt contains one star. Changing the size of the stars or the colours of the fabric does not result in a new name; it is still a Five-Pointed Star. In the late nineteenth century, one of the most frequently employed patterns was that of a log cabin. The log cabin connoted the image of home, its popularity as a central theme in quilts attributable to the expansion westward across America. At its centre, the quilt contains a square that is coloured either red to represent the hearth fire or yellow to signify a lantern that guides travellers to their destination. Surrounding the square are alternating arrangements of light rows and dark rows that convey the sense of life's joys and sorrows, as well as mimic the placement of logs on a fire. This pattern has been adopted and adapted within different cultural contexts, with the unique flavour of the local setting incorporated into its design, illustrating how a conventional pattern can be tailored, so to speak, in ways that an individual quilter deems appropriate to a particular place and time (Witzling, 2009).

Given that quilters can spend hours on a particular design, they have time to reflect on the name that they assign it. The name might reflect themes in history, politics, or religion, in nature, poetry, or romance. It could be chosen based on the distinct qualities of the quilt, such as its fabric or stitching. But often its name has a special significance to the quilter herself. By way of example, female pioneers integrated their social context into their quilts by giving them names like Pilgrim's Pride, Bear's Paws, Rocky Road to Kansas, and Texas Tears (Webster, 2008, p. 117).

One of her own quilts, which was draped over the banister, Amelie christened "Apples" (25-II). Having carefully mapped out its design, she had various stories, she said, about the process of collecting the materials that went into it. Rather than possessing a single linear story, in other words, there were multiple threads running through her narrative concerning it. Apples is a patchwork type of quilt, which historically served a practical purpose when, for example, limited resources made it necessary for people to use old clothing and other materials to put patches on quilts whose fabric was thin or torn (Webster, 2008).

The top of the quilt has twenty-eight squares, each one with an apple in the centre. The squares are arranged in seven rows and four columns, with a one-inch, dark border framing each one. Every square has a white background, a lime green trim on the left and right sides, and a central image of an apple surrounded by leaves. No two pieces are alike. Each is fashioned from its own fabric, has its own unique pattern (chevron, polka dot, plaid, or solid), and features its own distinct colour scheme (pink, red, or burgundy). To top things off, the quilt's batting gives the apples a three-dimensional appearance. Overall, it is a design created by Amelie herself – one that has enabled her to express facets of her own individual identity.

As I say, the making of such a beautiful, complex quilt is associated in Amelie's memory with a variety of stories. Many of them revolved around a trip that she and her husband, Frank, made across the United States, stopping at various locations en route to collect the pieces of fabric that would eventually become part of it. On one occasion during their travels, Amelie asked him to drop her off at a fabric store and to come back two hours later. When he returned to pick her up, he found her socializing with other quilters and noticed that, stacked on the table, were over twenty different bolts of fabric – a bolt being sixty inches wide and holding up to one hundred yards of material. As the two of them prepared to leave, the sales associate handed Amelie a small handful of fabric: fifteen pieces of one-quarter of a yard that had been cut from each of the bolts. Looking in shock at what was in her hand, having assumed that she had purchased all twenty bolts, he exclaimed, "You spent over two hours here and that's all you are getting?!" (26-II). "To him," Amelie explained, "that was perfectly logical. To the rest of us, we just about died laughing" (26-II). In fact, as she recounted the story to me, she enjoyed a good laugh once again.

Agency

In his analysis of the themes of agency and communion, power and intimacy, in how people narrate their life stories, Dan McAdams (2001b) claims that those who rate "high in power motivation emphasize agentic themes of self-mastery, status and victory, achievement and responsibility, and empowerment" (p. 112). Conversely, those "high in intimacy motivation emphasize communal themes such as friendship and love, dialogue, and caring for others" (p. 112). These latter individuals, says McAdams, tend to personify themselves as "the caregiver," "the loyal friend," and "the lover" (p. 112).

Even though Amelie used lots of "we" language during my interviews with her, which would suggest a strong communal orientation, she characterized herself, primarily, in agentic terms. She stressed, for instance, how she had come from nothing, married at a young age, had three children under the age of three, and worked as a teacher for wages so humble that she had to take on a second job year round to make ends meet. Student loans, a first mortgage, a second mortgage – all caused tremendous financial pressure. In short, "We had no money. We had nothing" (21-I). Nonetheless, she and Frank worked day and night to dig themselves out of debt until, eventually, through purchasing various real estate properties, they were able to generate additional revenue streams. "Sometimes you have to work 24/7 to get yourself out of the hole," she told me; "you're not going to do that for a week or two weeks. You might have to do that for three or four years" (25-I).

Emphasizing the importance of working hard to overcome obstacles in life, Amelie believes that her story conveys a powerful lesson that could offer encouragement to others who are struggling – younger people like myself. Her messaging is "You can do it!" (25-I). It was revealing, for instance, that when she discussed such hardships, she did not dwell on the negative aspects of them, nor seek sympathy from me because of them. Rather, and in keeping with her personal preference for positive stories and with the "positivity effect" (Carstensen & Mikels, 2005; Mather & Carstensen, 2005) that gerontologists have found evident among older adults in general, she shared it all in the form of a life lesson. This was especially interesting since, at the time, I was a twenty-something university student. I wonder whether she would have shared the same lesson in the same way had she been interviewed by someone closer to her own age, someone more settled in their life, who might not have appreciated, or benefitted from, the intention behind it.

Turning Points

Discussing the role of "turning points" in people's autobiographical narrations, psychologist Jerome Bruner (2001) defines them as "episodes in which, as if to underline the power of the agent's intentional states, the narrator attributes a crucial change or stance in the protagonist's story to a belief, a conviction, a thought" (p. 31). The injection of turning points into one's story, Bruner says, is "crucial to the effort to *individualize* a life" (p. 31; emphasis Bruner's).

One such turning point in Amelie's own life, it became clear to me, was when one day, quite unexpectedly, her right side became completely paralysed, a condition diagnosed later as multiple sclerosis (MS). Though she had had symptoms beforehand, she didn't know at the time that this was what she was experiencing and so had no way to prepare herself for such a dramatic decline in her health, which changed virtually every aspect of her life. Her career was over. She could no longer walk, stand, cook, or engage in any number of other ordinary activities. "The worst part of it," she told me, was that "my brain was affected ... I don't read directions very well ... I used to make muffins all the time. I couldn't even make muffins because I couldn't read a recipe and I could try and say OK, I'm going to take out all the ingredients and I'm going to put them away after I use them, but I'd be walking around with a bottle of ginger or something and thinking did I put it in? Or am I putting it away? Or am I taking it out? What am I doing? ... It was at least two years that I couldn't cook anything, that I couldn't really do very much of anything" (37-I).

But although Amelie had lost her independence, her positive, determined attitude remained intact, and with it her sense of (narrative) agency. No way would she play the "victim" card. Instead, each day she would ask herself, "What can I do?" (44-II). Deciding not to lie in bed all day long, for example, she set herself a goal – to get up, get dressed, and go downstairs. It didn't matter how long it took her to get downstairs or if, after doing so, she slept in her chair for most of the day. The key was to do something. As time progressed, she set herself other small goals every day and strove diligently to reach them. Rather than allow her limitations to stop her from being active, she adapted to them. For instance, she still loved to read, but having lost her normal vision, she elected to buy audio books instead.

Along with setting goals, she also sought medical advice regarding alternative options for treating her condition. One doctor told her that what she had would never get better and that she just needed to "get used to it" (45-II). Refusing to accept this assessment of her situation, she sought a second opinion from another doctor who suggested that she begin taking steroid injections immediately. Though she entered the hospital in a wheelchair, she walked out with only a cane following the very first injection. From that point on, her health steadily improved.

Amelie's philosophy during this period of her life was – and still is – that if she cannot do one thing then she will do something else instead; thus she often re-evaluates her abilities and finds new activities to pursue. "I still can't read patterns," she told me; "I just do my own. I do a lot of things my way. I have to" (40-I). As far as quilting is concerned, her belief is that if it gets so that she can't do it at all, then she will find something else she can do that affords her a similar sense of satisfaction.

As I say, Amelie's condition steadily improved. She still had limitations, such as not being able to read quilting patterns or follow recipes; nonetheless, she could walk and, in time, she recovered her strength to a remarkable degree. Indeed, she improved so much that after her neurologist retired, her new neurologist was convinced that she must be faking having MS at all. Rather than argue the matter, however, she agreed to be tested again and so proved her doctor wrong.

A particular news story that she saw once on television illustrates her dedication to such a positive philosophy. The camera shows a man standing on top of a structure, flood waters raging around him, holding onto a pole with one hand. Underscoring the importance of thinking and acting outside the box, she assured me that if she were in his position, she would remove her pants and tie herself to the pole. She would not be swept away by the water. Her choosing to tell me about her experience with MS, and about her response to this news story in particular, accords well with Bruner's (2001) view of turning points as episodes that "underline the power of the agent's intentional states" (p. 31) and, in her case, set her apart from others – that individualize her – as both creative and determined.

Intergenerational Narratives

Intergenerational narratives are stories that get passed down from one generation to the next (Merrill & Fivush, 2016; Ryan et al., 1999). They have at least four main functions: education about personal and historical events, the building of relationships, the transmission of values, and the expression of generativity (Norris et al., 2004). These four functions are eminently represented in Amelie's account of her family's propensity for storytelling.

She described her father, for example, as a "tremendous storyteller" (12-I), who had in fact left her audio recordings of himself telling stories that, at the time of the interviews, she was transcribing. These narratives constituted a complex web in which, in a sense, the narratives of her grandparents, parents, and children are all intertwined (Merrill & Fivush, 2016). To educate her on historical events and on his own life in the midst of them, her paternal grandfather, for example, had told a number of stories to her father, with whom he was not especially close. Amelie was thankful that her father had shared these stories with her because, from them, she learned a great deal about her grandfather's life that she would not otherwise have known.

For instance, as a soldier in the French army, he had been caught up in the Siege of Paris during the Franco-Prussian War where they had to eat, as Amelie put it, "I don't know what, but anyway, it was really … if you ever look up the Siege of Paris – it's terrible" (12-I). Though initially there was a two-month supply of food, the war continued for more than twice that time, which meant that fresh meat soon ran out and was replaced with tinned meat. Their meals varying little, the soldiers soon began experiencing scurvy, diarrhea, and dyspepsia (Gordon, 1871). This lack of proper nutrition, combined with exposure to freezing temperatures and general exhaustion, made up the horrific conditions that soldiers like her grandfather were forced to endure.

From stories such as this, Amelie also learned that in 1872, when her grandfather was eleven, he grew tired of living with his bossy mother and sisters and so left home to work on a ship. During this time, he learned seven languages and travelled the proverbial seven seas to such far-flung places as Japan and Cape Horn. Navigating around the latter was itself, of course, a major accomplishment. "Sometimes," Amelie explained, "it would take them a week to get around [it] because the winds would blow them back" (13-I). Still, her grandfather made the trip safely and successfully a number of times.

Despite the strained relationship between them, her father listened to his father's stories and, as I say, passed them on to Amelie, who for her part collected newspaper clippings that corroborated her grandfather's accounts. In all, she said, "I'm grateful because … his father had such … an interesting life" (13-I), a life, you could say, that she sought to emulate in her own. It was because her grandfather had been to China, for instance, that she travelled there as well, with her sister, and was able to walk along its famous Great Wall.

Amelie wanted me to know, though, that her father himself also told stories. That said, since his passing she has wished keenly that she had asked him more questions, because he too, she maintained, had had an interesting life. For example, at one point, he participated in a program where the government placed young men in make-work camps in order to keep them from starving. While she knew certain aspects of this experience, she lacked specific details, something that bothered her greatly. At the same time, it motivated her to focus on building her relationships with her own children and grandchildren so as to avoid repeating the same mistake. As one means of doing so, she set out to pass on to them her love of reading by writing short stories that they would enjoy reading for themselves.

"When I wrote the stories for my granddaughter," she explained to me, "I wrote them because she didn't like to read" (22-II). Amelie wrote them, in other words, in the hope of capturing the child's attention and sparking in her a love of reading too. One such story, which she wrote in a manner suitable to a child's reading level, revolved around a central character going on an adventure and travelling to various places throughout the world – a storyline reflective, you could argue, of both her grandfather's life and her own.

As a former teacher, Amelie outlined to me how she also uses storytelling to provide advice and teach lessons to her granddaughter, because she does not want her grandchildren to have to go through the sorts of things that she had to. "I would like to leave something for ... other people," she said, "not just necessarily my children and grandchildren, but I would like to leave something of what I've learned" (7-I) – a classic expression of a key form of generativity as passing on one's wisdom to the next generation (Norris et al., 2004), what psychologist John Kotre (1984) refers to as "generative transference" (pp. 30f.).

Both Amelie's mother and grandmother had been teachers, and Amelie followed in their footsteps. As a child, however, she had wanted to be a doctor. Being a woman, though, her only real option at that time was teacher's college, since the tuition was free. As for attending university, she was discouraged from doing so. "It's a waste of time, it's a waste of money" (55-I), others told her repeatedly. "You're just a girl. You're going to get married and nobody's going to care what your education is" (55-II). Through the stories she wrote, then, she promoted one of her own core values, or core life-themes, namely determination. "I am trying every chance I get to instil in my granddaughters [that] you can be anything you want to be, and don't settle. There are so many options out there" (55-II) – options that she herself was denied.

Stories can, in a sense, ensure a person's immortality by providing a concrete means to transmit values, ideas, and beliefs from one generation to the next (Ryan et al., 2004). Amelie's stories were primarily about family, supplying the members of her family with details that sketched a cultural and historical context within which they could better appreciate the lives of their antecedents. For instance, her maternal grandmother, who had six children aged two to fourteen, caught a highly contagious illness from the drinking water and so her whole household had to be quarantined for forty days. She took to her bed. Despite feeling terribly thirsty, she was denied food and water in order to "starve" the fever, which was a common but cruel practice at the time. She died a horrible death. Continuing to live under quarantine, her husband still had to care for the children and meet their needs, which among other things meant cooking and baking, tasks with which men in those days were typically not familiar (15-I).

Such stories from within her own family demonstrate the hardships that people experienced, hardships that seldom exist in the same way today. For instance, people still make bread from scratch, but it is not usually their only choice. Stories like these, then, are a means of connecting the family together across generations and of offering insight into the great strength that people can display in dealing with adversity. As such, they come under the category of "redemptive structures" or "sequences" – stories that involve negative events that are followed by positive outcomes (Norris et al., 2004, p. 362); stories of how people started with nothing, for instance, yet worked hard to reach their goals, something that, overall, Amelie's story demonstrates as well. Amelie's goal in writing such stories, in other words, was not to evoke sympathy from her readers but to transmit knowledge, and in doing so, to inspire.

Given the value she places on building and sustaining relationships, especially among members of her family, it is worth noting here Amelie's concerns around changing technology. She lamented to me how her older grandchildren are forever texting, something she herself is not adept at doing, and are uncomfortable speaking on the phone. This is a "different world," she said to me, somewhat wistfully, and people are losing out from not having "face to face, hands-on relationships" (28-II). She went on: "I think that's a big loss because … some of the … best things in my … life have happened, and the worst, because of relationships" (28-II). Intergenerational narratives are precious to Amelie, but intergenerational *gaps*, relationship gaps – between herself and her own grandchildren – exist nonetheless, gaps she hopes to help fill by continuing to write stories for them.

Final Thoughts

My great-grandmother's quilt has always had a special significance for me. In a real way, revisiting my interviews with Amelie has given me an opportunity to reflect more deeply upon that significance. "Once a story is given by the speaker and taken up by a listener," claims gerontologist Kate de Medeiros (2013), "it becomes a part of the listener" (p. 152). The stories and memories that all of the participants shared with me – especially Amelie – have indeed become a part of my story, too.

I sometimes wonder whether my great-grandmother made the quilt for someone special. And did she name it? Was it meaningful to her at all? Senft (1995) claims that information about a quilter can be uncovered upon close examination of the quilt itself, for its materials, design, and stitching reveal something about the crafter behind it. While it is true that these technical aspects may give some insight into the quilter, I tend to agree with Rogerson (1998) that quilts' histories are largely unrecoverable once the quilters have died – if, that is, they did not share the stories associated with them. This is the case with my great-grandmother's quilt. I have often inquired about these details, but sadly many of them are unknown. These stories are lost. As a result, I will attach to the quilt the stories I have learned about her from others in my life. And I shall give it a name: Autumn Leaves. But what right, if any, do I have to do this? It may be in my possession, but is it mine to name? Whether it is or it isn't, I believe that in doing so I'm adding to her quilt a piece of myself in hopes that I, too, might someday be remembered.

7 Labyrinth Ring: Identifying Our Stories and Digging Deep

WILLIAM L. RANDALL

We are in the middle of our stories and cannot be sure how they will end; we are constantly having to revise the plot as new events are added to our lives ... We live immersed in narrative, recounting and reassessing the meanings of our past actions, anticipating the outcomes of future projects, situating ourselves at the intersection of several stories not yet completed.

– Donald Polkinghorne (1988, pp. 150, 160)

The Autobiographical Connection

A core assumption underlying narrative inquiry, as I noted in Chapter 1, is that, strive though we might to remain objective, we inevitably hear, read, and interpret the stories of our participants through the filter of our own. The beauty of a book like this, though also perhaps its besetting sin, is that analysis gets mixed with autobiography, however veiled the autobiographical component may be. At best, and as proponents of "autoethnography" claim (see Bochner & Ellis, 2016; Ellis & Berger, 2002), it enriches our analyses; at worst, it undermines them. Either way, maintaining scholarly detachment from many of the topics that we're writing about has proven impossible to do. The fact that we each chose particular participants, or at least the particular objects that they refer to, as the focus of the chapter that we've authored suggests that we have sensed certain parallels between that participant's life and our own, and that we are curious what those parallels can tell us about *us*. This chapter is no exception. The more I think about it, the more the parallels between myself and Hermann, as I call him, seem uncanny. Let me begin by coming clean concerning them.

For one thing, Hermann is an academic, and so am I. He keeps a journal on a more or less regular basis, and so do I. He uses his journal to reflect on his reflections, to engage in "meta-reflection" and, in that sense, "live through the day twice" (2-I), and I do much the same. He sees himself as a writer, in the sense that writing is, for him, a way of thinking, one that can take you to new places in your thoughts, can lead to "surprises" and "discoveries" that you wouldn't experience if your kept your thoughts inside your head. I couldn't agree more. As he says more than once during his interviews with Jenn, paraphrasing the author E.M. Forster, "How do I know what I think till I see what I write?" More than this, and as is the case with me as well, he sees writing as a route not just to self-expression but to self-creation. "Writing," he says, "is about self-development" (14-II). Like me, then, he considers himself a life-long learner, for whom learning is a mode of spirituality almost. He certainly interprets a major part of his life as "a journey of continuous learning" (16-II) – a journey that, conveniently, the academic life supports. My sentiments exactly!

On the theme of journey, and judging from the first big story that he shares with Jennifer – the story of "my change in terms of worldview" (6-I) from "an adamant Catholic to an atheist in terms of not believing in a personal God" (12-I) – his own journey has been a complicated one. Again, though, its trajectory has been akin to mine: from a conservative form of Christianity while growing up (Catholic for him, Protestant for me), one grounded in the feeling that "I'm always doing something wrong" (13-I), to, at this point, a more wide-open, more inclusive form of faith – where "faith" is broadly defined, along the lines of a James Fowler (1981), who views faith as "a universal human concern" (p. 5), or of a Deepak Chopra (2014), as "wonder before the mystery of existence" (p. 252). And while he studied theology and *almost* became a Catholic priest, I studied theology and *did* become a Protestant minister. Reminiscent of Robert Frost's famous poem about two roads diverging in the woods, I took the road he didn't take. For ten years, I lived the life – the possible life – he might have lived.

Still more parallels are his habit of reading widely (autobiography, biography, fiction) outside his home discipline, and his attraction in particular to the writings of the author Hermann Hesse. From my mid-twenties to early thirties, I read as many of Hesse's works as I could get my hands on – everything (ironically) except *The Journey to the East* (Hesse, 1961), which Hermann viewed as having a huge influence on his own thinking. Another parallel of sorts is that he is from Germany, and even though I am not, I have travelled in Germany (West and even East) on numerous occasions, including one fateful summer evening when I got lost wandering the back streets of Berlin trying to find my hotel. Plus, I have German ancestry that I've always been intrigued about, my mother's mother having been a Kaulbach from Nova Scotia's south shore, a region settled by German families in the 1700s. And given this German connection I, like Hermann, have been prone to speculation on what might have been, on the road not taken: how I would have behaved, or how my values would have been compromised, and what sort of person I might have become if, for instance, I had grown up under Hitler during the Nazi era or, following the war, in the totalitarian world of communist East Germany.

Where the two of us part company, however, is that I don't wear a ring. In fact, I don't even own a ring. Nor has the concept of a labyrinth ever really caught my attention, whereas for him it was the image on which he soon settled when participants were asked by Deborah to sketch a lifeline of their lives – that is, the highs, the lows, the turning points. Many chose a river as an image to do so (I know I did), others chose a mountain. Hermann chose a labyrinth since, in his words, it "gives me a different access to my life story" (4f-II). So, with these two combined – a labyrinth ring – as the thing that holds special significance for him, there is a slim chance that I can shed light on that significance with a tiny bit of objectivity.

Storying Style

I'll come back later to the labyrinth ring and the meaning it holds for Hermann. First, though, a few comments are in order concerning what we have been on the watch for with all of our participants, as I outlined in Chapter 2. For one, the storying style that Hermann defaults to in responding to Jennifer's questions seems comparatively thin in terms of the level of detail and description he provides about his life, or about the specific experiences he recounts. They are also fairly sparse in terms of "I said-she said" dialogue, in terms of interactions with others in general, in fact; and this despite the fact that he claims early on that he could "sit here and tell stories for ages" (17-I). In truth, he does not stand out – at least in the interviews – as a particularly avid raconteur. And, on the surface anyway, he comes across as somewhat low in terms of what McAdams (1988) has called "narrative complexity" (pp. 105–132). In addition, I found his way of speaking during the interviews rather challenging to follow, characterized as it was by numerous stops and starts and self-interruptions, due in part perhaps to his first language not being English.

This factor noted, though, there was still something that I found difficult to read about him, something inscrutable, as if there were much between the lines that he was holding back. Not deliberately necessarily, because he answered the questions that he was asked. And, in fairness, the focus of those questions – in all the interviews we conducted – was not on the story of his life per se. Rather, it was on the role of storytelling *in* his life, on the impact the workshops had on his experience of his own story, on the difference between writing about his life and just thinking about it, and on what it was like to read what he had written to others. Nonetheless, there were "shadow stories" (de Medeiros & Rubinstein, 2015) that he alluded to only fleetingly and that left me wondering *who is this person, really?* – stories about his first marriage, for example, or even his second wife, or the skiing resort business that he and his second wife had that didn't work out (17-I), not to mention stories about his father and the relationship between them. We know nothing at all about his father. As for his mother, he refers to her only in conjunction with a story that he says "I have journeyed with for many years" – the story that Jennifer and Denise mentioned in Chapter 4 about him seeing two angels in the backyard at the age of six. And even at that she is cast in a negative light by laughing at him and saying, "The way you behave I don't think angels would come to you" (13-I). In this regard, you could say that he was the opposite of other participants in the project, whose lives, as Jenn probed them, seemed more like the proverbial "open book."

That said, while the narrative complexity of what he shared in the interviews was comparatively low, there appeared at the same time – perhaps precisely *because* of what he left unsaid – to be a multilayered quality to him, and a sophisticated level of autobiographical reasoning that was reflected, for instance, in his propensity for engaging in "counterfactual" speculation (Ferguson, 1997), as I'll be discussing later on. And he possessed a high degree of narrative agency as well, insofar as he was well aware that he indeed *has* a story, a very interesting one in fact, one that he'd like to be able "to morph into … an interesting novel" (10-II). And he was aware, moreover, of how "there is lots of potential for changing your story while you still live, up to probably your last breath" (18-II). When asked if there was a life lesson he'd want to pass on to others, he responded first with "life is never as simple as it seems" and second with "there's always another way of looking at [things]" (12-II). Here's a more extensive excerpt, expressed in his somewhat circuitous storying style, that illustrates his awareness of how *re-storying* is always a possibility:

> When you live, starting to live your life you actually commit to something and, uh, when you do that and you reflect about it, … you have the opportunity to change the story. Not necessarily what happened in the past, you can change your interpretation though … when you look at a decision-making process in the present and you reflect on how is that integrated or connected to something that you've done in the past then you reinterpret to some extent what happened in the … you can reinterpret that … and you

> can change how it affects your decision-making now ... So you know, really, that appealing opportunity to add something to the story that wasn't there before. Not just another day or another year, but to add a perspective, to add an emphasis or to make the story different. (17-II)

Let me continue on this theme: although, at fifty-seven, Hermann was the youngest participant in this project, he was mindful, too, that while the "breadth of opportunities" we have as we get older tends to narrow, "in terms of depth, there's probably more opportunities" (18-II) – depth as regards self-understanding. And for him "changing from breadth to depth" (20-II) has become increasingly important. This distinction between breadth and depth parallels the one that Jerome Bruner (1986) drew between the "landscape of action" that any story may be said to possess – in this case, a life story – and the "landscape of consciousness" (p.14). Simply put, the landscape of action concerns what happens in the story, or in other words the events, the plot, and the setting in which everything unfolds. The landscape of consciousness, on the other hand, concerns what various parties to the story *make* of what happens: their respective perspectives on or interpretations of "the action" – from the author to the narrator to each of the characters, and to each of us as receivers of the story, as listeners, viewers, or readers – each of whose "narrative positioning" is bound to be unique. While the landscape of action to our life stories tends, for obvious reasons (decline in mobility, autonomy, energy, etc.), to shrink as we age, the landscape of consciousness – our awareness of and reflections on the events of our lives – knows no intrinsic limit to its potential for expansion. In this connection, Hermann is someone whom we might expect to score high in terms of narrative openness, for he seems intensely aware of the multiple stories that run through his life, each of which, as Donald Polkinghorne (1988) would put it, is "not yet completed" (p. 160). Before looking at what these intersecting stories are, let's consider briefly what is known about labyrinths.

Labyrinths and Rings

Labyrinths, and images of labyrinths, have a long and venerable heritage. They can be found in numerous cultures across the centuries, going back to at least ancient Greece and the palace of Knossos in Crete. In Hindu and Hopi cultures, images of labyrinths abound, as they do in Christianity, the labyrinth embedded in the floor of Chartres Cathedral, circa 1200 AD, as a classic case in point. Combining the image of a circle with that of a spiral, the way laid out in a labyrinth is a meandering yet ultimately purposeful path. Indeed, walking through a labyrinth has served within several traditions as a spiritual practice for centring, contemplation, and prayer. It serves as a symbol for the spiritual journey, for a pilgrimage towards … God, truth, enlightenment, or whatever one desires most deeply in one's life.

Often, the term "labyrinth" is used synonymously with "maze," as Hermann himself does (21-II). However, researchers tend to distinguish between them. A labyrinth is commonly "unicursal" in nature, meaning that it features basically only a single path, meandering though it be, towards a single centre. A maze, on the other hand, is "multi-cursal," presenting us with numerous pathways to choose from and directions to pursue – some of them intersecting, some dead ends, but with no centre as such. Here is what Hermann himself has to say about the labyrinth, when asked by Jennifer if there were any exercises during the workshops that he found especially meaningful:

> There is one in particular which comes to mind and that's the, you know, the exercise about the – what was it? – river analogy. Or the labyrinth? … I still have [it] here [retrieves image]. I like that chaotic kind of thing because it really has all the notes and everything in there [he had inserted years at various points in his labyrinth drawing]. So we were told to sketch your story line. That's what it was. Yeah, sketch your story line and some people did a river, some did a tree, and I did this and I haven't even completed it yet. So I come back to that and look at it and say, "OK, that's one thing I want to go back to and go through the various stages of life, sometimes life goes, you know, further out and sometimes it's more straight lines up and down that way." So that was important. (4-II)

Interestingly, the diagram he drew is a hybrid of a labyrinth and a maze, as if his understanding of what constitutes each has a certain fluidity to it. He then goes on to talk about his ring:

> I wear a ring that has the same symbol and that's probably why I came up with this representation … it's a ring made by [a] First Nation with a, the, labyrinth and the, you know, little human being standing outside of the beginning and not knowing, you know, where this goes and it's kind of the same thing … that's where I got the idea. Except that the ring is round and, uh, so you're kind of, the whole ring is a labyrinth so that's where it came from. So it's in the back of my mind but I haven't done anything with this particular exercise. It's *still work to be continued* … (5f-II, emphasis mine)

Two or three things stand out from this excerpt. One is that he hasn't completed drawing the labyrinth, not just because there wasn't enough time to do so during the workshop but because he's still living the life that he sees it as representing. Also, as I said, the drawing itself has elements of both a labyrinth and a maze. Further, as in a traditional Navajo labyrinth ring, his ring features a "little human being standing outside of the beginning and not knowing ... where this goes" – a figure he presumably relates to himself.

This leads me to the thought that, "in the middle of the journey of your life," as Dante has famously expressed it in the *Inferno*, we understandably don't have the same perspective on the "whole" of our life as we might start to have in, say, our sixties, seventies, and eighties – as we shift into what McAdams (1996) calls the "post-mythic" stage in the development of our narrative identity. In other words, we can't know whether what we're in the middle of is in fact a labyrinth, with its unicursal design and its single path towards the centre, or a maze, with numerous pathways and no centre as such. In this regard, the observation made by Donald Polkinghorne (1988) concerning the narrative complexity of our lives, which I cited at the start, bears repeating: "We live immersed in narrative ... situating ourselves at the intersection of several stories not yet completed" (p. 160). "We are in the middle of our stories and cannot be sure how they will end" (p. 150).

The labyrinth ring as a cherished object, which interestingly he admits he only wears "sometimes" (5-II), serves as a visual reminder of the complexity of the journey of one's life, and the central importance of searching for meaning, for self-understanding, lest one forget this and allow one's life to become one of those "simple stories" (8-II), as he calls them, that many people's lives can trace. I'll return to these considerations a little later, but for now, what are the main pathways of Hermann's life, the main journeys he sees himself on, the main stories he sees himself living in the middle of?

The Faith Story

First, there is what we could call the faith journey or the faith story – and he uses these two terms, "journey" and "story," somewhat interchangeably throughout. As he outlines it for Jennifer in response to her question in the first interview about a "turning point" in his life, this journey, he says, goes from his being "raised Catholic" (6-I), to being "an altar boy for many years" (6-I), to "considering becoming a priest" (6-I), and to the point where he "started studying theology" (6-I). However, because he was "already married" (7-I) at the time and because "in the Catholic church that was a no-no" (7-I), he obviously couldn't become a priest. Though "it [faith] was always a strong part of my life" (7-I), he says that "at some point it started changing with my first marriage breaking down … and afterwards remarrying" (7-I), so "as a member of the Catholic church, you're really out" (7-I). With his second wife, a Lutheran, he thus began attending Lutheran churches, and found Lutheran theology more intellectually appealing and Lutheran congregations more "open and welcoming" (8-I).

When the two of them immigrated to a remote village in the interior of British Columbia, there was a church within walking distance of their house that was Presbyterian in name, and therefore comparatively conservative as far as mainline Protestant denominations are concerned. However, since it was one of only few churches in the region, it was attended by people of many different faith backgrounds. He describes it as "almost like the ideal of a Christian community" and they felt "really … at home there" (8-I). When the two of them moved to New Brunswick, they began attending a United Church of Canada in the area where they were living, the United Church being, as he put it, "one of the very liberal churches in Canada" (9-I). However, that particular congregation proved to be "extremely conservative" (9-I). As Jennifer and Denise noted in Chapter 4, when the pastor, who herself was "very open, very liberal," married a gay couple, "the rest of the congregation was more or less against that" in a "subversive" way. As a result, he says, he and his wife "sort of withdrew."

As Hermann himself admits, "this is getting [to be] a long story" but "it kind of shows a couple of stages that I went through." "The next big stage" (10-I), he explains, was when he began travelling each year to the Indian subcontinent as part of an internship program that he helped to coordinate between the university where he was teaching in New Brunswick and a college in Eastern Bhutan – a journey east par excellence. In the course of these annual visits, he was "exposed to the practices of Buddhism" (10-I) – in other words, to prayer wheels, flags, and other rituals that, in a sense, parallel what he grew up with as a Catholic, and most of all, to an "automatic kind of almost mystical understanding of if I do this, then this will happen" (15-I). "[W]hat it did for me," he said, "and I still haven't totally figured out how and why that came along," is that "it made me much more aware of … there are so many different beliefs in the world" (10-I). As he explains in one of the two stories that he wrote between the first interview and the second, entitled *Journey to the East,* this awareness of the many different beliefs in the world had been seeded in him much earlier in his life, during his teens, when he moved with his parents (we never learn quite why) from Germany to Jakarta. Besides attending Catholic church "on an almost regular basis," he also, as he writes in his story, "visited mosques, temples, and religious sites of many colours and cultures."

As for how these experiences affected him, he says that "in my mind all of a sudden it made me wonder much more about the importance of a belief system for me" (11-I). More than this, though, "I started all of a sudden much more seriously questioning the existence of a personal God" (11-I). In essence, "I started to differentiate … between what I thought was the substance [of a given belief system] and the kind of external accessories." The phrase "all of a sudden" could suggest that he underwent a conversion of sorts, to "seeing the light," concerning how "the ritual and the dogmatic content you have to believe" is "not the real faith" (11-I) – which he senses is bound up with "the message of love and of being loved" (11-I).

Here, in a more "unplugged" manner, is how he sums up what has obviously been a formative experience in his life, one which he hopes someday "to morph … into an interesting novel" (10-II).

> The long story short is [that] I saw myself going from an adamant Catholic … to an atheist. An atheist in the sense of not believing in a personal God. Believing in some of the kernel of the message, but not the personal God. And experiencing that transition was really something because it took some time and I'm still not sure I'm totally over it, to even be able to say I am an atheist … But I'm thinking, you know, if you think things through from my perspective, what really is at the essence of the messages that were important to me is something that is not necessarily connected to a personal God, let alone to a certain picture of a personal God or a certain story around a personal God. So, you know, that's where I am at in my life story right now, is trying to cope with and trying to understand what that does to my lifestyle, to my living, and what it tells me about my own past and history, and so part of what I'm trying to work through in terms of my autobiographical approach is how can I put that into a story? (11f-I)

A few minutes later in the interview, as he is about to recount the story of his immigration to Canada, he stresses that with "the faith story … there is more of a beginning [but] definitely not an ending because, you know, I'm not at the end yet" (17-I). In support of this assessment, he makes an interesting distinction during the second interview when answering a question about a time that he came to a "crossroads" and had to choose which way to go. He is telling Jennifer about an academic position that he might have taken at another university, one that adheres to a conservative version of Christianity and would probably have required him to sign a statement about his beliefs before issuing him a contract, and this at a time when he was still "a believer in terms of a personal God" (25-II). With his tendency towards speculation on the road not taken, he wonders "how would have that story gone on, in terms of would I have gone through the same thinking process that I did" – that is, from believing to not believing in a personal God (25-II). What would have happened "had I gone through the same process and lost my faith," he wonders aloud, immediately interjecting that "I don't like that term because it always implies … that the one who loses faith is at [a] disadvantage." In his words, "I don't think so; I think it's a journey thing. It's a different kind of perspective … but it's ['lost my faith'] a very common kind of label." He then offers an alternative label for his experience: "When I *changed* my faith" (25-II), he says (emphasis mine).

So, this central storyline in Hermann's life does not appear to be finished. His "faith," which is the term that he employs, has clearly changed from his days as an "adamant Catholic." And it continues to change in terms of content and structure – in keeping with theories about "stages of faith" proposed, for instance, by researchers such as James Fowler (1981) – but it has not stopped. "Freedom from religion and the opportunity to freely engage in the worldview of my choice" – which is language he uses in his story *Journey to the East* – may be what he feels he enjoys at present. But he is not free from faith. In a real sense, he is still searching for the essence, for the centre, for "the real faith."

The Immigration Story

Next is what Hermann would call the immigrant story. After tracing the story of his journey of faith, and after telling Jennifer that he "could sit here and tell stories for ages" (17-I), he volunteers what he bills as "another really transforming kind of a story," namely "my, our, immigration to Canada" (17-I). Compared with the faith story, which "definitely [has] not an ending," this second story is "more of a complete changed story" (17-I), in part because it is linked to actual geographical locations – Germany, Canada, British Columbia, New Brunswick. Yet it, too, he says "still keeps on going" (17-I), in the sense that New Brunswick doesn't feel like his final destination. Rather, he continues to be pulled back to BC, and the mountains. In the meantime, he'll to "hav[e] to be content with" the "three-to-four-hundred-metre hills" of New Brunswick and "call them mountains" (18-I).

As he says to Jennifer, with a certain wistfulness in his words, "that valley in BC was kind of where I had that feeling of I always belonged here, even if I never was there before" (17-I). A certain portion of that feeling is linked to what he calls the "immigrant's dream … in terms of not seeing neighbours, being just in nature" (18-I). Part of it, too, is linked to the mountains, which obviously New Brunswick does not have. Indeed, the move to New Brunswick, he admits, "was much more of a practical perspective because [in BC] you're in the middle of nowhere." Plus, with only part-time teaching and consulting work available, plus a business venture that didn't pan out, "we just didn't have enough income there" (17-I). So, when a full-time faculty position opened up in New Brunswick, they made the decision to make the journey east.

While a tenured position, a steady pay cheque, and proximity to the ocean are positive features of life in New Brunswick – and indeed he and his wife have purchased a second property in the province to be even closer to the sea – there is still something missing that life in New Brunswick can't provide, something that if he could afford to he would return to BC to experience again (18-I). It is the feeling he reports experiencing as he flew into Vancouver (18-I) and saw the mountains for the first time, the feeling that he and his wife would get "driving up and down that valley [in BC] all the time" (18-I). It is the feeling of "I always belonged there," the feeling of "having arrived" (17-I), the feeling "that this is just it, this is it. This feels right" (18-I). So, if the first big story of his life is centred on faith, then this one, we could say, is focussed on the feeling of "rightness" – or the feeling of home. And "the story for me," he says, "has not ended yet" (17-I).

The German Story

Third, there is the German story, which Hermann refers to as "the other big story framework" in his life (19-I). In fact, he takes pains to stress to Jennifer that "it's not a story but it's a framework" (19-I). If you will, it could be considered a meta-narrative or master narrative, insofar as his faith story, his immigrant story, and even his learning story are each in a sense rooted within it, or rather it is the overarching context within which these other stories unfold and are entwined. But as a "framework" for these other, more individual story strands, it is concerned less with the facts than with "counterfactuals." As the historian Niall Ferguson (1997) writes:

> We constantly ask ... "counterfactual" questions in our daily lives. What if I had observed the speed limit, or refused that last drink? What if I had never met my wife or husband? ... It seems we cannot resist imagining the alternative scenarios: what might have happened, if only we had or had not ... Nor are such thoughts mere day-dreams. Of course we know perfectly well that we cannot travel back in time and do these things differently. But the business of imagining such counterfactuals is *a vital part of the way in which we learn.* Because decisions about the future are – usually – based on weighing

> up the potential consequences of alternative courses of action, it makes sense to compare the actual outcomes of what we did in the past with the conceivable outcomes of what we might have done. (p. 2, emphasis mine)

Researching the history of the Third Reich as a doctoral student back in Germany, he found himself delving into the issue of how and why people at the time – people of his parents' generation, for instance – either collaborated with Nazism, appeased it, or actively resisted it (see Marks, 2011). As he puts it, "I always find it very interesting to play with the thought of going back in time and placing part of my life in that context and just to see what happened if I was going to do whatever I did" (20-I). He wonders, for example, "how would that have played out" if he had studied theology in the days of Hitler. "Would I have continued with that? Would I have found a way to adapt to that? Would I have been part of a resistance movement? I'm not sure ..." (20-I). He continues: "and then the same thing, transporting part of my life into Eastern German[y] before the wall came down, [in a] similar kind of totalitarian context, how would I have made out?" (20-I).

Harking back to his distinction between framework and story, he concludes that "it's not a story because I wasn't living there" (20-I). To the extent that it is a story, though, it is a virtual one, or rather a web of possible narratives – of "multiple fluid narratives" as the anthropologist Mary Catherine Bateson (2007, p. 213) would say, possible narratives peopled with the "possible selves" (Markus & Nurius, 1986) whom he might have been, and the "unlived lives" (Alheit, 1995, p. 65) he might have lived. The psychological power for him of this framework-story is evident, though, in the vigour with which he responds to one of the last questions Jennifer asks him during the second interview: "If you could reinvent yourself, what stories would you tell?" (28-II).

His response begins like this: "to reinvent myself ... I don't know whether I would call it reinvent but ... part of what I was talking about earlier, playing with putting myself into a different kind of context like National Socialism, there's always been that question to me, how would I have behaved if I would have been in that particular situation" (28-II). He notes, however, that this question is not one he wrestles with in quite the same immediate way his fellow countrymen would have had to some seventy years ago, in the midst of a war. "No wars here," he says, referring to life in Canada, "no existential kind of threats" (29-II). Yet the energy impelling him here could suggest otherwise, for he then goes on to list nearly two pages of sub-questions that this possibility, and others like it, raise for him. These include "how would I react if I got the verdict that I have cancer ... or have ... just half a year to live?" (29-II) and "what if I would have been the son of a millionaire?" (29-II). It's his comments on what this kind of speculation "tell[s] me about my own thinking process" that I feel are especially revealing, though, and they point us towards the fourth big story that is central to his sense of self: the story of his life as a learner, which I'll turn to in a moment.

He takes pains to stress to Jennifer that the millionaire storyline, for example, is not a matter of "wishful thinking" for him (29-II), or of "putting myself into a context that's making up for what I didn't have," or of "reinventing in terms of I would like to be another person" (28-II). Rather, "it's more [a matter of] reinventing in terms of I'd like to try to, to try out what different perspectives that probably I don't or won't have the chance to, or not now, and I want to know it now so I'm going to put myself into the position ... and then play with that" (29-II). It's a matter of "reinventing myself ... in terms of learning and, and journeying" (29-II). And it's a matter of wrestling with an essential existential question, namely "what type of person am I, at heart?"

The Learning Story

The fourth and, by his own admission, most fundamental storyline in Hermann's life is what we could call the learning story. In the second interview, he tells Jennifer that he "interpret[s] a major part of my life as a journey of discovery, a journey of continuous learning" (16-II). This, he notes, is "one of the big upsides of being in academe, of being a teacher," because "you're continually expanding your learning journey" (16-II). When she asks what themes are part of his story, he takes a few more seconds to think and then responds with two strong phrases: "the journeying for sure. The learning for sure" (18-II). He follows this up immediately, however, by clarifying that "I like learning better than discoveries" (18-II). As he puts it: "[I'm] not necessarily a discoverer. I'm a learner" (18-II). Pressed by Jennifer to explain what he means by this distinction, he says, "It's more about the process than the product. Discovering is about a product. You've discovered something. It's not that it's not important. And, you know, by learning I discovered a lot. But to me, *it's more about the ongoing process* as opposed to the claim of discovery" (20-II, emphasis mine).

Hermann's distinction between discovering and learning corresponds broadly, I suggest, to his distinction between "breadth of opportunity," which he notes tends to decrease as we age, and "depth of opportunity," which he hints has no inherent limit. This in turn, it may be argued, parallels Bruner's (1986) distinction between the landscape of action to our life stories, which begins naturally to narrow in with age, and the landscape of consciousness, which in theory can widen out indefinitely. Although he is the youngest participant in our study, as someone nearing the end of his sixth decade, he is shifting, we might say, from "the morning of life," to quote Carl Jung (1976), to "the afternoon of life" (p. 17), a shift that brings to mind the observation made by the philosopher Arthur Schopenhauer (2004): "The first forty years of life furnish the text, while the remaining thirty supply the commentary; ... without the commentary we are unable to understand aright the true sense and coherence of the text, together with the moral it contains and all the subtle application of which it admits" (p. 94).

Schopenhauer's use of the terms "text" and "commentary" is in keeping with the metaphor of "reading our lives" that Beth McKim and I have made central to our reflections on "the poetics of growing old" (Randall & McKim, 2008). To me, Hermann is someone very much committed to reading not just academic texts or literary texts but "the commentary" dimension to the text that *is* his life, with its multiple, intersecting story-strands, whether actual or counterfactual in nature. As far as the counterfactual kind is concerned, his intuition mirrors that of Peter Alheit (1995), a professor of adult education at the University of Bremen who uses the term "biographicity." Alheit argues that "the main issue" in what he calls "biographical learning" is "to deepen the 'surplus meanings' of our biographical knowledge," which "in turn means to perceive the potentiality of our unlived lives" (p. 65). And for Hermann, whether it be in his "double entry journal" (3-II), in the workshops themselves, or in the various projects they've inspired him to undertake so that he can "dig deeper" (21-I) into himself, writing is how he goes about doing so (14-II), how he *reads* the complex, internalized text of his own life, his "texistence," as Beth and I have dubbed it (Randall & McKim, 2008, p. 95–113). As a means of helping him, in his words, to "see things you haven't seen before" (6-II), it is a prime medium for what Pierre Dominicé (2000) calls simply "learning from our lives." The act of writing, more than mere thinking, in other words, opens up pathways of which he otherwise might not be mindful – a theme that the chapters in Part 3 will be exploring further. It pins your thoughts down, gets them outside of your head and onto the page so that you can *see* them, work with them, develop them further. For such reasons, and as expressed by children's author Juanita Havill (cited in Wahlstrom, 2006), "writing is an act of discovery" (p. 70). Notwithstanding Hermann's ambivalence about that particular word, writing involves "discovering what haunts you, what you need to return to in your life, what you want to say" (p. 70). For him, writing is thus a holy act almost, surrounded by the sense of ceremony it deserves. Witness his need to "still write with my pen in hand" (3-I), with "a special kind of a book" and "a special kind of pen" (4-I).

Reading and writing, writing and learning, learning and developing – for Hermann, these activities are tightly intertwined, as are the four central stories that I've tried to outline here – not at all, though, in a static manner, but as an "ongoing process" (20-II). Such an open-ended perspective on his life overall is reflected in these enticing words from narrative psychologist Mark Freeman (1993): "Our lives," he proposes in his book *Rewriting The Self*, "[are] like richly ambiguous texts to be interpreted and understood ... whose meanings are inexhaustible, whose mysterious existence ceaselessly calls for the desire to know, whose readings cannot ever yield a final closure" (p. 184).

Concluding Reflections

During the second interview that Jennifer did with him, Hermann refers several times to the ways that the workshops have reinforced for him how much writing about his life enables him to make sense of things that resist sorting out when he's only thinking about them inside of his head. Accordingly, writing requires more discipline, more commitment, and more risk, since what is at stake for him in it is nothing less than "self-development" (14-II) – development, I would suggest, of both the social-cognitive and social-emotional types that were mentioned in Chapter 2. For Hermann's, I would further suggest, is pre-eminently a narrative of growth, not security (Bauer & Park, 2010, pp. 66–71). If anything, particularly through the counterfactual speculation that they've led him to re-engage in, these workshops have stirred up once more for him certain core existential questions, most centrally "Who am I?" and "What kind of person am I, really?" In that respect, they have been not just invigorating but, we could say, unsettling as well, in terms of fuelling his drive to "dig deeper" (21-I).

Asked what life lessons he would want to pass on, he answers that "life is never as simple as it looks," and "we often have to look much deeper to get a sense of what's really going on" (12-II). As for his own life in particular – and writing about it makes him that much more aware of this – it is by no means a "simple story" (12-II), not the kind that, he says, he is "often disappointed by" (27-II). Instead, what he favours are "the stories that lead you through those subtleties that you don't see at first sight and that make you think about, okay yeah, that's another way of looking at it" (12-II) – in short, the sort of stories that invite you to dig deeper. His own life story, with its multiple, intersecting plotlines – the faith story, immigrant story, German story, and learning story, none of which is either simple or complete – is just that sort. This, the workshops have helped him to see and, in a sense, to celebrate. To quote Freeman (1993) again, it is "a richly ambiguous text … whose readings" – and writings! – "cannot ever yield a final closure" (p. 184). It is a text, in other words, that abounds in "depth of opportunity," whose landscape of consciousness possesses no intrinsic limit, and towards which it is most fitting to take an attitude of not-knowing in an "open-ended" (28-II), even wondering, way.

In many cultures and traditions, the labyrinth is a symbol for the spiritual journey, which is inevitably and primarily an inner journey, perhaps the most difficult of any we might make. In the words of former UN secretary-general Dag Hammarskjöld (1964), "the longest journey is the journey inward" (p. 48). And "does the journey ever end?" Hermann asks, rhetorically (27-II). "Yes, it kind of does," he answers, "but the ending of one journey is the beginning [of] a new" (27-II). Concerning the labyrinth as a metaphor for the journey of his own life, then, he is still in the middle of that journey, and to echo Polkinghorne (1988), "cannot be sure" how it will end (p. 150). Nor, to be honest, can he know for sure whether it is a labyrinth through which he is journeying or a maze instead, with multiple pathways and multiple centres. Indeed, he seems unclear on this question. While his instinct is to believe that there is unity amid the multiplicity, he admits that the diagram he began working on during the lifeline exercise is "still work to be continued" (5f-II). It's as if he is simultaneously *inside* the labyrinth-maze of his life yet *outside* it too, like the little figure featured on his ring. Writing about our lives permits, even promotes, this dual sort of stance towards our lives. It enables us, at once, to enter more deeply into the complexity (not simplicity) of our self and our story yet to hover outside it as well, looking in, keeping open to the multiple perspectives always possible towards it. Hermann's ring reminds him of this paradoxical but beguiling quality of his own mysterious existence.

A few final words of a more personal nature … I admitted at the outset that I see a lot of myself in what Hermann says about himself. His stories and my stories are not so far apart. And there is certainly much more in these interviews that I could have dug into in the course of exploring the parallels between us. A case in point would be his story of seeing the two angels at the age of six, and its enduring power for him as a "signature story" (Kenyon & Randall, 1997, pp. 46–49), a story that he reports having "journeyed with for many years" (13-I). What has that journey entailed for him, I'd be curious to know, in terms of his experience of "belief"? I admitted too, though, that I did not always find him easy to follow; partly because of the meandering nature of the interview process itself, partly because his first language is not English. But, for certain, it was also because of the layered and, dare I say, labyrinthine quality of his narrative world, fraught as it was, for me at least, with all manner of back stories and shadow stories tucked between the lines.

As with all of the participants whom we're highlighting in this book, and as with all people period, there is more, always more, than meets the eye, and more to the objects that hold special significance for them too. Writing about the difference between characters in novels and people in "real life," famed biographer André Maurois (1986) observes that "living human beings are dangerous enigmas" (p. 4). "As we stand before our friends or our enemies," he explains, "it is as though we stood watching a drama of infinite complexity of which we know not, of which we shall never know, the end" (p. 4). While I might dispute the word "dangerous" in Maurois's remark, the "enigmatic" element – the puzzling or (forgive me!) a-maze-ing element – is one that I could hardly agree with more. Certainly, this brief foray into the world of Hermann's story, tentative as that foray is, has triggered questions concerning my own life that I expect I'll be pondering for quite some time. Or, to use a metaphor more in keeping with the thrust of this chapter, it has opened fresh pathways of self-understanding that I'm excited to explore.

8 Torn Page from a Textbook: The Story of the Violinist That Wasn't

ERIN WHITMORE

No one lives all the life of which he [*sic*] was capable. The unlived life in each of us must be the future of humanity.

– Florida Scott-Maxwell (1968, p. 139)

Trilobite Cookies

One summer afternoon a few years ago, I was sitting in the public archives of the New Brunswick Museum in Saint John, New Brunswick. While working on a project about women in late nineteenth-century Atlantic Canada, I had stumbled across the papers of the Ladies' Auxiliary of the Saint John Natural History Society. My interest in how women were involved in what we now refer to as social justice movements had led me to these papers by a somewhat circuitous path. In keeping with the gender norms of the time, the meeting minutes of the Ladies' Auxiliary were focussed not so much on natural history per se but on their activities in organizing events for the "real" (male) Natural History Society. As a feminist scholar interested in accounts of women's everyday lives, I knew such records often contained much more nuanced engagements with the world outside of the everyday than might initially appear (Fuller, 2004; Smith, 1987; Ulrich, 2001). And, indeed, it was often through the many "things" that appeared in such records that it became possible to connect with these more subversive narratives.

As I read through the meticulously detailed plans about where social events would be hosted, who would prepare what dish, what could be sold to raise money for the Society, and so forth, I stumbled upon a reference to the "trilobite cookies" that apparently the Auxiliary's president, Katherine Matthew, regularly prepared for meetings of the Society. Baked by the wife of George Matthew – a prominent New Brunswick geologist – Katherine's cookies seemed to me the quintessential "thing" to represent the complex position that white, affluent women held in late nineteenth-century Atlantic Canada as part of, yet separate from, the major economic, social, and political changes that were going on around them (Morton & Guildford, 1994). In this case, she was surrounded by an intellectual world of scientific exploration. Yet as a woman living in 1890s Saint John, New Brunswick, she could engage with that world only in limited and specific ways – in this instance, by baking cookies (Whitmore, 2005a, 2005b).

I have often wondered what Katherine Matthew might have been thinking as she prepared these trilobite cookies. Was this her way of protesting the domestic constraints of her life? What did she know about trilobite fossils herself? Had she lived in a different era would it be she who was the famous geologist and her husband the one baking cookies? Or perhaps there was no subterfuge about it at all, and she took immense pride in the cookies she shared with the Natural History Society members. Whatever the answer, the trilobite cookie, it seems to me, was a thing that harboured within it innumerable other "possible selves" (Markus & Nurius, 1986) that she may have been relating to or imagining for herself, were it not for the gendered constraints of her time.

I would love to have spoken to Katherine Matthew and asked her these sorts of questions myself. But her story – and particularly the trilobite cookie itself – sparked in me an interest about the ways (and things through which) women's lives envision and engage with all manner of possibilities, however circumscribed those possibilities may be by the norms and conditions of the day. The record of Katherine's life – limited as it is to the bits one can cobble together by reading the minutes of the Ladies' Auxiliary – allows us only to speculate on her own hoped-for, and lost, possible selves. However, the spoken and written accounts generated by Harriet, a seventy-eight-year-old participant in our project, provides us not only a much more detailed picture of her life but also a more extended contemplation of this theme of possibility, and of the possible *selves* that she has carried with her throughout her life. Specifically, her account of what she labels "the story of the violinist that wasn't" (13-I) – a story for which the thing I focus on in this chapter serves as both a key plot point and a provocateur for a broader telling of the social conditions that shape Harriet's life – presents an opportunity to take up what Katherine's story can only hint at. It permits us to delve more deeply into the role of things as entry points into the theme not just of possibility, but also of ambition, achievement, and resistance as vital if largely overlooked parts of women's stories in general (Heilbrun, 1988), and those of women in later life in particular (Ray, 2000).

Lost Possible Selves and Feminist Reminiscence

I begin with this story of Katherine Matthew's cookies as a way into Harriet's story with its evocation as well of a specific thing – a page torn from an Italian-language textbook – for two key reasons. First, it illustrates the potential for things in the narratives that women author to serve as windows onto the complexity of their lives and the layered ways in which those lives are storied (Carney, 2018; Hannan et al., 2019). As feminist historians of material culture have argued, "objects tell stories" (Ulrich, 2001, p. 6). Moreover, these stories are often ones that have been largely left out of dominant historical and sociological records. For instance, historian Laurel Thatcher Ulrich (2001) studied nineteenth-century New England through the lens of such everyday objects in women's lives as spinning wheels, tablecloths, baskets, and (harking back to Jennifer's chapter) quilts. In so doing, she revealed women's largely hidden yet transformative role in shaping the economy of the time. As she and other feminist scholars have argued (Fuller, 2004; Smith, 1987), the everyday things in women's homes that they mention in their diaries, write about in their letters, note in the minutes they take, or – as is the case here – refer to in their reminiscences appear on the surface to be markers of a woman's adherence to conventional gender norms and roles. At the same time, they are routes into a more subtle "counter-story" (Nelson, 2001) about how women have wrestled with and resisted the limits that such norms and roles have placed upon them.

Second, I've begun with this story because of the way that Katherine's trilobite cookie – like the textbook page in Harriet's story – demonstrates how things referred to in women's accounts of their lives also provide portals onto, and at times monuments to, the "possible selves" (Markus & Nurius, 1986) that they have imagined for themselves but that, for a variety of reasons, remain hidden and suppressed. For those unable to realize the hopes contained within these now "lost possible selves" (King & Mitchell, 2015), storing, sharing, writing, and talking about things that signify such possibilities become the only – if often severely limited – ways of honouring the hopes they once held for their lives, and may continue to hold. While it is not always possible for women to draw attention to stories about resistance, ambition, and achievement, precisely because of the gendered norms that silence them, introducing a thing that signifies these stories into a conversation, a diary entry, or a reminiscence becomes a subtle way to invite an exploration of those norms without explicitly doing so. For older women, who for various reasons may not be comfortable with overtly voicing what feminist theorist Sarah Ahmed (2017) calls their "feminist story" (p. 19), the inclusion of such things can signal to practitioners of narrative care that a feminist "shadow story" (de Medeiros & Rubinstein, 2015) is lurking underneath and yearns to be told.

In what follows, I suggest that these two functions of things in women's later life narratives, as signifiers of (1) the complexity of their lives in relation to the social conditions in which they have lived and (2) the possible selves that they have imagined for themselves, are at the heart of a process, and a framework, that I describe as *feminist reminiscence.* We see this mode of reminiscence modelled in Harriet's review of her life, particularly in its centring of the thing that she mentions in the first interview with Jennifer and then in the story she writes between the first and second interviews, and that she in fact shows to Jennifer in its physical form, namely a page torn out of an Italian-language textbook. Feminist reminiscence, I propose, is an approach to autobiographical reasoning in later life that sees the author explicitly grapple with the ways in which her life story – and, in Harriet's case specifically, the lost possibilities *within* that story – has been shaped by the broader systems and structures within which she has lived.

In the example afforded us through Harriet's narrative reflections upon her life, we see that reminiscing about the lost possible self that she has memorialized in the textbook page dynamically transforms the act of reminiscence itself. It shifts it from a process content with individual meaning-making to one focussed on politicizing, and rendering visible, the systemic ways in which her hopes and dreams were denied her, and on her efforts to resist and reshape these systems. Through feminist reminiscence, I will suggest, Harriet produces a powerful counter-story to prevailing understandings of later life for women as a period of disengagement and decline (Calasanti et al., 2006; Phoenix & Smith, 2011). Instead, she shows it to be a time of personal transformation, of activism and influence, in which, rather than acquiescing to the conditions that work to discount them, women demand that these conditions be acknowledged and accounted for (Hooyman et al., 2002; Ray, 2000, 2004; Woodward, 2003). Finally, in addition to being a framework through which she tells her own feminist story, feminist reminiscence, as Harriet engages in it, is a process that can be utilized and mobilized by others.

Some Theoretical Considerations

Although the page does not appear as a thing in Harriet's life until midlife, its effect upon her has been present since age eight. In her early forties, she is enrolled in an Italian language class while obtaining her degree at university and finds herself using the very same textbook that she remembers her brother using as a schoolboy, back in post-war 1940s England. More than this, she comes across the precise passage that, decades earlier, had been the catalyst for what she labels "the story of the violinist that wasn't" (13-I). The English translation reads: "God protect you from a bad neighbour and from a student who is learning to play the violin." As she explains to Jennifer, the sentence printed in the textbook – which is accompanied by a picture of a young girl playing the violin and a boy with his hands over his ears – is the exact same sentence that she recalls her young brother reading aloud to her mother. As a result, the woman forbade Harriet from playing the violin again, thereby effectively ending her cherished dream – her hoped-for self – of becoming a concert violinist. At the time, both Harriet and, apparently, her mother believed that her brother's complaint was serious and not, as Harriet suddenly realizes looking at the textbook, a schoolboy prank in which he was merely repeating a line from his studies in an attempt to impress their mother.

Deciding to photocopy the page in question, Harriet transforms the ephemeral phrase spoken by him so many years before into a tangible thing, thereby underscoring the significance of this moment in the story of the violinist that wasn't, and in the story of her life as a whole. More than that, when she refers to the page in the interview, and then writes about it between the first interview and the second, its significance is underscored still more. She reveals it to be a thing important enough to have held on to for over forty years, and to offer as the centrepiece around which, from her vantage point at seventy-eight, she begins to construct a new and more politicized version of the story of the violinist that wasn't.

Seeing the stories that older women tell about significant objects in their lives as gateways into a larger exploration of their (lost) possible selves, as well as opportunities for feminist reminiscence, holds particular relevance for researchers operating on the border where gerontology intersects with social work, narrative theory, anti-oppressive feminist theory, and material culture. Dovetailing with the work of feminist historians of material culture (e.g., Auslander, 2005; Ulrich, 2001) is a small but growing body of research that examines the significance and function of "things" in the lives and stories of older women (Hannan et al., 2019; Krasner, 2005; Lively, 2013; Thompson & Chatterjee, 2014). Such research suggests that things function like markers of the complex tensions that women negotiate between adherence to and resistance against dominant stories concerning gender and ageing alike. For example, in their examination of the role of significant objects in the biographical narratives of older women in Ireland, Hannan et al. (2019) found that "objects offer a useful, tangible means of articulating and communicating the complexity of women's longevity" (p. 51). In particular, they "shed an important light on the intensely complex and personal struggle that it is to be a woman, trying to make one's way in the world, particularly after many decades of life where one's personal history mirrors the historical and social changes one has lived through" (p. 54). It is the potential of things to support older women in "express[ing] a range of identities," and "mak[ing] connections between their experiences and larger social and cultural currents" (p. 63), so Hannen et al. argue, that signals their relevance as focal points for feminist analyses of women's experiences in later life.

Although gerontologists interested in the function of things in the stories told by older people have yet to zero in specifically on their function in supporting stories about possible selves, research on this concept has firmly demonstrated its relevance to studies of ageing (i.e., Hoppmann, Gerstorf, et al., 2007; Hoppmann & Smith, 2007; Smith & Freund, 2002). First introduced by Markus and Nurius (1986), the theory of possible selves, as I hinted earlier, contends that the images that individuals hold about themselves in the future are a vital and exciting part of their whole self-system or self-concept. Our "repertoire of possible selves" include those we fear becoming, those we hope to become, and those we expect we will become (p. 954). As cognitive manifestations of our aspirations and hopes, possible selves provide insight into the little-studied area of what Markus (2006) calls "the space of what might be" as a critical dimension of human development (p. xi). At the same time, despite being oriented towards the future, possible selves also provide important information that can help us understand "why we do what we do" (p. xi) in the past and present.

The implications of all this for working with ageing populations in particular, as I say, have been receiving increased consideration. For example, in their study of the possible selves of adults aged seventy to one hundred-plus years, Smith and Freund (2002) found that not only were such selves a "dynamic part of the self-concept in very old age" (P499) but they were also "highly personalized and varied" (P498). In contrast to dominant ideas of old age as a period of "disengagement from future planning" (P498), their study demonstrated, in other words, that people in later life continue to generate and imagine versions of possible selves, something that holds the potential to affect their health behaviours, their level of motivation, and their well-being overall (Hooker & Kaus, 1992; Hoppmann, Gerstorf, et al., 2007). As such, possible selves research is contributing to the broader goal of both critical gerontology and narrative gerontology, which is to problematize the limiting "narrative of decline" (Gullette, 2004) that is usually linked with later life and instead to profile more positive sides of ageing. Harriet herself seems to confirm this contribution when she reflects on the value of the workshops in helping her to shift her future-oriented thinking:

> We especially at this age, we think ... rather negatively of the future. What is the future going to hold? ... It's, it's, a large fear and I find that fear is very crippling ... This [participating in the writing workshop] gives you – now I have to think of the word for it – it, makes you realize somehow that your life did have worth, and that it still has worth ... by the nature of ... what the stories substantiated in you. (18-II)

Given my focus here on the story of the violinist that wasn't, particularly pertinent is a smaller body of possible selves research that examines what have been called "lost possible selves" (King & Hicks, 2007; King & Mitchell, 2015; King & Raspin, 2004). Lost possible selves are "representations of the self in the future, which may have once held the promise of positive affect, but which are no longer a part of a person's life" (King & Mitchell, 2015, p. 319). Nonetheless, they can continue to have an impact on one's sense of identity and subjective well-being. Evidence provided by King and Mitchell (2015), however, suggests that intentional narrative engagement with lost possible selves can be a means of freeing oneself from potentially crippling regret and instead fostering greater personal maturity, and of generating new, more helpful stories that enhance one's sense of meaning in life. Such evidence connects well, of course, with research outlined in Chapter 1 concerning the role of integrative reminiscence in fostering "narrative resilience" (see Randall et al., 2015). Indeed, "acknowledging the value of the multitude of selves left behind along the way," write King and Hicks (2007) – anticipating what, I believe, is Harriet's experience as well – "may serve as a means to develop a complex understanding of the self and the world" (p. 634). More to the point perhaps, "recognition of the losses that have led to one's current place in the life story may open one up to a number of valuable and rich experiences, including a paradoxical sense of gratitude for loss itself" (p. 634).

Building on the early work of Robert Butler (1963), researchers have greatly deepened our understanding of reminiscence in general by identifying the various functions of reminiscence (Webster, 2002), plus the various types (Wong & Watt, 1991), which Bill noted briefly back in Chapter 2. Few studies to date, however, have brought an explicitly *feminist* understanding to both the process of reminiscence and, as it were, the "product" – an oversight that I believe Harriet's overtly feminist approach to that process shows us can result in missing the social justice elements that run through her oral and written accounts. Indeed, while in the second interview Harriett does claim that the opportunity to reminisce about "the story of the violinist that wasn't" "really did help in a very therapeutic way" (5-II) – a statement that indicates the positive benefits she has derived through what has been called "integrative reminiscence" (Wong & Watt, 1991) – the full meaning and the politicized dimension of this statement are eclipsed if we do not see her involvement with reminiscence as an explicitly feminist act.

Weaving together the above insights from feminist material culture, feminist gerontology and narrative gerontology, and possible selves research, I will now examine more closely what feminist reminiscence looks like through the prism of the "thing" of the Italian-language textbook page. More specifically, I'll be exploring five core elements – or, if you like, stages – of feminist reminiscence, as Harriet models it for us:

- Telling the story of lost possible selves and bringing them "out of the shadows"
- Revisiting the contexts in which these selves were lost
- Naming strategies employed to resist and revise possibility despite these contexts
- Realizing how these strategies were extended beyond the individual to the collective
- Recognizing and honouring later-life expressions of, and allegiances to, lost possible selves

The cumulative effect of these elements, I believe, shows feminist reminiscence to be a politicized act that allows Harriet – and potentially older women in general – to understand how her stories, much like the "thing" that she has held onto, conceal powerful strategies for transforming the systems that have limited her own life and the lives of other women with her.

"Scarred It Over": The Thing as a Way into Lost Possible Selves

Towards the end of the second interview, Jennifer asks Harriet to comment on what she found particularly helpful about her participation in the interviews and workshops. In response, Harriet highlights the therapeutic benefits she has derived from having the opportunity to talk and write about her life. As she explains, "therapy is when we write about our lives. It's an act of writing that moves us toward change" (5-II). In particular, the opportunity she has been afforded to revisit a story that "had come out of the shadows" has proven especially beneficial. In her words: "It made me give a great deal of thought to the violin which, um, before I had just scarred it over, uh, but I really did *look and analyse* what happened and [it] really did help in a very therapeutic way" (5-II, italics mine). As would-be practitioners of narrative care, we are invited by Harriet, then, to consider what is involved in "really ... look[ing at] and analys[ing] what happened" in stories that "come out of the shadows," above all, stories that have previously been "scarred ... over."

Although, as Harriet admits, "seldom ever, uh, do I tell or speak of the story of the violin" (2-II), it is a story that she reveals, in both the two interviews and the piece she wrote between them, she has at least privately revisited and tried to make meaning of throughout her life. Moreover, it is a story that she has to a certain extent memorialized in the textbook page itself. Her formulation of a concert violinist possible self first appears at age eight when, as I outlined earlier and as Jennifer and Denise explained in Chapter 4, she was given a violin to play while at school and fell instantly in love with it. She describes how she "felt in my gut that I was going to be a violinist. I loved it" (12-I). The violin, she goes on, has a transformative effect on her psyche as a "timid" and "terrified" girl recently returned to post-war London after being evacuated to the countryside at age two and living for six years with another family "where I had been afraid of everything and withdrawn and didn't know ... I knew this." Following her brother's "complaint" that her playing distracted him from his studies, however, her mother takes the violin away, initiating the "story of the violinist that wasn't" in which Harriet's strongly held possible self is lost.

If we trace her relationship to this lost self, we find that despite being forbidden the necessary means to realize it at age eight, Harriet has not – even at seventy-eight – forgotten this once hoped-for identity. For instance, although we don't hear the details of how it happened, Harriet somehow gets her hands on a violin as a young woman living in the United States. She describes "playing the violin for a long while" (13-I), albeit as "always a very solitary kind of thing" (13-I) and not fully in keeping with her original dream of "want[ing] to be in an orchestra" (13-I) – something that she feels is out of reach because of not playing it as a child. Again, in her early thirties, she embarks on another attempt to resurrect this possible self when she receives a scholarship to study music therapy in California. She begins at the conservatory yet is thwarted once more in her effort to transform herself into her hoped-for violinist self:

> I'd always loved music and wanted to study music, but ... by that time I was thirty-two years of age. And [I] got a scholarship to study music therapy, and went to university, to [the] conservatory actually. But the children, the

> young people there had studied music since they were three and four and I felt terribly intimidated really ... There were very few jobs in music therapy, and so I changed over and went into nursing. Seemed much more practical. Became a nurse. (7-I)

Having chosen the more "practical" route, Harriet seems at this point to let go of any further efforts to realize her violinist possible self and takes on, instead, the identity of "the violinist that wasn't" – a descriptor that simultaneously centres what has been lost and signals her ongoing loyalty to it. To be sure, as Harriet begins to dig into this story that has "come out of the shadows," it becomes clear that, though she may title it the "story of the violinist that wasn't," her once hoped-for self has not entirely disappeared. She tells Jennifer, for instance, that just the previous New Years' Day, she cried while watching the Vienna Philharmonic Orchestra. "I watched the violinist," she explains, "and I think yes, there I am. Yes" (13-I).

As I mentioned already, a key turning point in the story of the violinist that wasn't occurs when she discovers the precise sentence that her brother had spoken to their mother so many years before. Accompanied by a picture of a little girl playing the violin, it appeared in an Italian-language textbook that she is using for one of the courses she takes while pursuing her nursing degree. As a seventy-eight-year-old woman recalling the revelation that her brother's "complaint" was made in an attempt to show off and thus was nothing more than a misunderstood joke, Harriet initially offers this detail as a "funny story" (12-I). Yet as she "look[s at] and analyse[s] what happened," she realizes, in making sense of the fact that her mother's reason for forbidding her to play "wasn't for real at all" (13-I), that it is perhaps more than merely a "funny story." To be sure, the fateful sentence that her brother recited – now enshrined in the textbook page – is the beginning of what she variously characterizes as the "unrequited love story" (1-II), the "tragedy" story, the "comedy" story, the "silly" story (14-I), and the "ultimate story" (13-I) of the "violinist that wasn't." As she wrestles with how to characterize it, in other words, the story's significance for her remains unsettled. Her struggle to assign it a genre in turn indicates, I would argue, the limited scripts available for women's lives overall (Heilbrun, 1988), and the unique complexities that reminiscence poses for women whose lives do not fit neatly into conventional "forms of self-telling" (Bruner, 1987, p. 16).

"I Thought It Was My Fault": Revisiting and Revising the Context of Loss

In explaining how participation in the workshops and the interviews "moves us toward change," Harriet observes that in "really look[ing at] and analys[ing] what happened," she has previously, and perhaps erroneously, "thought [for] many years that it was my fault that I didn't follow through on it [playing the violin]" (5-II). With this observation, she articulates one of the ways in which she has made sense of the story throughout her life, namely by viewing herself as blameworthy and as lacking in dedication. Having opened herself up, though, to "really look [at] and analyse what happened," she signals – both with this statement and with the introduction of the textbook page – that she may wish to revisit and re-evaluate how she has previously interpreted her inability to become a concert violinist. Despite having "thought [for] many years" that she was to blame, her engagement in a mode of integrative reminiscence that has been called "dynamic reminiscence" (Chandler & Ray, 2002, pp. 80–92) – in other words, reworking the meaning of key memories in the moment – has itself cast doubts on her prior ways of making sense of events. She readily acknowledges that her age at the time prevented her from disobeying her mother. However, her detailed descriptions of the deeply gendered context of her girlhood – in which her brother's interests take precedence over her own – point to an effort on her part to express how larger social conditions in fact played a central role in this loss. While the textbook page depicting a little girl being told to be quiet is perhaps the most obvious example of this context, Harriet's analysis of it as such opens up into a more complex process of feminist reminiscence in which she articulates multiple instances when her pursuit of her violinist possible self was challenged by the societal constraints with which she grew up.

When invited by Jennifer in the first interview to tell one or two stories about her life, Harriet begins with an account of how it was that she came from London to live in rural New Brunswick. Her very first sentence is revealing. "When I was very young," she says, "my parents, my mother specifically, was very afraid that I'd become a nun ... and she would never have grandchildren and that sort of thing" (6-I). As Harriet supplies more details, it becomes clear that by "that sort of thing" she is alluding to the gender norms of the time, according to which she would be expected to marry and have children of her own. Her mother's concern that she follow this path results in her being "shipped to New York City" (7-I) at age eighteen or nineteen – the motivation behind it being for her to find a husband and, accordingly, pursue the path available for women that is set out in what has been described as *the marriage plot.* The marriage plot, writes feminist scholar Carolyn Heilbrun (1988), "demands not only that a woman marry but that the marriage and its progeny be her life's absolute and only center" (p. 51). In Harriet's description of her childhood, and the circumstances that led to her being shipped to

New York, it is easy to see how the master narrative outlined in the marriage plot permeates the expectations she is told she should have for her future. For example, she describes how as a child her mother changes the stories of the operas that they listen to so that "they all had a happy ending. Every single one" (4-I). Referring to *La Bohème*, "Mimi married Rodolfo and they lived happily ever after" (4-I). "As a child," she tells Jennifer, "I had been told all these stories that every single one of them, um, lived happily ever after" (5-I).

The pressures of gender norms in post–World War II Britain – and the constraints they place upon Harriet, her mother, and women in general – are manifest in other subtle ways in the descriptions she shares of her girlhood. Although she does not discuss in depth the impact of the war on her mother, separated from her children for over six years, she hints at several shadow stories – including that of her father, whom she mentions in passing as "never home" – that point to the distinct ways in which the war intersected with these gender norms to create additional limits and indeed trauma for women like her mother. For instance, in a conversation Harriet recreates between herself, her brother, and her mother, she imagines the guilt her mother must have experienced in not somehow fulfilling her role as a parent:

> She had all these questions posed [to her by us] like, "Why, um, why did you leave us for six years?" You know. "What a terrible thing to do." And, you know, "Our house wasn't bombed so why couldn't we have stayed here?" And she said, "Well, the house across the street was bombed, we didn't know." (12-I)

In the story she writes between the two interviews, Harriet alludes to her mother's attempts to atone for the trauma and abuse suffered by her son at the farm where he was placed during the war:

> My brother was ten or eleven years of age. I can only imagine what his life had been like for he was never, ever to speak of it with me. Was it perhaps the fact that my mother felt guilty at what my brother ... had endured during those terrible years of war on the farm in Peterborough ...? I was acutely aware from the start ... [his] every aspiration was to be granted him whenever and wherever possible from then on.

Remembering this through the lens of what her mother might have been experiencing at the time is important for Harriet in understanding the layered ways in which the gender expectations of her girlhood played out in the options she was presented with for her own future. Recounting at seventy-eight the “completely dysfunctional” (2-I) situation of her family in the years following the war, she offers explanations that subtly shift the blame away from both herself and her mother – “the dark, strange, woman,” as Harriet hauntingly expresses it in her story. Instead, she acknowledges the enormous limitations that have been placed on her mother’s life as, seemingly alone, she tries to navigate raising two children within a world in which intense violence has made them “all strangers” (2-I). Nonetheless, as the following excerpts from her story attest, Harriet clearly had certain core beliefs communicated to her as a young girl that her brother’s development and desires are ultimately of greater importance than her own:

> Teachers taking me aside would look aghast when I explained there was no use of my studying because my brother was much brighter than me and I could never compete (as I’d been told) and that, too, I was a girl and therefore of less worth.
>
> I excelled at sports and was questioned if I would like the chance to go on in the field, I asked if I would need my mother’s help because she had stated she could not afford to educate both of us and that it was boys needed an education, girls didn’t need one since they only “married.”

Harriet also includes subtle details that demonstrate that, in spite of her mother’s efforts, she has her own suspicions early on concerning the promises of the marriage plot. Relating to Jennifer her job as an usherette at Covent Garden Opera House, which allowed her to watch the opera while handing out programs, she discovers, for instance, that the happy endings promised in her mother’s stories of women’s lives were not necessarily true.

> I would see that Mimi didn’t marry Rodolfo. Mimi got tuberculosis and died this horrible death … Tosca, you know, um, jumps off the parapet and kills herself. She didn’t get to marry her boyfriend either, um, and on and on it goes … in one opera after another. (5-I)

Harriet paints a stark portrait of herself as a young girl awakening to what it might mean to be a woman and, as such, to what possibilities were (and were not) available to her: “And me with my eyes just pouring down with tears because it happened to every single one” (5-I) – a realization that Harriet sums up during the first interview as “learn[ing] early that life wasn’t always what it appeared” (5-I).

At another point, Harriet shares the story of her grandmother, which seems to demonstrate anything but the happiness Harriet has been led to believe awaits her in marriage. Though it was "considered not proper ... for ladies to be on the stage" (10-I), the woman had herself been an opera singer. However, her wilfulness in doing what "was considered not proper" is similarly punished:

> When my grandfather married her, the first thing he did was to take her off the stage and ... I think she was very, very unhappy. My mum said she used to sing outside when she put the clothes outside to hang in this little London row house and you could imagine all the little people in London hearing this Grand Opera singer singing in the backyard, but that was my grandmother and yet it just wasn't done for women to be on stage. (10-I)

Despite her best efforts, Harriet's mother's attempts to secure a "happy ending" for her daughter by encouraging her adherence to marriage fall through. Shortly after Harriett is sent to New York, her mother dies unexpectedly of a brain aneurism, and although Harriet does in fact get married to a professor, he "ultimately," she says, "fell in love with one of his students" (9-II). "So that," she says succinctly, "was the end of that" (9-I).

The implications of these gender norms are most harshly felt – and, as we will see, most vigorously resisted – in what Harriet says about her relationship to the violin. In her written account of playing it as a young girl, the language and imagery she employs emphasize self-expression, disregard for social norms and appearances, and an unwavering commitment to her self-defined path, all of which contrasts sharply with the stifling expectations of femininity that she is being told she must perform:

> And then it happened. Violins were brought into the school. I held it as though all the world had been placed into my arms. I loved it from the moment I saw it. The bow on the beaconing four strings, G, D, A, and E as I was told, made sounds of the sweetest nature and these sounds seemed all mine because I had made them! They were of my own creation and sweet beyond any imaginings. I couldn't get enough of the studies. The violin teacher gave me more and more hymns which I played at Morning Assembly, while insatiably begging more. Little Mozart pieces were added. A taste of Beethoven! At home I studied by the hour, improving quickly but still of course needing more practice and indeed maturity.

In one particularly well-developed scene that she relates to Jennifer in the first interview, she provides a touching portrait of herself playing the violin:

> So when I went to school, um, they had, they had somebody came in and taught violin and we played the hymns for morning prayer. Um. And I

> apparently, I can still remember it, the last verse of … the little hymn was played and I carried on playing because I just loved it so much and the whole school congregation said, "Didn't you almost die of embarrassment?" "No," I said. "It was wonderful." You know, "I'd do it again. (12-I)

Indeed, when she is ultimately barred by her mother from playing at all, she fights desperately for a compromise that might allow her to continue to play by volunteering to practise in the attic. She vividly recalls her memory of this moment:

> And my mother came to me and said, "You've got to stop practising the violin." And I said, "No, I can't," you know. "I, I have to play." "No, you have to stop; it's bothering your brother." And I said, "Well that doesn't matter, I'll go to the top of the house … and I'll play." "No, you can't, you can't play anywhere; you've got to stop. You've got to give the violin back and you've got to stop." (12-I)

The detail and immediacy with which Harriet relates this dialogue, which took place some seventy years before, speaks to the importance she places on articulating, making visible, and putting her resistance on the record. This offer to restrain herself, to put her brother's needs above her own, and to be less obtrusive so that she can continue to play the violin becomes a tactic she will utilize throughout her life: looking for ways to subvert and resist dominant systems through appearing to adhere to them, yet at the same time remaining committed to her own values and goals. As an eight-year-old girl, however, Harriet is still learning this mode of navigating the world as a woman, and sadly is denied even the right to practise her beloved violin in the attic. That said, in re-examining the context of the loss she suffered in this moment, she resurrects a story that proves a formidable challenge to her earlier understanding of her own passivity and blame in that loss.

This impulse to blame herself for the unfolding of the story of the violinist that wasn't is one that feminist critics ask us to problematize as a form of erasing the complex social conditions that are often at work in women's lives. Feminist narrative theory and therapy has long emphasized the vital role of "bringing in the social" (Brown, 2012) when exploring challenges in women's lives. Dominant, master narratives seek to individualize and pathologize women's failings or "problems" (Brown, 2012; Burstow, 2003). However, a narrative strategy that makes room for a context-specific understanding of that "problem" can play a powerful role in shifting away from themselves the blame that women are often made to carry so that they can, more rightly, see the "problem" as a consequence of the circumstances of their lives within patriarchal systems. To be sure, as Harriet begins piecing together the circumstances in which her mother took the violin away from her, she finds that the dominant narratives in the deeply gendered world of post-war Britain harbour little space for stories in which young girls can grow up to be concert violinists. In this sense, the textbook page with its overt representation of societal pressures for women to remain silent, docile, and agreeable becomes a catalyst for many other more subtle stories that come "out of the shadows" as Harriet reminisces about the starting point of the violinist that wasn't. Collectively, these reveal a narrative of resistance that counters previous interpretations of her own passivity.

"What Does One Do?": Grappling with the Setbacks of Lost Possible Selves

Having unearthed the "story of the violinist that wasn't" and considered the gendered context in which it began, Harriet goes on to revisit other turning points in her life with a particular focus on how she copes with this loss. In doing so, she moves into the third stage in her process of feminist reminiscence in which, in light of the various ways she responded to this loss, she critiques her previous characterization of the story as something intrinsically "tragic" (5-II). In the process, she unearths another story – the story of her resistance to this loss and of how in fact it is this loss that has made her "the person [she] later become[s]" (6-II), a person "very happy with the way my life turned out" (15-I). Insofar as that life, as we will see, has been filled with numerous accomplishments, Harriet is forced to re-story, to re-genre-ate, the "tragedy" of losing her hoped-for violinist self in favour of a genre more reflective of the life of activism and resistance that she has gone on to live.

Having left her musical therapy program, she pursues a degree in nursing. This is yet another turning point that takes her on a "more practical" path, one that eventually finds her and her friend, "Lisa," living in rural New Brunswick where she creates for herself a new and satisfying life. She describes to Jennifer, for instance, the pleasure she takes in the beauty of the New Brunswick landscape – a landscape that is reminiscent of the countryside where she stayed as a girl during the war and makes her "feel like I'm living in a Walt Disney movie because the deer come and we feed them and the birds and the squirrels and the chipmunks" (16-I).

Harriet describes yet another turning point, though, in her process of fashioning a life other than the one she had imagined for herself as a child. After seven years of working as a psychiatric nurse at a local hospital, she once more begins questioning her life's path. She remembers vividly, for example, the moment when she asks Lisa, "This is all very lovely and everything, but what does one do?" (8-I). Here again, she uses the opportunity of being interviewed to identify various examples of her lifelong resistance to any storyline for her life that has her unquestioningly accepting the path laid out before her – a path that, in spite of being "very lovely," chafes against what she knows at this point to be the much more complex stories unfolding around her and in her.

As a means of answering her question "What does one do?" she travels back to England to spend time at a retreat centre run by nuns, from whom she seeks counsel. In the context of Harriet's story of her childhood, nuns – along with women opera singers and concert violinists – belong (at least in her mother's view) to a group of women who, in rejecting the marriage plot and thus challenging traditional gender scripts, pose a threat to current systems and structures. Harriet's choice to explore this spiritual path can be taken therefore as another example, discovered in the process of reviewing her life, of her authoring a life story for herself that resists conventional narratives. Indeed, as she recounts to Jennifer this experience with the nuns, it becomes clear that they – like Harriet – demand of themselves an involvement with the world around them that allows for neither the passive comfort of an unexamined life nor the option of wallowing in the tragedy of a lost dream. Witnessing how the many people attending the retreat seem to be confronting a similar crisis of meaning to what she is, Harriet experiences an epiphany of sorts. She decides that what she will "do" is to create a retreat centre on her own property, back in New Brunswick, that will allow people the same opportunity that she has had to "get away from the world and think about what it is that's happening in their life and what they want to do" (8-I). She goes on to explain how, on her return to Canada, she and Lisa establish a centre that, for the next sixteen years, will become their shared life work – work that allows her to become a powerful activist, community figure, and teacher all in one.

Reading Harriet's questioning around "what does one do" through the lens of feminist reminiscence positions it as a sign of her ongoing commitment to exploring models for female life outside of the limited ones offered by prevailing conventions and scripts. Her creation of a physical space in which others can undertake the same kind of questioning represents, I would argue, a radical intervention in the dominant discourse, one that casts this as not just an individual challenge but a societal one as well. Harriet's storying of what she does in fact *do* in response to her questioning is an exemplar of how older women can use the process of life review to unearth previously unavailable or unspeakable stories of resistance in the face of losing hoped-for possible selves.

At the same time, it demonstrates the complex, careful ways in which women have had to – and continue to – negotiate and, at times, subvert overarching conventions and scripts in order to fashion for themselves more meaningful futures and more fulfilling possibilities. Importantly, inspired to "really look [at] and analyse" the process she has undergone from the "tragic" (5-II) realization at age forty that she will not be a violinist to becoming "the person you later become" (6-II), she also seems to find it fitting to adopt a more "ironic stance" (Randall, 2013, p. 3) towards her failure to live out a prescribed vision for her future, one that was supposed to see her as as miserable as the tragic heroines she witnessed as a young usherette at Covent Garden Opera House. By engaging in what I'm calling feminist reminiscence, her vacillation among many potential ways of framing the story of the violinist that wasn't – as a tragedy, a comedy, a funny story, a silly story – is a reflection less of her own uncertainty about how to make meaning of her life at this point than of the absence of a suitable genre within which to situate her unique experience.

"A Gentler Way of Life": Generativity as Feminist Resistance

In "look[ing] closely [at] and analys[ing]" the particular form that her resistance takes – the development of a contemplative retreat centre and, as we shall see, involvement in anti-war activism – and in recognizing the connection between this resistance and her girlhood dream of being a violinist, Harriet's review of her life reveals a fourth stage of feminist reminiscence. In this stage, we witness her articulating how, in authoring a new and original script for her own life, she facilitates the authoring and offering of a similar script for others. Given the connection she senses between her lost possible self and "the person you later become" (6-II) – in her case, a widely respected peace activist and owner and host of a retreat – Harriet emphasizes that grappling successfully with life's setbacks entails not just making meaning for oneself but extending beyond oneself to others the lessons thereby learned. As she explains to Jennifer, referring implicitly to the theme of "generativity," it is in the extension of these lessons outward that growth and transformation occur. The "hurts that bring about scars," she says, are embraced in ways that allow for "formulating an even better human being in the long run" (6-II).

The lessons she has learned by revisiting the story of her lost possible self – and those she offers to the next generation through her activism and her retreat – are distilled into what she describes as "a gentler way of life" (6-II). By this, she means an ethic that is open to all who willingly engage with life's setbacks and, in so doing, evolve into "an even better human being," one who has "empathy towards other people whose lives ... also didn't follow a rigid path" (6-II). On the surface, a retreat that allows people to "get away from the world" (8-I) and carve out a "gentler way of life" (6-II) might seem to embody the very apathy that has caused Harriet to question her life path in the first place. But, as she demonstrates in her descriptions of the retreat and its significance, her decision to build it is on multiple levels a refusal to accept the systems, structures, and scripts that insist she should follow traditional paths. And it is an invitation to others to similarly resist conditions, norms, and stories that they might otherwise take as given.

As Harriet reflects further on the path she has pursued, following her final decision to give up the violin, she stresses to Jennifer that what she is most proud of is "speaking out against the horrors of war" (23-II). This is a form of activism she has practised in multiple ways, through protests, speaking at universities, and, of course, constructing her retreat itself, an activism that, while seemingly distant from her violinist possible self, is in fact another important context for her process of "look[ing] closely [at] and analys[ing]" this story. Through her oral and written accounts alike, her discussion of the retreat focuses on the significance of its location directly across from a large military base. Deeply distressed by the bombing and training that happens on the base – and seeing in it reflections of her experience of war as a child – Harriet, we learn, has dedicated herself to anti-war activity and other endeavours that promote peace and community, and to inspiring such activity in others. Indeed, while her mid-life question "What does one do?" is centred originally on her own life, she appears to believe it her role to pose this question to a much broader audience as well.

Constructed with the purpose of providing a peaceful setting "to think about things and why they do things," the retreat is itself a powerful symbol of how Harriet's ethic of a gentler way of life contrasts starkly with the base adjacent to it. Creating a space in which people can stop and ponder how their lives are implicated in the systems that the base represents is a subversive intervention in those very systems. It is not, as it might initially appear, a space for escaping from the world, for disengaging from it. Rather, it is very much one in which people are engaged – engaged in asking "what does one do?" in "thinking about what it is that's happening in their life" (8-I). And it is a space in which they can reorient themselves in a manner that allows them to participate in the world in new ways – ways that question the systems within which they live. Viewed through the framework of feminist reminiscence, then, Harriet's commitment to nurturing a gentler way of life exemplifies how she revises the understanding she has of her life to show not only her resistance to such systems as an individual but how she has empowered others to practise a similar resistance as well.

"Stories That Are Life Giving": Honouring Later Life Allegiance to Lost Possible Selves

At the time of her participation in this project, seventy-eight-year-old Harriet, now retired from her work at the retreat, is still deeply involved in negotiating tensions that she has dealt with all throughout her life – tensions between war and peace, between hierarchy and community, between oppression and equality, between violence and love. Towards the end of the second interview, she returns to a consideration of the story of the violinist that wasn't, offering a more nuanced explanation of how, as a young girl and young woman, she had once imagined that she could transcend these tensions to promote a gentler way of life through music. In doing so, she makes important connections between music and the ethic such a way of life involves that reveal the meaning her hoped-for violinist possible self has held for her to be far deeper than simply the desire to be an accomplished concert violinist. For Harriet, music communicates "innate love" (11-I) and possesses the capacity to create among people an "immediate bond" (15-II) that can challenge the sort of suffering and divisiveness that she has witnessed in her life.

As a young girl, playing the violin was a means of healing, of self-expression, and of coping with the trauma of war. It was a means of fostering connection, peace, and community in an environment that, for several reasons, left her little power to shape the world around her. As she reaches the end of the second interview, though, and thus the final stage of her process of feminist reminiscence – in which she recognizes how she has honoured her violinist possible self all through her life – she makes a significant realization: that though she was unable to achieve these goals through music, she has not given up on nurturing the values they bespeak. Her retreat, her anti-war activism, and the many other activities through which she has pursued the ethic of a gentler way of life have in fact become the vehicles through which she has held on to the very ideals, and possibilities, that she saw in herself as a violinist at age eight.

In discussing the experience of reviewing her life through the interviews and workshops, Harriet expresses how revisiting the story of the violinist that wasn't has been not just a therapeutic process ("the scar tissue was opened up and sealed again" [2-II]) but a form of meaning-making as well. "It gave meaning to those years," she tells Jennifer, "because this was such an important part of my life that I had simply cast aside for more necessary things of life and forgotten about a childhood dream" (2-II). Having had the opportunity to reflect on this lost dream, she underscores in her written story the importance of revisiting such moments: "Dreams crushed at any age are difficult to cope with," she writes, "but children's dreams and desperation in such matters are seldom given the credit they deserve and children, after a while, have hearts that bleed." More than simply returning in an obsessive manner – or via obsessive reminiscence – to the story of her lost possible self, however, Harriet's distinct engagement with the story of the violinist that wasn't through the framework of feminist reminiscence allows for the discovery that she is not, as she puts it, "just a bundle of worthless cells" but someone who "had a life and … hopefully somewhere along the lines it was worthwhile" (18-II).

For Harriet, telling "stories that are life-giving" (14-II) lies at the heart of feminist reminiscence. Without doubt, she demonstrates the "life-giving" potential of this fifth step, a step in which she draws connections between her lost possible self and the person she later becomes, in what is essentially a final and profound act of resistance, one that makes clear that, notwithstanding the outward limitations placed on her life, she has by no means contentedly accepted them, nor will she. In doing so, she has not only honoured her vision of a lost possible self, but – perhaps more importantly – she has come to "*like* the person that I have evolved into being" (6-II; emphasis mine). By this, I would argue, she means a person who has held onto and fought for her vision of a possible world that runs counter to the world marked by patriarchy, inequality, and environmental destruction that denied her, as a young girl in 1940s Britain, the realization of her possible self as a violinist and of the values hidden therein. In this sense, "things" and, more importantly, the *stories* of "things" function as powerful tokens of yet-to-be revealed histories and understandings of older women's lives – histories and understandings that, more often than not, are contained within lost possible selves.

Concluding Thoughts

By holding onto and, more to the point perhaps, sharing with trusted others objects of significance to them, women in later life are also holding onto stories that demand careful attention and analysis. It would be easy, for instance, to write off Harriet's treasured textbook page as merely a reminder of a "funny story" (12-I), as she herself does when speaking initially of its significance. However, as she says about the experience of sharing the stories that have lain hidden and layered within this otherwise benign item, a single page from a textbook, "in the stories you see the core, the heart beat that makes them, them" (9-II). Indeed, as I hope

I have shown, by supporting women in revealing the various stories, and *layers* of stories, that are contained within significant things in their lives, feminist reminiscence can support them – perhaps for the first time – in telling the full story of their (lost) hopes and dreams. It can support them in developing an understanding of the complex contexts in which these hopes and dreams were lost. And it can support them in naming the strategies by which, despite such contexts, they have revised their lives in the face of these losses and ultimately honoured those original hopes and dreams. In this way, feminist reminiscence becomes a political act that practitioners of narrative care can use to co-create with women an understanding of how their stories harbour within them – much as do the things that they cherish – powerful strategies for resisting and revising the systems that have limited their lives.

In closing, I return to Katherine Matthew's story and the question of what other possible selves may have been lurking in the trilobite cookie. Though unable to ask this question of Katherine herself, I imagine the response she'd have given being closely akin to the one Harriet has provided. Although the times and circumstances of their lives differ widely, there are several similarities. Both were engaged in social movements of their time. Both lived close to, and with awareness of, the natural world. And both displayed immense creativity in supporting their community and relationships. Finally, as I have been exploring in this chapter, Harriet, like Katherine too might have done, offers an account of her life that, at multiple points, illustrates her ability to simultaneously adhere to and yet subvert the norms of her time that shaped both the selves that she could realize and those that she lost. Taken together, their stories remind us that the things in women's lives can signify far more than they may seem to, and that honouring the stories latent within them means honouring the transformative vitality of women themselves.

9 Packet of Letters: Legacy Narratives and Serendipity Stories

MARCEA INGERSOLL

The truth about stories is that that's all we are ... So you have to be careful with the stories you tell. And you have to watch out for the stories that you are told.

– Thomas King (2003, p. 10)

Recollecting

It occurs to me that neither of my children has probably ever written a letter. Not really written one, anyway. They have not sat with a box of stationery and matching envelopes, carefully crafting sentences that then walk neatly onto the page. They have not tasted the gum of an envelope as a literate kiss whispering its message to a distant lover. They have not walked from the bus stop to the post office to select just the right stamp for the season, the contents, the recipient. Or written playful notes or coloured the envelopes or put stickers and coded messages on the outside of letters, wondering what the postal carrier might think as they slipped the bulky length of a sixteen-page missive through the letter slot miles away from the writing desk where those thoughts were inked on paper. Letters are an artefact of time cherished by those of us who sent them back and forth, lacing up friendships and pulling them tight across the years.

Personal letters are quickly becoming a thing of the past. Few of us remember what it *really* means to write a letter. For real. In cursive handwriting. My children have probably written letters for school, for assignments, for their teachers or classmates. They would not, however, have written letters *for real.* Not in the way that I used to sit in church as a young girl and write pages of detail about the events of my days to my kindred spirit (yes, that is how we called one another, we were Anne and Diana; thank you, L.M. Montgomery).

But before I tell you about my kindred spirit (I'll get back to her later, I'm that kind of storyteller), let me tell you about Joy. That's the name

I've given to the participant known in our study as LS29. "Joy" is not her real name, but I've given her that moniker because it reflects the light and essence of her storied self. I am a researcher who reads many, many transcripts, often in concert with other researchers, to seek the insights revealed in the storied words of others. One of the things we note when reading and discussing transcripts is the differences in how people speak when interviewed, their storying style, as it were. Some interviewees respond directly to the question, never varying, never straying, always asking, "What was the question again?," making sure they've got it right. And others will stop and seek reassurance: "Am I answering your question?," they will say very earnestly, or "Is that what you were looking for?" Still others speak in fragments, backtracking, talking as though there is a virtual cursor, paused, flickering, waiting to see whether to backspace over their previous commentary and delete, rewrite, delete. Joy is a woman who pours out story. Her transcript reads like the clear water of a sunlit stream, flowing over smooth stones, magnifying them, illuminating the riverbed as memory dances steadily forward.

Serendipity Stories

The story that Joy wrote between the first and second interviews brings to light some essential questions about life as a journey of encounters tinged with possibilities and opportunities that we might experience or miss out on. In her seventy-four years of living and storying, Joy has had many experiences, many encounters, and as she looks back on her life one chance encounter is central to her recollections. The act of reliving and re-storying her life has brought her to the place of memory where one event in particular rises up, comes forward, takes up valuable space in the bank of memory past and is continually cashed in as a cheque for the (re)membered present. Joy circles back to a chance encounter on a train when she was in her twenties. It is a story that calls to mind the significance of chance encounters in other narrative work that I've done. Joy's recollection of her chance encounter on the train is marked by a kind of serendipity that others have also highlighted when telling stories of experience.

Along the journey of life, we have encounters that are completely by chance yet are incredibly formative, and that affect our experience moving forward. Joy's story suggests to me, as a researcher who has encountered this type of story before (and who continues to move forward on my own journey of understanding the role that narrative plays in our lives), that these encounters deserve a label of their own. So I'll call them *serendipity stories* and define them as stories about chance encounters that bear significance for our lives, redirect our journeys of experience, and become deeply threaded into our life narratives. The first interview Joy did with Jennifer centres on an encounter that illuminated the sky of story that she shared with us. Lit it up. "Expansive" is a word that occurs to me because of the way the encounter expanded her life and illuminated her perspective, and also because of the way the connection expanded across her lifetime, remaining bright even at the time when life, we might say, begins to dim. Her encounter on the train became a light filling up space and travelling across time, bearing significance across the life course. A serendipity story.

As has been explained earlier in this book, each participant in our project took part in two interviews, attended a series of writing workshops, and wrote a story about a significant event in their lives. In her first interview, Joy shares that "life is sort of coming around full circle" (1-II) for her, and that looking back is "uplifting" (1-II). A focal point for her central reminiscence, as Jennifer and Denise hinted in Chapter 4, is a collection of cherished letters. Joy's chance encounter turned into a cherished lifetime friendship with a man whom I will call "Scott" (because of her reference to him being from Scotland). It was an unlikely association, she being in her twenties and he in his seventies, but poetry is a powerful connector. After "hours of uncomfortable silence" next to an "elderly gentleman," while taking an interprovincial train trip, Joy recounts in her written story how the silence was broken when he remarked on the "dismal rain" and she agreed (p. 2). More small talk followed, and before long the mutual discovery that they both wrote poetry was a point of commonality that erased the silence and filled the journey, leading to a prolific correspondence and a reunion when Scott appeared at her home the following year. A serendipitous encounter on a train began a significant and enduring friendship, captured in letters that she carefully kept.

We keep things that we treasure, that mean something to us, hold value for us in our lives. Joy refers to a "pack of letters" (18-I) she retained from the two decades of correspondence following that chance encounter on the train. She recounts how "I don't have the ones I wrote to him, but … we corresponded twenty-some years because … he was seventy [when they met] and he was ninety-some" when he died (18-I). Joy returned to the pack of cherished letters, a record of that lifelong friendship, to frame her reminiscence and the story that she wrote concerning it, a story she intended to leave behind.

Leaving Things Behind

The desire to leave something of our selves behind, to pass on some kind of legacy, is innately human. Gravestones are an assertion of our existence on the planet – a permanent marker of lives lived. This impulse to leave things behind begins in youth, and if you've ever been in a high school bathroom and seen "So and so was here" etched into the stall door, you have witnessed adolescent evidence of this very human urge. Legacy, that desire to record and transmit evidence of our existence for generations future, is a complex and largely understudied yet inherent part of the ageing process, according to gerontologists Elizabeth Hunter and Graham Rowles (2005), who examine its role and significance in the latter stages of life. They interviewed fourteen participants ranging in age from thirty-one to ninety-four, all of whom were near death due to cancer diagnoses or age, about the importance to them of the idea of legacy, and about what they believed their own legacy might be. Three overarching themes, or forms, emerged from Hunter and Rowles's analyses: biological legacy, material legacy, and what they describe as the legacy of values. Such a typology provides interesting reference points for understanding how some of the participants in our own study, including Joy in particular, talked about their memories, their lives, and the stories they were writing and might want to leave behind.

The first, biological legacy, involves the passing on of genetic heritage and health conditions to biological children, or the donation of the body or organs to others or for medical research. The second, material legacy, includes three main subgroups of things that people were concerned about passing on: heirlooms, possessions, and symbols. Heirlooms, write Hunter and Rowles (2005), "carried with them the weight and responsibility of history and quite often in-depth family stories," and it was "important not to break the multigenerational chain of family ownership" (p. 335). Possessions included non-sentimental items such as household goods, but participants did not carry the same kind of expectation as to whether objects of this sort would be cherished. Symbolic material legacy was associated with public symbols or societal markers, and "the transmission of the self through the creation of a lasting testament to one's existence" (p. 338). For the majority of participants in Hunter and Rowles's study, however, the third form of legacy, and the one they deemed most important, was a legacy of values.

Cherished Objects

I want to hover for a moment over the second form in this typology – material legacy – and touch down on heirlooms in particular, those cherished objects or stories that have been passed down through generations, and that carry an intergenerational expectation of care, regard, and continuation. In Chapter 14, Deborah Carr refers to stories as gifts. "They're gifts of intimacy," she writes, "and even though questions remain unspoken, the stories you tell provide clues to the answers," and they hold value. Objects, or things, are the concrete anchors for the conceptual. It is the memory or the story that is the thing that is cherished, and the object is the concrete representation of the concept we are cherishing: the memory, the story, the person.

Cherished objects are material manifestations of our lives, giving tangibility to the encounters we have had and the connections we have shared with others along the way. In this book as a whole, it becomes clear that objects can serve as concrete catalysts for recollection. In this chapter in particular, letters are another example of cherished objects that capture or reveal our stories of identity and experience. As with the cherished objects that are passed down from generation to generation, with the hope that the next generation will gain from the value they hold, whether material or sentimental, stories are also passed on. These stories form our identity; they are "the stories we are" (Randall, 2014). One participant in a workshop that Deborah led in Haiti "summed it up well: 'May we go home and write our stories so that our children's children will know who we were and what we did on this earth.'" "Writing," says Deborah, "had given them a means of leaving something of themselves behind" (see Chapter 14, this volume).

In Helen Humphrey's (2000) novel *Afterimage*, the main character, Annie Phelan, is an Irish orphan with no parents and no heirlooms. The only thing Annie has as a legacy is the story of a locket and a ring that had been given to the family who took her from Ireland to England. Annie knows these objects were sold in order to survive, but "each time she was told of the locket and the ring, it was as if the telling itself was solid, was something she could turn over in her hands, hold up to the light to see it shine" (p. 50). Even as I write this chapter, and read Humphrey's novel, the interaction of text with reader and content and context emerges to highlight how fiction illuminates how stories themselves are cherished objects: "Annie's mother is a story. Her mother is a far-off feeling that she sometimes falls out of when she wakes. She has nothing real left to her from that life. Only stories ..." (p. 51). And yet stories are real, they are *things that matter.* The stories comfort Annie, the "words of the book cover her as comfortably as a blanket on a cold night. She can wrap herself in the warmth of them" (p. 58). In our stories we find our truths. In our fiction we find our reality. And from our reality, we craft our legacy.

Gerontologists Warner Schaie and Sherry Willis (2000) use the term "legacy creating" to describe the developmental phase in which older individuals enter and review the entirety of their lives, and I see sense-making as a part of that process. For Joy, the chance to write things down meant a weight lifted. "Telling your story and really going in depth," she said, was "healing for me and problem solving" (3-II). Letters are commonly cherished objects that people frequently return to when problem solving (Sherman, 1991b). While the urgency of this legacy creating might increase as we enter the later years of the life cycle, legacy curation begins long before we are older. The recent popularity of the CBC show "Grown-ups Read Things They Wrote as Kids" represents our tendency towards the curation of things, and specifically of things we write, as evidence of who we were and are across the life course (Rak, 2018). These collections of written memorabilia are both nostalgic and anticipatory: they reveal a nostalgic looking back to see who we were and an anticipatory hope that we will continue telling our stories forward. Telling our stories to and of ourselves and others, after the moments might otherwise be forgotten, is part of the legacy we leave behind, and cherished objects are an integral part of our narrative sense-making.

Sense-Making

There is something about not just proximity to later life but also immersion in a global pandemic that nudges folks towards making sense of their lives, a kind of draft form of a legacy narrative. When the world as we know it came to a halt in early 2020, people were confined to their homes to avoid the threat of a novel coronavirus. In isolation during COVID-19, my mum was one of many folks who occupied themselves with the sorting of old photographs. Taking them out of the chronological albums she had curated over the years, she sorted them into boxes for each of her children and grandchildren. This act of sense-making for the future considers a shift in both ownership and audience – deconstructing the chronology of the albums yields a movement towards legacy. Establishing a thematic approach that is audience specific and future focused, one generation recognizes the instincts of the next to curate their own experiences individually. As they are disassembled and dispersed, passed on to the next generation, the albums are no longer contained objects that reflect a family unit, but individual photos that diffuse outward to other places, houses, directions.

Considered this way, acts of sense-making can be seen as strategies for establishing a legacy narrative, part of the legacy creating that Schaie and Willis (2000) describe. Joy seems to want to make sense of her story, to establish chronological coherence perhaps as much for her own understanding as for the desire to pass the story down. As she unspools the memories, we see her unthreading to rethread, dismantling to reconstruct. And in this reconstruction, this anticipatory passing onward, there is also omission. Some photos never made it from my mum's albums into the boxes that she distributed to us, and some wouldn't have made it into the albums in the first place. As Bill noted in Chapter 2, there are always shadow stories, stories left untold. There are always dimensions of the past that are not recorded or preserved because they are either forgotten, deemed unimportant, or intentionally hidden. Stories of pain, loss, or shame are not always preserved for the telling (Ingersoll & Whitty, 2021), and omission is a dimension of our sense-making.

Legacies of Omission: Critically Revisiting Normative Narratives

In the outline for this book that Bill and Matte initially submitted to the publisher, here's how they described the thrust of this chapter:

> **Love Letters: The Lure of Other Lives**
>
> An unexplored possibility for romance on a train trip as a young woman is archived in a collection of love letters one participant has held onto that spell a complex tangle of relations between the self and others.

In that reading of Joy's story, filtered through one type of lens, the fifteen-year letter-writing friendship between her and Scott contains an unrequited romantic interest. There is, both in Joy's story and in Scott's poetry, ample allusion to this interpretation. It is a logical reading that is familiar, probable, acceptable. In his intriguing book *Love Is a Story*, psychologist Robert Sternberg (1998) explains that throughout our lives we are subtly but continually pressured into creating only stories that are culturally acceptable.

According to Sternberg, there is a larger cultural matrix, "some sort of text, which exists outside the relationship, and which is prescriptive of the way in which the relationship should go" (p. 46). A classic cultural narrative, he notes, is the fantasy story in which the prince and princess meet and they live happily ever after. As Joy pulls together the threads of her story with Scott and tells us about the poetry he wrote in adoration of her, we can neatly fit their relationship into the fantasy story of a prince meeting his princess, with the barriers of age and distance thwarting their happily-ever-after. Or we could read their relationship as an "asymmetrical story" (p. 46) in which an older individual takes on the role of teacher and the younger is the learner, with the pair connected by their shared interest in poetry. In the story that Joy wrote, Scott is depicted as a prince in pursuit, caught up in a whirlwind of infatuation.

According to Amanda Smith Barusch (2008), whose work nicely integrates theory and research concerning love on the one hand and ageing on the other, infatuation is a multidimensional experience with an "ecstatic, almost spiritual intensity. The infatuated lover becomes obsessed with the beloved" (p. 65). Barusch notes that "recent work by anthropologists (and any reading of love poems from other cultures)" reveals that infatuation is a universal cultural notion, and humans are hardwired for it (p. 71). The connection between Joy and Scott could align neatly with a fantasy story or an infatuation story, either of which becomes interrupted by a story of unrequited love.

In another reading of their relationship, however, different details surface to frame a line of thinking that highlights how normative cultural scripts affect our life stories and how contemporary cultural scripts are changing. For a young woman travelling alone to have an immediate sense of security with a male seat companion, her interpretation of their connection and her willingness to exchange contact information at their parting may not have been colored by a sense of romance at all but by the sense of comfort that comes from a perceived lack of romantic possibility. As an unmarried older gentleman of means, with a love of poetry and a refined sense of fashion (including a lifted heel on his shoes), Scott may have immediately created with his demeanour a sense of security for Joy, a young unmarried woman alone on a train. She may have felt safe believing that his interest was purely platonic, because perhaps it was. Joy shared in her interview that as a young woman she was unsure if she wanted to marry but did not want to risk a reputation as a "spinster" (39-II). The heteronormative pressure and socio-economic constraints of the time may have led Joy to marry and raise a family even if she may not have been so inclined. In her story she refers to Scott as a "bachelor," and if we read this through a different lens, the question of romantic love might be answered quite differently.

Katherine Ott (2014), curator in the Division of Medicine and Science at the National Museum of American History, considers the role of objects in revealing historical values and how those objects hide or reveal counter-heteronormative histories. She points out that discerning meaning is difficult when considering past objects, and that "retrospective recognition is nearly impossible with people who lived in a time when it was dangerous to go against gender norms or a place where this kind of difference could not even be imagined" (p. 1). In circumstances where heteronormativity is the only acceptable option, that becomes the life lived and the lens applied. In Chapter 14 where Deborah outlines the three workshops she led, she highlights the power of social narratives to influence our own journeys, and her question to participants is a powerful one: "What story did the world you grew up in tell you about who you should or could become?" The example she shares is relevant to a critical revisiting of Joy's story and gives us insight into how romantic fairy tales perpetuate normative narratives.

Identities of possibility are limited by the fairy tales and family tales that tell us who we should or could become. Fairy tales frame a young girl's search for prince charming, heteronormativity is an intergenerational inheritance (Ahmed, 2006), and the family tree is a genealogical legacy that enshrines this goal. A family tree, "whilst not an absolute guarantee of heterosexual coupling," as one source explains, "places male/female pairings at the heart of the home and also functions to highlight those people who did not get married" (Sandell et al., 2018, p. 42). At the same time that family trees omit same-sex relationships, that omission can "sometimes lead to people being marked out by virtue of their single status – 'spinster aunts' and 'bachelor uncles' – full of queer possibilities" (p. 42). Our family trees tell a predominantly heteronormative story, while also identifying spinster aunts – like the one Joy didn't want to become.

The words "spinster" and "bachelor" have a long history of being "coded terms for gayness" (Chudacoff, 2000, p. 273). Joy notes in her recollection during the interview that she is looking back on this relationship, these letters, this part of her life, with a different perspective now that she is older. As scholarly observers, we are also called to reinterpret and revisit normative narratives with a consideration of other possibilities and interpretations. The work of Karen Blair, professor at St. Francis Xavier University, reveals possible insights into the friendship between Joy and Scott. Blair (2019) notes that a "lack of anxiety related to gay men's sexual intent increases women's comfort" (p. 1; see also Grigoriou, 2004). In an alternative narrative, this could explain the immediate comfort that Joy felt, perhaps unaccustomed to bachelors whose attentions were predisposed to the literary and fine linens. An intellectual intimacy between the two is another possible interpretation. Even as some of us may read into Joy's words that there was a romantic connection, in a critical revisiting of this encounter we could also suggest platonic or other non-heteronormative possibilities. The point of a critical revisiting is not actually whether there was or was not a romantic love interest. The point is understanding that, as with all things, value is assigned (or not) by those who create, possess, pass along, or inherit them. Value is tied to what is acceptable according to larger cultural scripts (Bohn, 2011; Sternberg, 1998), and as Joy notes, she found herself "editing things out that I knew to be true and maybe replacing them with something that was more acceptable" (16-II). Value and meaning are created by and in the transactions between readers and texts and influenced by the larger societal stories that affect these transactions. The person whose sense-making prepares a narrative for leaving behind may do so with one intention for the reading and telling of the story, but intended interpretations reflect the values and perceptions of the teller and are not always aligned with or reflective of those of the recipient.

Legacy Narratives

While some other chapters in this book focus on the materiality of cherished objects, I focus here on the narrative itself as cherished object that is performative and symbolic rather than material in nature. I invite readers to think of the story as *the thing* that is cherished, that is itself an heirloom (Hecht & Tyrell, 2007).[1] And in suggesting that the story is a thing cherished, I also propose the term "legacy narratives" to capture those stories that participants choose to pass on to future generations, and assert that legacy creation involves a process of sense-making that includes omitting or revising details according to whether or not they are acceptable within our cultural scripts.

Stories containing value to tellers who have a desire to pass them on to others are a performance of meaning and value that, as I say, can be considered legacy narratives. As with beauty, meaning is in the eye of the beholder or the reader. Just as objects are cherished because of the meaning they hold for those who keep or discard them, so the meanings of the stories that we keep, tell, hide, or discard are determined by the teller and the told. The story as object does not change, but the performance and interpretation do. The object may not change, but its value does. This brings to mind literary debates where some argue that a story is what it is, and others argue that a story is as widely interpretable as the perspectives of those who hear it. In the 1960s, literary theorists began to challenge previously held notions of an immutable text with a fixed or singular meaning, making way for forms of response that recognize the lenses that inform our readings. Stanley Fish (1980), for instance, asserted that it is various "interpretive communities" – or narrative environments, to use the term introduced in Chapter 2 – that produce meanings rather than either the text or reader. In a similar vein, Louise Rosenblatt (1986, 1994) suggested that the meaning of a text is a transaction encompassing the author, the reader, and the text itself. This same understanding might be brought to the idea of legacy narratives.

1 *Editors' note*: See Chapter 3 on the written narrative as a thing distinct from the object depicted in it (e.g., letters), and see Chapter 15 for further discussion on this topic.

Rosenblatt insisted that words on a page do not contain meaning until they are read, and that it is the reader who creates meaning as they interact with the text that an author has transmitted. Meaning changes over time, as does language, and I use Merriam Webster's 2019 word of the year, the singular "they," very deliberately in the previous sentence to illuminate this point. Rosenblatt's (1985) transactional theory sees the "reading act as an event involving a particular individual and a particular text, happening at a particular time, under particular circumstances, in a particular social and cultural setting, and as part of the ongoing life of the individual and the group." This harkens back to Hunter and Rowles's (2005) reminder that "understanding legacy involves exploring the personal beliefs that underlie leaving something behind, be it memories, photographs, grandma's ring, children or bequests to charitable organizations" (p. 331). Joy's story is written with careful attention to these dimensions, and with an anticipatory hope that her story will be read with an understanding of its intended value and meaning. Understanding is one dimension of the legacy narrative transaction, and valuing is another.

A legacy of values, or beliefs that are passed on as a type of personal legacy, is one component of Hunter and Rowles's typology. Value can only be created by a shared understanding of the meaning of a thing. Legacy narratives have actual or intended value and anticipate a transaction between teller and inheritor. They are stories of things cherished, or cherished stories, that are passed on in a transaction of hope between the author and recipient – a hope for a shared understanding of the thing, or of understanding that comes from having the thing. Legacy narratives also have the potential to represent or transmit in symbolic or performative ways the types of legacy identified in Hunter and Rowles's typology, or to reproduce normative narratives.

Normative ideas and their impact on life narratives have been described by narrative scholar Annette Bohn (2011) as cultural life scripts. According to Bohn, the "cultural life script is semantic knowledge about an entire life span within a culture that is acquired across childhood and adolescence"; and it is a "prerequisite for autobiographical reasoning because it facilitates the connection between the self and the culture beyond the individual life story" (p. 28). Bohn notes that "the cultural life script should be considered the overarching organizational principle of autobiographical memories across the lifespan" (p. 29). Normative cultural scripts – which we might think of as "narrative templates" or "forms of self-telling," terms that Bill introduced in Chapter 2 – present a schema for sense-making, and the legacy narratives we leave behind reflect our adherence to such scripts and the potential reproduction of singular, normative narratives. "The single story creates stereotypes," says author Chimamanda Ngozi Adichie (2009), "and the problem with stereotypes is not that they are untrue, but that they are incomplete. They make one story become the only story." The possibility of a love story fits the stereotype of unrequited romance. And this revelation of the danger of a single story highlights another dimension of the complexity of narrative, which is that a single story is nearly impossible if we consider the subjectivity associated with memory and story recollection and composition.

For anyone whose family members have interrupted them at a family gathering where they're recounting a memory and been told that "that's not how it went at all!," it is clear that our stories are framed by the memory of the beholder. Joy told us that she realized, through the workshops, "that aging can complicate your memory." In other words, "I thought I knew exactly what happened, and I would have bet money on it, and yet I now was thinking did that really happen like that?" As she put it, "you start to doubt your memory or yourself" (12-II). Memory, experience, subjectivity – these complexities focus or expand the lens of interpretation. For anyone who has had poetry written for them by older men, the notion that this was a literary connection and not a romantic one might ring true. For any woman who has experienced the freedom of sharing intellectual intimacy with a man whose interest in her was poetically romantic, the connection between Joy and Scott rings true. For two strangers who have shared an instant connection that is the foundation for a lifelong friendship, their story rings true. Not all of the details of it are clear, however, for as Joy writes, "time dims the memory or what I choose not to recall" (p. 5). In composing it, she creatively interlaces Scott's published poetry with her own recollections of both their initial encounter and their ensuing relationship. She travels back in time, through memory, to the moments of their meeting, with the reflective gaze of nostalgia and "the realization that I had been allowed a special friendship which manifested itself in various expressions of love" (p. 6). Not a single story of love, but love in various expressions, with various interpretations and complexities: multidimensional. In other words, it is up to us to determine how we might interpret Joy's words, and Scott's. After all, any story left behind is a legacy for us all.

Connecting

Legacy narratives are stories that are both *about* "things that matter" and *are* the "things" that matter, and they are part of our individual, familial, and social legacy. Like Joy and Scott, I have had a brilliant lifelong friendship whose origins lie in a mutual love of poetry. My kindred spirit, Amy, and I first met when we were thirteen and twelve, respectively. We had both entered a poetry contest sponsored by a local peace group, and our winning pieces were published in a local paper, *The Quoddy Tides.* I loved her poem and a chance meeting gave me the occasion to tell her so. That encounter is our serendipity story. Amy lived in another province but summered on the island of my youth – and during the summer of our chance meeting we vowed to be friends forever. And we have. We conversed by letter for many years, having grown up just on that edge of time before letters were replaced with phone calls, then emails, then texts. We never dreamt that the shoeboxes of letters we kept in closets would one day be replaced by carelessly sent and rarely archived iMessages and emoticons. And while today we enjoy the instant ability to connect when we want to share a thought with one another, these digital exchanges raise questions of what will last, what will endure. With the expediency of the instantaneous there is also an accompanying loss of the material object where care, connection, and continuity were made visible. The immediate connection of a *Hey there, just thinking about you and hope you're having a good day!* flashes on the black mirror of the cellphone screen, tightly tucked into the text bubble, there and then gone again. No envelope still faintly scented with sparing sprays of Love's Baby Soft or Polo by Ralph Lauren. No Benetton ads from *Seventeen* magazine taped to the page to conjure the spirit of the age. And yet here those memories are, recorded now, tucked tightly into the text of this page.

Amy and I speak often about the letters we once laboured over, addressed with flourishing care, and sent off in anticipation of a reply. Just last year we pulled out some of these past missives and read them, travelling back through time to visit our younger selves: two teenage girls who met by chance when they entered the same poetry contest and formed a friendship that is now reaching towards its fourth decade. We both have shoeboxes of our correspondence, settled deep in the backs of our closets, kept with other precious garments and keepsakes and memories of time gone by. Will our children cherish these envelopes of time past and lives lived? Will they read them to know who their mothers were and what preoccupations of youth connected them across provinces, then across countries, and always across the years? Will these letters be a light living beyond our time, leaving a legacy for those who loved us? How will members of our family trees engage in acts of legacy creating in a digital age? Today's children do not know a time without the Internet, are less likely to live in small rural communities, and are more likely than their grandparents were to grow up in urban spaces. There is a generational disconnect in the ways we curate what we value. The tactile and material act of keeping cherished letters, scrapbooks, hope chests, and china sets is an heirloom of the past. The immaterial and digital nature of cloud-based communication raises interesting questions about the role of objects in legacy creation. Legacy is a curation of experience deemed fit to transmit, inspire, inform, sustain. In the age of the digital, of rising transience and dwindling attachment to objects and items of sentimentality, how might future generations leave things behind?

Towards a Conclusion or Two

Legacy narratives are reflective productions that require the teller to recall, select, and make sense of events in order to produce the retelling. By incorporating the narrative strategy of sense-making, legacy narratives are productive recollections intended to function as stories told from a particular point of view about the past and the present that can be passed on to future generations. Critically revisiting narratives can help us further understand the values of the teller and the told, and to understand how normative narratives structure life stories and the legacy narratives we leave behind. In an essay entitled "The End of the Story? Narrative Openness in Life and Death," Bill describes how we are always operating *within* some sort of story about our lives, and our stories are inseparable from our lives, our selves, and our identities (Randall, 2019). He points out how we compose our self-stories in relation to others, those people who are influential co-authors in the continual and communal storying and restorying of our lives. And then he takes us into the knowledge that our individual and communal stories are also part of larger societal narratives or metanarratives. In Chapter 2, he alludes as well to the stories that are not told, those that are concealed. Because legacy narratives reveal our personal beliefs about and perceptions of value, some stories are legacies of omission, deliberately hidden from the narratives that we choose to pass on, because they do not adhere to normative cultural scripts.

Finally, as the case of Joy, I believe, illustrates, narrative is its own form of legacy: story itself is an inherently human phenomenon. It is biological, material, and laden with values, passed on through the millennia. We are predisposed as a species to genetically transmit a sense of story, to etch our narratives in ways that immortalize the form, and to record our values for the next generations of humanity. "Of all the ways we communicate with one another," writes Canadian journalist, Robert Fulford (1999), "the story has established itself as the most comfortable, the most versatile ... Stories touch all of us, reaching across cultures and generations, accompanying humanity down the centuries" (p. x). I like to think of story as being deeply interwoven in the patterns of our lives in a way that we might call *ecological,* and perhaps others have already called it this. Our stories exist like our species: in contact, collaboration, and sometimes conflict with ourselves and others as we manifest our existence on the planet, where all of our cellular compositions of selves abide. In an ecology of symbiotic interaction, our stories are our *symbolic* interaction – in an integral and integrated system of existence. Stories told forward are the DNA of our species, splicing, replicating, and reproducing in and for future generations. As a living and dying species, we have a perhaps biological pull to tell our stories forward, so that they might be a legacy of our living. We hope that our symbolic manifestations will live on beyond the time when our unique cellular and corporeal combinations diffuse. We are wired with a human hope for the reconfiguration of our selves in other forms, a hope predicated on a spiritual belief and cellular belief alike that, in death, we do not disappear. We diffuse.

10 Beer Stein: From Trauma to Fairy Tale

WILLIAM L. RANDALL AND ANTHAZIA KADIR

It matters how we tell the story.

–Janet Ruffing (2011, p. 93)

The Mystery in My Story

Some years ago, a student in a course that Bill regularly teaches called "Narrative Gerontology" commented on how the various reflection exercises that he had the class engage in weekly were helping to her appreciate "the mystery in my story." Her comment recalls the observation by André Maurois (1986) that Bill cited at the end of Chapter 7 that to be in the presence of a fellow human being, even one we imagine we know rather well, it is as if "we stood watching a drama of infinite complexity of which we know not, of which we shall never know, the end" (p. 4). The adventure our team has had of employing our "narrative imagination" (Andrews, 2014) to enter the lives of our nine participants supports these two observations – even if, for all of us except Jennifer, our entry point has been second-hand. Our experience of Joan, the participant we're focussing on here, and whom we've affectionately dubbed "Princess" (for reasons that will soon become clear), is no exception. If not the word "mystery," then certainly "complexity," has resonated with us strongly as we've made our way, line by line, into her distinctive storyworld.

Our aim in this volume is not to psychoanalyse our participants. Rather, with gratitude for their willingness to let us in on some of their dearest memories and deepest thoughts, it is to understand how they "story" their lives (Kenyon et al., 2011), and within that, to try to understand their connection with the objects that they have singled out as holding special meaning. For Joan, that object is the one she wrote about in the story she composed between the first interview and the second – the story of a "roots trip" (Yngvesson, 2003) that she made with her daughters, and (ironically!) her ex-mother-in-law, back to the village in the south of England where her life began, and to the house where she was born.

This trip, which we'll come back to in more detail below, was a sort of coming-to-terms exercise for her, for she had hopes of reconnecting with her childhood in tangible ways, revisiting her grandfather's home, and finding things more or less as she had imagined them. This desire to find both family and familiarity signals a journey that she had in fact been on ever since leaving England as an infant. She expected it to afford her that "full circle" feeling. As we learn more about her, however, we realize that her longing for "home" was not focussed on a physical place alone, but is a search with no end in sight. For her life has always been in flux, a feature that only enhances the complexity of her story and, in our view, makes it so powerful overall.

According to Thomas Moore (2000), author of *Care of the Soul*, "there are places in this world that are neither here nor there, neither up nor down, neither real nor imaginary. These are the in-between places, difficult to find and even more challenging to sustain. Yet they are the most fruitful places of all. For in these liminal narrows a kind of life takes place that is out of the ordinary, creative, and once in a while genuinely magical" (p. 34). Joan had thought that, somehow, her return to England would make amends for a family scandal that, on some level, she felt it was her responsibility to wash clean. What she found instead was a place that had changed radically without her. Having viewed "home" as a place that one longs for just as it was, she found that the very concept of "home" can, in reality, be fraught with uncertainty and fluidity, in keeping with its status as a "cultural imaginary" (Synnes & Frank, 2020). She set out looking for a place as she (dimly) remembers leaving it, but what she found instead was newness. The place, the people, and the things she had associated with "home" had, quite literally, moved on, yet this, in a sense, gave her permission to do the same. As Moore's words suggest, "in-between places" can be "the most fruitful places of all" (p. 34), for they allow us – as the experience of returning to this particular place allowed her – the room to grow into herself. It allowed her the licence to go some place inside of herself that had refused to go away no matter how difficult her life so often was. If you will, it allowed her to return home to her own self. We'll come back to such possibilities later, and to the story of the trip itself, which is the story she chose to write out between the first interview and the second. Here, though, is how it starts:

> My grandfather had passed away twenty years before in 1967. I had been named in my grandfather's will, thus the reason for our present trip. His

second wife had just passed away over the last year and I had received funds from his estate. It's a long story, though, as it goes back to when I was born. My mother was an only child; however, she too died in 1967 – one day before my grandfather. So here I was at last in England checking out my roots.

As Jennifer and Denise outlined in Chapter 4, the thing that Joan brought back with her from this life-altering trip was a beer stein. It had been stumbled onto by a neighbour, quite by chance, half-buried in the vacant lot where her grandfather's manor house once stood before being bulldozed in the middle of the night under what were apparently quite suspicious circumstances. But this is no ordinary beer stein, for it bears the crest of her family of origin, thereby confirming her identity as being "of gentry" (39-II), an identity that in the minds of teachers and others throughout her life who accused her of having "delusions of grandeur" (38f.-I) – and at times in her own mind too – has been seriously in doubt. While she tells Jennifer that "every little trinket up there [on her mantelpiece] means something" (49-I), the beer stein is in a class of its own. That said, there is yet another thing in her possession that is closely linked to it in significance. It is a handwritten letter that she received around the time of her fifteenth birthday from her grandfather, the man behind the stein, who somehow managed to keep track of her whereabouts during what we shall soon see was an incredibly chaotic youth. She reads aloud from it to Jennifer:

A short while, you'll be fifteen. Doubtless you will be leaving [school?] but do stay on as long as you possibly can. There is little better in this world than a good education and it is only after you are fifteen or sixteen that you really begin to learn. (60-I)

Once Upon a Time

With these essential elements – a fairy grandfather, a princess, and a holy grail (in the form of a beer stein), not to mention an ogre or two! – we have the makings of a story that would enthral most small children – *The Princess and the Beer Stein,* if you like. But the real tale would be a fairly harsh one for most children to have to live, not to mention far too tangled to follow. For Joan's own storying style, at least as it comes across in these interviews, has a chopped-up, stop-start quality to it that makes it challenging for a reader (certainly for the two of us) to keep things straight, chronologically, thematically, and the like. It has elements of what Arthur Frank (2013) calls a "chaos narrative" (pp. 97–114). Yet her various forays into the past are nonetheless significant and worth exploring: reading from her grandfather's letter, keeping the beer stein in a special place of its own, mentioning her grandfather's second wife and how things turned out differently in the end, hiring a solicitor in England to look into her inheritance but not going through with it, and so on and so forth.

While these stories of needing, wanting, and desiring are scarcely told in a straightforward manner, she nonetheless tells a lot of them, with lots of detail and dialogue. She would score high, we can therefore assume, on narrative complexity, and on narrative agency as well, with an indomitable sense, despite the troubles she has faced, of being in control of how she responds to them. "I choose my own path" (14-II), she asserts to Jennifer, by way of example. And she exudes a sense of excitement almost at how intricate, how interesting, and how powerful (painful, yes, but powerful too) her story is, confusing though it be both for her to tell and for us to track. She portrays herself not as the victim of circumstances but as the heroine of her life narrative who wherever possible "choose[s] life" (7-II, 37-II). Jennifer and Denise have sketched her story briefly already, but let's let Joan outline it herself, as she summarizes for Jennifer what she wrote in response to one of the prompts that Deborah used to get participants' narrative juices flowing. It is the classic story-opener, "Once upon a time ..."

> Once upon a time ... a little princess was born in England ... [she] took a trip on a big ship to North America with her mommy. Soon after, mommy met up with daddy, and they all moved into a big castle ... Soon new babies arrived and they moved to a little bungalow ... mommy had to do the best she could by herself in Canada. Then the struggle began and mommy took the little princess, but it didn't work out, so finally mommy left the princess with daddy and all his kids and then she went away. Now at nine years old, little princess [was] in [a] strange home [a foster home] and on her own ... By this time, she was thirteen. She left and ended up in three more homes. By the time she was eighteen she was engaged and got married at age nineteen, had two little princesses and made a good life. (7f.-II)

Of course, this is just an exercise in a workshop, its aim being to invite participants to step back from their lives in a light-hearted vein and envision it in the typically positive way that words like "once upon a time" invite. With Joan, though, you have the sense that it was particularly potent as a means of beginning to corral together the countless bits of "narrative debris" (McKendy, 2006), many of them pretty hard-edged, that might otherwise resist integration into her story as a whole. It is a means for her to tackle what gerontologist Peter Coleman (1999) calls "the task of reconciliation" – in other words, assimilating into the story that one entertains about one's life the difficult episodes and traumatic times one has endured, a task that, according to Dan McAdams (2001a), "is one of the most challenging tasks in the making of life stories, especially in midlife and beyond" (p. 664). It is a means of envisioning the trajectory of her life as constituting a *story*, with a beginning, a middle, and – ultimately, hopefully – a happy end. As a "narrative pathway," to borrow from researchers Schofield et al. (2017) in their study of the stories told by youth who leave residential care, it is one of "Love, Loss, and Moving On" (p. 785).

Innocuous as the exercise may have seemed on the surface, then, we can be confident in saying that it enabled her to wrap her mind around her life and, as she herself puts things, "ma[k]e a fairy tale" out of it (8-II), both the bits in it that she can tell and those so traumatic that part of her prefers not to tell them at all. For there are any number of experiences in the middle of her little composition – or in the "muddle," as Robert Atkinson (1995, p. 26) refers to it in his lovely book *The Gift of Stories* – that get glossed over. The muddle, writes Atkinson, "is when things don't go smoothly ... when things involve conflict, chaos, and disorder" (p. 26). With Joan, her muddle has several "shadow stories" (de Medeiros & Rubinstein, 2015) that get alluded to, ever so lightly (so as not to disrupt the fairy tale "feel"), with ominous phrases like "then the struggle began," "it didn't work out," "she went away." Yet, staying true to the genre, Joan winds up her fairy tale with the proverbial happy-ever-after ending: "[she] had two little princesses and made a good life" (8-II).

We'll offer a sense shortly of some of these more shadowy episodes, those she hints at during both interviews with enticing comments like "that's a story in itself" (15-I, 20-I, 28-I, 49-I), "there's a story in there" (24-II), "my story could go on and on" (52-I), or simply "there's too many stories" (27-I). In the meantime, though, the mere thought of these stories, one can imagine, must overwhelm her with the sense of how tough will be the task of reconciliation, of gathering them together under one neat, narrative arc. For many are the very sort of skeleton-in-the-closet tale that most of us, somewhere along the line, will have among our "family stories" (Stone, 2008) – the kind of stories that, in agreement with the writer Thomas King (2003), Joan might say she has "been chained to all my life" (p. 9). But for now, we can ask, how does one go about pulling together such a litany of troubles? "Trouble," insists Jerome Bruner (1999, p. 8), is exactly what a story – any story – requires for it to be a story at all. A story with not just a happy ending and a happy beginning but a happy middle as well would not make a terribly satisfying narrative to hear or watch or read. No trouble, no tale, in other words. "[I]f the story is *trouble-free*," says Bruner, "it is likely to run out, to bring on death" (p. 9; emphasis Bruner's). But for Joan, it's precisely the trouble – the muddle, the chaos – that resists clear narration, as in *this happened, then this, then that.* So, the challenge for her at this point in her life – a challenge that both the workshops and the interviews have perhaps brought her closer to tackling – is to organize this trouble within a single overarching tale. Casting it within a "once upon a time" framework is how, initially or provisionally, this could be accomplished.

The Hero's Journey

Joan is an older adult when she composes her little fairy tale in response to Deborah's prompt. It is possible, however, that such a tale has been at the back of her mind in nascent form ever since she was a child, as a silent script, or a "believed-in imagining" (Sarbin, 1998, pp. 15–30), that helped her hold things together whenever the world around her was flying apart. Whether they be time-honoured ones like "Hansel and Gretel" or "The Princess and the Pea" or ones that we make up on our own, as Joan has done here, fairy tales have that kind of power (see Randall et al., 2022). In the words of Bruno Bettleheim (1989) in *The Uses of Enchantment: The Meaning and Importance of Fairy Tales*: "while it enters the child, the fairy tale enlightens him about himself and fosters his personality development" (p. 12). "Fairy tales," he writes, "are so meaningful to children in helping them cope with the psychological problems of growing up and integrating their personalities" (p. 14).

The whole topic of fairy tales is a complex one in itself, of course, and raises many more questions than there is time or need to delve into here – including the question of the effects of fairy tales on little girls' imaginations in particular. But at this point, we want to draw on the thinking of well-known mythologist Joseph Campbell, author of (among many other books) *The Hero with a Thousand Faces* (1949).

In *The Power of Myth*, based on a series of televised interviews with Campbell on PBS, he tells interviewer Bill Moyers that there are two kinds of heroes within mythological tales, those that choose the heroic journey and those who are "thrown into" it (Campbell & Moyers, 1988, p. 129). As very much, in our view, the hero of her own story, with a vigorous sense of narrative agency, Joan – or "Princess," as we shall call her from now on – is clearly in the latter category. She did not choose the chain of horrors and misadventures that her life, certainly in its first fifteen years or so, turned out to be, but through it all she chose life (7-II; 37-II). By whatever route the hero's journey is embarked upon, says Campbell, the typical trajectory – not unlike what Arthur Frank (2013, pp. 115–136) calls a "quest narrative" – has three main stages: "Departure, Fulfillment, and Return" (p. 129). We'll use these stages as reference points for making sense of Princess's life, at least as she has spoken of it during the interviews that Jennifer conducted with her. In her case, though, we'll insert a fourth stage between departure and fulfilment. For want of a better term, we'll call it *disaster*.

Departure

The departure stage begins with her leaving England as a nine-month-old child and coming to Montreal. The leaving happens under a cloud, however, for her mother had given birth to her out of wedlock and, as was sometimes the custom with young women who brought disgrace upon their families in this manner, was sent out to "the colonies" (i.e., Canada), albeit with a dowry. The sense of disgrace is lessened somewhat by the knowledge – which she clings to religiously for the rest of her life – that the two of them are from a background of privilege, that she is "of gentry" (39-II). With this in mind, the observations made by Canadian memoirist Sharon Butala (2005) concerning her own mother provide a parallel to the experience both of Princess's mother and of Princess herself:

> My mother clung to her one story all her life. It was that she was "of good family," by which she meant a family once, long ago, connected to aristocracy, a family of means, a genteel family, a family of people with decent hearts and minds ... in whom, therefore, a sense of superiority to the common run of humanity had been bred. She was wedded to that story, saw no possibility of another. She had been taught that no circumstances could diminish her, because being "of good family" held within it the requirement that she always be better than any such circumstances. (pp. 43f.)

The sense of disgrace is also reduced by Princess's assumption that her real father – who was never a tangible presence in her life but only a ghost, as it were – had been a British naval officer. (A half-sister whom Princess never really got along with told her later, however, that her father was not a naval officer at all but rather the family chauffeur! [49-I, 24-II]) As well, in their early days of being in Canada, before her mother married and therefore brought a step-father, plus more siblings, into Princess's little life, she recalls enjoying the special favour of her mother. She describes the woman as having "sacrificed her life for all of her children" (28-I, 12-II) and, specifically, making sure that Princess was "the best-dressed baby in Montreal" (17-I).

Disaster

Although the chronology of events, not to mention the events themselves, are difficult to be certain about, given the chopped-up nature of Princess's narrations, her mother "left [her] forever" when she was two years old. Here's what she says about that fateful day:

> The day my mother left forever, and I told you I was two years old, you know, with my grandmother, and I have in mind, like I guess whenever we write some of this stuff I had in my mind my mother's suitcase where she had all the photographs of, of all the years of us as babies, you know, she took that with her that day. Yeah ... that was ... Handcuffed in front of me and arrested for kidnapping me. Crazy. He [her step-father] said I was not his child, but my mum was arrested for kidnapping because he told me at a young age, at nine years old, he wasn't my father. I'm like, I was in shock I guess and I said, "Oh, I already knew." Or something as a little kid would answer and [uh] but in the meantime he'd been, how would he do it? Calling the police and when she would leave with me, tell them she kidnapped me and I wasn't his child. So one minute he was telling me I'm not his child then putting me up that he, I am his child, and charging her for kidnapping me. (12-II)

The higgledy-piggledy style of her narrative here, not to mention the confusion surrounding certain key facts (for example, was she two or nine when her mother "kidnapped" her?) brings to mind the observation made by novelist Margaret Atwood (1996) in *Alias Grace*:

> When you are in the middle of the story it isn't a story at all, but only a confusion; a dark roaring, a blindness, a wreckage of shattered glass and splintered wood; like a house in a whirlwind ... It's only afterwards that it becomes anything like a story at all, when you're telling it, to yourself or to someone else. (p. 298)

It's as if this most traumatic of traumatic incidents that any child could possibly endure – her mother being arrested right before her eyes and being taken away "forever" – an incident that catapulted her into an unbelievably unstable, unpredictable life in foster care, is still, sixty-plus years later, "a wreckage of shattered glass," not yet a story per se. It is still too real, too raw.

From abandonment to abuse, trauma of any kind, of course, possesses untold potential to cause "disruption" in our life-narratives (Fireman et al., 2003, p. 9). But alas, for Princess this was but the beginning. From this event on, other incidents she underwent during the muddle of her early life included having a foster mother who was such a horrible parent that Social Services pulled her own children out of the home and yet left Princess there. Another mother (or perhaps the same one – it's not clear) shoved Princess's head into the toilet and might have held it there had Princess not managed to slam the door on her and knock her out (42-II). Still another, though again perhaps the same one, was so troubled, mentally and financially, that she tried to get her own daughter to become a sex worker (42f.-II). Then there is the incident of running away from one of the three foster homes she was placed in from age nine to sixteen, and sleeping overnight underneath a nearby house, and at another point (perhaps the same one?) "snitch[ing] things out of the garbage in order to survive" (43-II). At Christmas time in one of these homes, she reports that she and her foster siblings "were put out like dogs and then brought in to eat scraps from the table" (43f.-II).

One can only imagine the despair she must at times have been tempted to fall into, let alone how she envisioned "the story" of her life would ever turn out! As she tells Jennifer, "I was the most depressed kid" (39-I). To make matters worse, she had teachers and other persons in authority over her telling her that she was a "juvenile delinquent" (9-I), "would never amount to anything, would not go to university," and would "be a woman of the streets" (8-II). At one point during these crazy years, she had a boyfriend whose "family broke us up because I was a foster child" (40-I), an event that to this day, she admits to Jennifer, "brings tears to my eyes" (40-I). Indeed, she continued to be discriminated against – for example, by a mother-in-law who tried to dissuade her son from marrying Princess because "you don't know where this girl came from" (30-II) and who at one point accused Princess of "doing favours" for the woman's husband (39-II), and then being falsely accused by the woman's son, Princess' husband at the time, of "running around" on him (45-II).

When asked during the interviews about turning points in her life, she went on for several pages of transcript citing one turning point after another – so many, in fact, that she eventually asserted that "mine's all turning-points" (43-I, 46-I). Such turning points were not turning points, though, in the sense of plot twists in the unfolding of an otherwise "normal" life-script (see McAdams & Bowman, 2001). Rather, they might more accurately be called trauma points; certainly, they were change points – points when life took her here rather than there, though neither "here" nor "there" might have seemed to her at the time as being a better option – points that very likely seemed downright pointless, as in the definition of life attributed to Mark Twain as "just one damn thing after another."

No wonder that, with so many experiences of chaos, of discrimination and rejection, of abandonment and abuse, of seeming pointlessness, she admits to having felt "pretty much alone … all my life," having to "find my own way" (56-I). No wonder that she felt she was "the most depressed kid," living for so many years never "knowing my roots" (17-I), never feeling "acknowledged" (50-II), and never knowing who her father was – whether naval officer or family chauffeur?! Yet she longed for him all the same, her longing captured by an old-time country tune made popular by Kitty Wells, "How Far Is Heaven?," which she suggests became her personal theme song from age four on (9-II). Certainly, it was one of the pieces in the repertoire that she would draw from later in her life as a stage entertainer, playing for nursing home residents, charity benefits, and so forth. The song's refrain asks, "How far is heaven?," followed by a suggestion that the singer wants to go to heaven "to-night" and also have her "daddy" hold her "tight" (Davis & Franks, 1950).

Despite these nagging questions as to "who are you, or where did you come from?" (1-II) and what are "my roots" (17-I), she held on, amidst all the instability and unpredictability, to the conviction that such uncertainty was not her ultimate lot in life, the conviction that she was "of gentry" (39-II) and that, somehow, things would turn out for the best. Despite being told she had "delusions of grandeur" (39-I), she did not give up hope. Helping to keep this hope alive were her grandfather's letters, a fact in keeping with what Campbell notes is a common feature of fairy tales: "Even though there's a happy ending for most fairy tales, on the way to the happy ending, typical mythological motifs occur – for example, the motif of being in deep trouble and then hearing a voice, or having somebody to help you out" (Campbell & Moyers, 1988, p. 138). The voice that Princess heard was that of her grandfather, encouraging her from afar not to lose heart – motivated, perhaps, by his own load of guilt for letting his second wife, Princess's step-grandmother, talk him into having Princess and her mother sent away in the first place.

Whatever the case, buoyed by Granddad's letters and by fond memories of her mother – whom she views as a victim of circumstances, whom Princess visited in prison and even tried to get pardoned, and who, she believed, continued to love her dearly throughout her own disastrous days (7-II, 37-II) – Princess could exude a feisty determination. She could "choose life" (7-II), could pick herself up and soldier on. And she could keep control of herself amid the mayhem of her world, not allowing alcohol to rob her of it, for instance, while partying with her friends (41f.-I). She could, as women historically have so often done, endure; she could let go and move on, or otherwise find the grace to live with the unbearable. "I'm considered to be a survivor" (7-I), "I was a survivor from the get-go" (7-I), she asserts to Jennifer within the first minutes of the first interview, and "I was independent" (8-I). And, as she remembers asserting when asked by her mother who she will be when she grows up, "I will be me" (8-II).

Fulfilment

Harbingers of fulfilment are already obvious in the departure stage, with the innate sense of manifest destiny that she brought with her to Canada in the company of her mother, a sense of being "of gentry" (39-II). But elements of fulfilment are evident even in the disastrous stage.

In their study of identity development in young adults after they've done time in foster care, Heather Mulkerns and Carol Owen (2008) talk about the "lack of a safety net" such children routinely report having experienced, and the "self-reliance" that gets forged within many of them as a result. Princess fits this pattern well. The sorts of statements that Mulkerns's and Owen's participants made could easily have been made by her: "it is only me I can count on ... There is no safety net except myself ... I still have a strong sense of not belonging" (pp. 438f.). But this aloneness and guardedness and self-reliance, while it has come with a price (her depression), has helped steel her to "be me" (8-II). Evidence of this is that, even amid the pandemonium of her foster years, she still managed to excel at school, despite the fact that, in order to prove a point to one of her teachers, she intentionally failed Grade 8. Yet she returned the following year to lead her class.

Her subsequent performance, she says, "prove[d] wrong" (14-II, 27-II) the nay-sayers who were possibly prejudiced against her from the start simply because she was a foster child, teachers who were convinced that the "academic" path was not for her and that she should settle for "commercial" instead (14-II, 27-II). Following her (then) husband to New Brunswick, she bypasses the usual route of earning a high school diploma and enrols in a bachelor's program in psychology as a mature student. Even after she and her husband divorce (37-II), leaving her to raise their two daughters on her own, she successfully completes her degree. Although, once more, the chronology is unclear, as is the matter of what exactly she worked at afterwards, she moved (with her children?) to Ottawa and, fulfilling her grandfather's hopes that she get "a good education," she completes a master's in counselling. As she repeated proudly throughout the interviews, as if summing up her sense of self, "I'm a high school dropout with a master's degree" (7-I, 10-I). Thereafter, though yet again the sequence of her jobs, involvements, and relationships (e.g., a second marriage that she says her "gut" told her she shouldn't have gone into) is difficult to trace with confidence, she carves out for herself and her daughters the kind of stable family life that she herself had never known. *She comes into her own*, we could say, as a parent, as a counsellor, as a functioning, contributing member of society. As she had told her mother years before, "I will be me" (8-II).

Return

The return phase has a specific event at the heart of it that focuses things wonderfully, and that one could say encapsulates the fulfilment phase, with which it is entwined. It is the literal return, or the roots trip, that she made with her daughters and ex-mother-in-law in 1987 and that we referred to at the start of this chapter. That this actual-technical return symbolizes a deeper sort of psychological-emotional return is supported by the fact that, out of all the other stories from her life that she might have chosen, this is the one she picked to write about between the first interview and the second. Here are some key excerpts:

> The day we arrived at [name of town in England] … to go view my grandfather's estate, I got the shock of my life. I drove back and forth on [name of lane] but could not see my grandfather's home, based on my memory. Finally, I stopped the car – one of my daughters asked, "Mum, why are you stopping?," to which I answered, "I just have a feeling … this is my grandfather's place" … But then … where was my grandfather's home, the front entrance, the windows etched in my memory, was nowhere to be seen. Instead there were three modern-type homes and two garages and no one seemed to be home, so I wandered about for a bit in shock … Then I looked around to where I saw some overgrown grass and said, "there used to be a fish pond right here." The girls moved the grass and sure enough the fish pond was there …
>
> The next day we went back … to have a bit more of a look around. I decided to check with neighbouring homes … We were well received by one of my grandfather's neighbours right next door and were invited in for tea. Of course I had explained who I was, my name, and was very open with them. I can't say I knew what I was looking for from them aside from confirming that I was right, that was my grandfather's estate next door and then I could go back to Canada with some peace of mind.
>
> But what happened next blew me away when his wife said, "We knew you existed but we did not know where you were." Those were the most powerful words anyone could ever have said to me. Then they shared some of their memories, as well as explaining how shocked they were when my grandfather's house was bulldozed down in the middle of the night, unbeknownst to the local heritage society as well.

> … my grandfather's neighbour said he was so torn up about it and that next morning went over to view the damage and found himself shuffling his feet through the debris when he kicked something "metal," bent down to pick it up. He looked at me and said, "Wait a minute" and came back saying to me, "I wondered why I ever picked it up," then handed it to me, saying, "Of course, it's yours." My grandfather's beer stein – I will always remember that visit.

Aided by her memory of "that visit" and by now possessing the beer stein itself, she must, we can imagine, have experienced not just a tremendous sense of comeuppance towards those who had mocked her delusions of grandeur but, more profoundly, an enormous feeling of acknowledgment and affirmation – *We knew you existed …* In its materiality, the beer stein is a vindication of her struggles to know her roots, and a confirmation of her long-held sense of identity. *I am, after all, who I always, deep down, believed I was.* As both metonym and symbol of a life denied her and an identity that is her own, it endures, on display.

Identity issues are seldom settled once and for all: for instance, in our adolescent years. They can haunt us all life long, later life included. They would certainly seem to have done this with Princess. But the act of finding the site of her birth home, and with it the beer stein of her grandfather, took her to another level inside herself, affording her at long last "some peace of mind." And that same peace of mind, we would offer, is kindled anew each day in her current life, where she is more at home within herself, as she enjoys the company of her cats in what she refers to with affection as "my English cottage" (34-I, 15-II).

Redemption, Generativity, and Life Review

The plotline at work in Princess's fairy tale reflects what McAdams (2006) would call a story of "redemption," which he defines broadly as "a deliverance from suffering to a better world" (p. 7). In her analyses of the narratives of former foster children, which draw on McAdams's thinking, Lindsey Thomas (2014) distinguishes among those whose self-characterizations are those of "victims," "survivors," and "victors." In terms of these distinctions, although she speaks of herself as "a survivor from the get-go" (7-I), Princess, we believe, is clearly a victor. It is only victors, Thomas says, whose narrations betray strong themes of redemption; victims and survivors "are unable to narrate their experiences in a way that allows for redemption" (p. 89). Instead, they "seem caught in 'contaminated plots,' unable to break free from a cycle of negative events" (p. 89).

Individuals whose narratives are filled with redemptive sequences and who can see their life as a whole in redemptive ways tend also, says McAdams (2006), to be highly "generative" individuals (p. 7). Highly generative people are committed to making some sort of positive difference in their families, their communities, their society, their world. When asked to complete instruments like the Loyala Generativity Scale, people in the helping professions – such as counselling, which has been Princess's own vocation – score particularly high. Certainly, Princess embodies this quality in spades. Her energetic personality, her career as a counsellor, her pride in her daughters and grandchildren and all their interests and accomplishments, her insistence, as a senior herself, on assisting fellow seniors to live as positively and productively as they can and to continue to contributing to society (4f.-I, 27-II), not to mention her passion around influencing children by encouraging them and not punishing them, a passion borne, no doubt, of her own experiences growing up – all of these testify to a strong strain of generativity running through her life. Once again, by way of proof, the mantra she keeps repeating to Jennifer is "choose life" (7-II, 37-II).

In fact, she is still living that life. "I'm not the retiring type" (36-I, 20-II), she announces to Jennifer on more than one occasion, and indeed she seems to resist the whole concept of "retirement," certainly in relation to herself. As far as ageing in general is concerned, she says, "it's about keeping on for as long as you can" (5-II). Thus, not only does she not see herself as "a writer really yet" (3-II), but as she says a number of times throughout, she's not yet really ready to write about her life. "I've got to live my life first before I know how to write the story" (55-II). While she reports having attended various life-writing classes and workshops, including the three offered by Deborah ("I never missed any one of them," she proudly announces [6-II]), she has not yet, according to her, worked her way sufficiently through "issues ... that go back over years" (7-II, 30-II) to have acquired the necessary emotional detachment (see Randall, 2013) to pull the story together either on the page or in her heart. Such detachment is provisionally permitted her, however, by referring to herself in the safety of the third person in her "once upon a time" tale. She is, as Erikson might say, squarely in the midst of "life review," a process he deems essential to achieving "ego integrity" and to avoiding, therefore, the pitfall of "despair" – a pitfall that we can imagine was frequently a possibility at several junctures in her life. The purpose of life review is to attain a sense inside ourselves that, all things considered, the positives and negatives alike, our life has been worthwhile; that, bearing in mind the circumstances we were born into, the genes we inherited, the personality we were assigned, and the slings and arrows with which we've had to contend, our life has been what it had to be and, "by necessity, permitted of no substitutions" (Erikson, 1963, p. 268).

The "issues" Princess refers to, we can suppose, revolve around her life-long sense of being alone – "all my life I've been pretty much alone" (56-I), "an outsider" (10-II), she confesses to Jennifer – and her deep-seated feelings of confusion, identity-wise, that come from not knowing "who are you or where did you come from?" (1-II). They revolve as well, we can suppose, around her relationships with mother figures in her life (e.g., foster mothers, mothers-in-law), relationships that have been fraught with negativity; and, very likely as well, her relationship with her own mother, for having abandoned her at such a tender age, yet whom she professes to love deeply and in no way appears to begrudge. Indeed, just the opposite: a key motive in her writing is, as she says, "to set the record straight and clear my mother's name" (25-II), and a core theme that guides her life is "forgive them for they know not what they do" (36-II).

Her little fairy tale is a start, however – a temporary scaffolding, we might say – until a more comprehensive, more coherent version of her life can assemble itself solidly within her imagination, if not in a piece of writing. It is a means for her of simplifying the sprawling complexity and psychic pain of so much in her formative years, not to mention the residual pain she has borne throughout her adult years, with so many stories inside of stories, in order that she can break through to a sense of her life's overarching shape. It is a means of beginning to clarify what is her unique personal "myth" (Atkinson, 1995; McAdams, 1996). Nonetheless, although on the cusp of a satisfying sense of narrative coherence, she's not quite there yet. She's not yet ready to write about her life, because she's still living it, and still dealing with issues that – ironically – perhaps only *writing* about her life will help her to face (see, e.g., De Salvo, 1999; Lepore & Smyth, 2002; Pennebaker, 1990).

That said, writing about it in the context of these three workshops, particularly the story of her trip to find her roots and certainly her Once Upon A Time tale, composed as it was in the third person, has begun to give her the emotional "distancing" (3-II, 8-II) that she has sought from many of the troubling details of her real life – a distancing she has craved so that she can see her way forward to a positive assessment and acceptance of all that her life has involved, the good, the bad, and the decidedly ugly. Conveniently, her tale is replete with victors (herself above all), victims (her mother), and villains (foster mothers, etc.); with a Prince Charming (the boyfriend whose parents broke them apart) and a fairy grandfather; with a happy (enough) ending in her English cottage; and, as the pièce de resistance, with a Holy Grail, the beer stein with the family crest – the ultimate proof that her "delusions of grandeur" were not so delusory after all.

One final thought is prompted for us by author Carol Pearson in her book *The Hero Within* (1989). In a chapter entitled "The Hero's Journey," she picks up where Joseph Campbell leaves off and outlines six "hero archetypes" – the Innocent, Orphan, Wanderer, Warrior, Martyr, and Magician – which she summarizes as follows:

> The Innocent and the Orphan set the stage: the Innocent lives in the prefallen state of grace; the Orphan confronts the reality of the Fall. The next few stages are strategies for living in a fallen world; the Wanderer begins the task of finding oneself apart from others; the Warrior learns to fight to defend oneself and to change the world in one's own image; and the Martyr learns to give, to commit, and to sacrifice for others. The progression, then, is from suffering, to self-definition, to struggle, to love. (p. 4)

As for the Magician archetype, Pearson describes it as

> a mode of heroism available to everyone. After learning to change one's environment by great discipline, will, and struggle, the Magician learns to move with the energy of the universe and to attract what is needed by laws of synchronicity, so that the ease of the Magician's interaction with the universe seems like magic. Having learned to trust the self, the Magician comes full circle and, like the Innocent, finds that it is safe to trust. (p. 5)

Despite its New Age-ish feel, Pearson's schema, we propose, possesses an intuitive (if untested) appeal. And it opens up a line of thinking that, fleshed out more fully, could be pursued to advantage in exploring the complexity of Princess's world. We will end here, though, by suggesting simply that, in being catapulted so abruptly from Innocent ("best-dressed baby in Montreal") to Orphan ("she left forever"), Princess might easily have remained, psychologically and emotionally, within the Orphan mode for much of her life, or perhaps at best the Wanderer mode, that of one who never really finds her way. But neither scenario has been the case. Fortified from within by her fairy tale, by the material proof of the tale's validity in the form of a material talisman, and by her "believed-in imagining" (Sarbin, 1998), plus all that it implies about her resilience and her destiny, she has moved through both the Warrior and the Martyr modes as well – as the high school dropout who has a master's degree, as the motherless-fatherless child who has raised two fine children of her own, and as the caring professional who has devoted her life to helping others with a passion that even retirement can't curtail. But more than this, signs of the Magician mode, we would submit, are also beginning to emerge, in her having conjured up for herself the kind of satisfying, meaning-filled life that, in the end, only choice and not chance can make come true.

11 Frozen Red Currants: Textiles, Memory, and Symbol-Making

BRANDI ESTEY-BURTT

We think of our lives – and of stories – as spun threads, extended and knitted or interwoven with others into the fabric of communities, or history, or texts.

– A.S. Byatt (2008)

If I had to use two words to describe Susan, as I'll be calling her, I would choose "active" and "connected." Now retired, she participates in two writing groups, attends numerous art and writing workshops every year, writes both fiction and poetry prolifically, spins her own yarn, and maintains an energetic interest in genealogical research. She wholeheartedly embraces new opportunities for learning and creating, and part of her openness to new experiences comes from her positive view of her own life story as dynamic and continuously unfolding. Her story's resilience – her *narrative* resilience – ties directly, in no small degree, to her sense of herself as a maker and as an artist: she actively stories her life in a variety of forms, including painting, writing, and crafting.

Throughout this book, we are exploring how older adults story their lives in connection with objects that have acquired special symbolic meaning for them. Sometimes – and this aligns with the theory that, with age, we become more capable of post-formal thought, which includes the ability to make metaphorical connections (Randall, 2023) – these objects surge to the forefront of the person's reminiscence as a tactile indication of major themes in their stories. In other cases, they quietly retreat, and more work must be done to tease out their symbolic implications. In all cases, these objects offer significant opportunity to reflect on the exciting diversity of ways in which people hold, interact with, and tell stories about things that matter in their lives.

In this chapter, I want to think about Susan's storytelling and the symbolism of her object through the lens of textiles. As A.S. Byatt (2008) observes in the epigraph above, storytelling has always had a tangible connection to the crafts associated with fabric-making. Most often, this history has been tied to women as producers of the fabrics necessary for daily family life, though Clare Hunter (2019) points out how these accounts of gendered labour have been deemed unimportant and all too frequently obscured in historical records. But textiles are things that have tied relationships together in powerful ways. Textiles are texts – stories of care and love shaped into fabric – as well as objects.

For Susan, textiles and stories form important connections that repeatedly emerge in her descriptions of her activities, her discussion of her particular object, and even in the metaphorical language that she uses in her interviews with Jennifer, as well as in the written submission that she wrote between the workshops at Deborah's request. Moreover, the contributions that her mother, grandmothers, and aunts have made to textiles are an important part of her own awareness of family history. The rug her grandmother made, for example, is an object that can be handed down to other family members. Susan is a weaver – a weaver of stories as well as of things – and the metaphor of a fabric that knits people's stories together runs throughout her thoughts on human history and legacy.[1] But the symbol that stands out for Susan is a painful one, one that points towards the grief involved in thinking about legacy and intimacy: it is a batch of red currants that were picked by Susan's mother before she died, and that Susan has kept frozen for over twelve years.

Perhaps now ready to, in part, process[2] her grief over her mother's death, Susan plans to use the currants to dye fibre and spin it into yarn to be used for different projects. No longer wanting to keep the currants in stasis, Susan has found a unique way to craft them into new objects – into textiles – and thus to create new symbols, even as she maintains a profound connection to her mother. Her complicated relationship with the currants raises interesting questions about living symbols, how they can be woven into new forms through storytelling, and how they can be passed along to future generations. In what follows, I'll first discuss women and craft and explore how Susan forges a genealogy through textiles with the women in her family, even if some of this work has been painful. I then turn to the links between storytelling and the construction of narrative identity before concluding with how Susan employs a poetics of genealogy to envision a cosmic tapestry of human story and belonging.

1 *Editors' note*: See Chapter 6 and consider the difference between patchwork/collage and the weaving of text/textile.

2 *Editors' note*: in a double sense of the word!

Women and Craft

I opened this chapter by describing Susan as connected. As I'll discuss later, she is deeply connected to her family history through genealogical research and to friends through her writing groups. For her, connection involves immersing herself in the process of reflection and creation as well as situating herself within a lineage of others who have done the same. Susan models this approach by exploring subjects like fabric-making from all points of the process, from gathering materials to later writing about her experiences in a poetry manuscript.

One particular manuscript project – one of many she has on the go – focussed, she told Jennifer, on "going out, picking a plant, cooking it up in a pot, sticking some wool in it, and then I write a poem" (6-I). Susan goes into more detail about the process, her reminiscence sparked by a basket of yarn on hand that she has dyed with such plants as old man's beard lichen, blackberry, lily of the valley, goldenrod, and beets. These plants are all locally available to her, and she has gathered many if not most of them herself. Next, she tells of how she "learned to spin ... I did a lot of stuff with this project that I'd never done before" (7-I). She further describes the process of first gathering the plants and preparing the wool with a solution called a mordant because "you have to basically soak the wool in alum first in order to make it take up colour properly" (8-I). Then she learned how to use a drop spindle, ultimately spinning all the balls of wool into yarn that she now keeps for personal use.

Throughout this poetry project, Susan adopted a hands-on, do-it-yourself approach to learning about her materials and the procedures for making yarn in order to better understand the labour that past generations put into making basic necessities. However, the project unintentionally became a way to explore her own, more intimate connections with her family. For Susan, the main family relationship evoked by the dyed yarn is with her mother:

> I wrote a poem about my mum during the last years of her life. She would pick currants, and so I used currants [to dye fabric] and I kept her last bucket of currants that she picked and she had given it to me because she wanted them for food ... So, I put it in my ... deep freeze in the fridge and so I've had it for like twelve years and so for this project I took it and it's actually still soaking out there. I've got the ... jar with the currants in it and I'll get a piece of cloth out of it basically and then I'll probably put that into a quilt. (9-I)

The red currants have become a complicated symbol of connection for Susan. They are wrapped up in the grief of losing her mother, a woman who had also obviously enjoyed doing things, like foraging for food, for herself. There are a number of questions arising from Susan's attempts to freeze the currants for twelve years – do they suggest difficulties in processing her grief? Is she trying to "freeze" her relationship, so to speak, with her mother? Why focus on the currants and not other objects that her mother may have passed on to her as well?

By virtue of having been touched and then gifted by her mother, but then having been frozen for so long, the currants have transformed beyond food to being objects in limbo. They were living fruit, and Susan's mother intended them to be eaten. In other words, they had a nourishing function as food, one that was to be shared with her daughter. The currants also bespeak the outdoors activity necessity to find and pick them and suggest an ecological relationship with gathering one's own food. All of these implications link the currants to life, vibrancy, and shared family meals.

However, currants are fleshy, organic entities that undergo inevitable decay as they age. Rather than being an object that can be physically handed down through generations, like a watch or a photo, the currants have an expiration date. They are short lived, and the count-down clock of their existence is irrevocably tied to the moment they are picked. In this way, the moment of picking becomes a fraught event, tied both to nourishment and gift-giving and to the stark realization of impermanence and decay.

This fact posed a problem for Susan, which is why she put them in the freezer; the cold has temporarily halted biological processes of rot and decomposition. She has stored them in the freezer part of her fridge, both an essential and central part of her home, but also an ambiguous one. In the freezer, they are food but also not-food, as Susan cannot bear to digest the fruit of one of her mother's last outings. The freezer represents a space of limbo, marking both an attempt to stop time but also an avoidance of the currants' inevitable transience – and the fleeting nature of one of her last encounters with her mother.

The currants, and their associations with her mother, have occupied a pivotal space in daily life since her mother's death, even if Susan has not yet felt able to do anything with them. Regardless, twelve years is a lot of time to put away such a powerful symbol of her mother's passing. Susan mentions that part of her reticence about her mother's death stems from its being accidental: the shock and surprise surely compounded what was already an incredibly difficult situation of bereavement. Carol Shields and Marjorie Anderson (2001) use the term "dropped threads" to describe the "holes" in women's talk and stories about the "defining moments [of their] lives" (p. viii). Such holes or gaps often appear in relation to events that are still too painful to talk about, and they act as snarled or dropped threads that aren't usually revealed as part of a person's tapestry of stories. In their *Dropped Threads* anthologies, Shields and Anderson discovered that many women possess such threads that they are unwilling to speak of for fear of judgment or causing more personal pain to themselves or others. The red currants represent one such hole, one such dropped thread, for Susan.

Part of the issue of this particular symbol for Susan lies in how the currants are highly susceptible to decay. Writing about spirit and community in the work of French philosopher Simone Weil, Diogenes Allen and Eric O. Springsted (1994) discuss materiality and its inevitable links to rot and deterioration: "we are material, and as pieces of matter, we are vulnerable to injury, illness, and decay" (p. 64). Matter as *thing* here becomes deeply enmeshed with its own implications of mortality, insofar as part of being human is to realize the finitude of our own matter. Allen and Springsted suggest that "to realize this ... is to come to terms with necessity" (p. 64). The currants offer one such inevitable reminder that things decay and die. Their organic matter shows us in a highly visible as well as visceral way that our bodies are vulnerable to time and change.

Death inevitably forces us to confront our own mortality as well as that of our loved ones, to confront that our bodies are open to injury and ageing. Bill Randall and Beth McKim (2008) observe that the changes produced by ageing unavoidably affect bodies and relationships: "Even if disease and disability fail to take tolls of their own, our resiliency, immunity, and mobility are all eventually affected" (p. 119). The currants are clearly an object tied to decay and suffering for Susan. They represent an event of mortality – her mother's death – over which she had no control and for which she had little time to prepare herself. Moreover, she has experienced blocks in her usual outlets of reflection – writing, art, and craft work.

These psychological obstructions are deeply connected to issues of intimacy and mortality. Acknowledging that she avoids certain topics in her own writing and work, especially the deaths of her parents, she says, "I really haven't written about their deaths. I've written about them ... but I haven't really written about their deaths and they were kind of horrendous [as] they were accidental deaths" (13-I). Gayle Letherby and Deborah Davidson (2015) speak about bereavement as a biographical disruption, a narrative disruption, that touches upon every aspect of a person's existence. "The experience of grief," they write, "is multidimensional and embodied ... it is a personal, social, political, intellectual, emotional, and bodily experience" (p. 347). They suggest the concept of "good grief," which involves work so that the "experience of love and loss is integrated into one's life in meaningful ways that continue bonds with the deceased" (p. 348). This kind of good grief further relies on the "shar[ing] and negotiat[ion]" of grieving "between and among grieving and supportive others" (p. 348), and, moreover, often depends on artistic activities as an essential part of the grieving process.

In addition to arts-based interventions and supportive communities, gerontologist Gary Kenyon (2011) has highlighted the element of time as an important part of gaining perspective on past experiences. He observes that "there is a gap or a space between what happens to us and the meaning that we place on it ... It is this space that allows for the possibility of restorying the experience toward less suffering" (p. 242). Often it takes time to step back and, through hindsight (Freeman, 2010), assess the meanings we attach to events and to process the emotions with which we have imbued a given situation. Hopefully, this temporal interlude can help one work towards acceptance. Kenyon (2011) emphasizes that acceptance is a "necessary condition" for being "narratively open" (p. 242) to change and for offering new ways of understanding painful events in our stories. Our stories are dynamic, and Kenyon underlines the work of re-storying lives as a significant practice of ageing well. This work often continues unconsciously, at the back of our minds, while we go about our daily lives.

I wonder if this is the case for Susan. At the time she is interviewed for this book, she has the jar of currants soaking close by in preparation to dye fabric. Twelve years after her mother's death, she is now ready to thaw the currants and re-examine her relationship to them and to her mother. In the ensuing years, she has immersed herself in literary, visual, and textile arts, forming deep bonds with her writing community and reflecting on her own genealogical and personal history through her various writing projects. She has literally and figuratively picked up the dropped thread of that part of her story in order to work through its implications. As Shields and Anderson found for the women with whom they worked, perhaps Susan has simply needed time to process the emotions and thoughts connected with those difficult events.

Randall and McKim (2008) offer the term "texistence" (pp. 5, 95–113) to point to how, among other things, we continually think about and revise our stories. Our texistence – or, if you like, our "biographicity" (Alheit, 1995, p. 65) – encompasses how we read, reinterpret, and re-evaluate our lives at different points. The idea of texistence demonstrates an important way of understanding our lives as a richly layered, continuously unfolding set of stories that we shape for ourselves and others. It is an especially apt word when considering the close etymological and historical links between storytelling and textiles, connections that go back as far as recorded history. In writing of one famous textile produced by women – the Bayeux Tapestry – Clare Hunter (2019) emphasizes how the women attended to "weight, movement, texture, expression, character, emotion, place," and she tries to "understand the choices they made – this pattern, that colour, this stitch" in order to see "how they made their story tangible, truthful and intimate" (pp. 31f.). Textiles are touchable stories that contain their own vocabularies woven of things like colour and texture and emotion. When one holds a piece of fabric or a skein of yarn, that object possesses a story that has a veritable weight to it, a presence that can be felt as fingers sensuously linger on the fibres. The stories of generations of women are embedded in those textiles.

Fabrics are therefore more than "just" clothing – they are stories in and of themselves that further function as an important point of visual and physical contact between people. Often considered mundane necessities of everyday life, textiles have a physicality that shapes everyday interactions. The fabric Susan is in the process of weaving from her mother's red currants will most likely be used for the quilt she mentions, which will always serve as a reminder of her relationship with her mother. It represents a new element in her texistence – her willingness to re-open the story concerning her mother's death and her intention to construct that story in transformative new ways. She is in the process of weaving a new narrative from the emotions, memories, and textures of her relationship with her mother. When she is finished, she will be able to hold that story in her hands as the currants have been given new life and fresh meaning.

Moreover, Susan's transformation of the currants into fabric – an object with a much longer lifespan and different uses than the fleshy, transient berries – offers an important meditation on change and impermanence. In a sense, she has reconfigured the idea of seemingly inevitable decline by seeing new opportunities for using the currants. It's a useful example of reconsidering the metaphor of decline in ageing – that people as well as things deteriorate (physically at least) as they age. A necessary part of being human is, of course, thinking about one's mortality and finitude (Gawande, 2014). But finitude is not the same thing as decline. There are rich new possibilities for living when one has accepted one's vulnerability, and challenging situations can provide important moments for reflection to help expand and deepen our stories (p. 118). Uncritically holding fast to a single story of our own selfhood or of who we see others to be risks inhibiting the potential for change and growth. In repurposing the currants for fabric, Susan dismisses the negative interpretation of decline in favour of an outlook that highlights the value of change as an opportunity for continued growth.

A.S. Byatt (2008) mentions that many classical stories of weaving "associate [it] and sewing with enclosure and fear" (n.p.), like Penelope in *The Odyssey,* Ariadne, and the Lady of Shalott. But for Susan, weaving actually becomes freeing: it indicates that she is, on some level, ready to emotionally deal with the currants that are part of her mother's legacy. Susan has taken the currants out of the freezer, where they were simply taking up space, and is ready to hold them, touch them, and transform them into new objects, creatively rethinking and repurposing their inevitable rot and decline. Moreover, rather than being a solitary endeavour, the process of soaking the currants, dyeing fibres with them, and spinning yarn connects her in a tangible way to her mother, who had picked each currant with her own hand. There is a beautiful point of contact here between mother and daughter that continues far past the point when one has passed.

The red currants are one noteworthy example of how textiles are important for Susan, and especially significant in thinking about her relationship with her mother, but she notes many other instances throughout her interviews. Often, these examples stand out because they also unite her with a female family member. She remembers a rug that had belonged to her great-grandmother, of which she thinks "it was definitely some hand-dyed stuff and it would have been from plants" (9-I). She also has a great-aunt, a dressmaker who, Susan surmises, "must have been interested in colours of fabrics" (10-I). Though they hadn't regularly spoken while her aunt was alive, Susan's great-aunt "has been such a big part of my life" through the diaries she left behind, and through a little quilt that "she made when she was in her last couple of years and that's the quilt I have on my ... bed every night" (27-II). In other words, textiles have been an important part of her family history, in a sense even offering a gendered genealogy of objects.

Looking at things through a gendered lens – as Jennifer, Marcea, and Erin have each done in their chapters too – highlights the kinds of labour that go into everyday objects, such as a handmade quilt or a knitted scarf, but that often become erased or taken for granted. These things have a genealogy that, when uncovered, points to gendered traditions of care and intimacy that quite literally stitched together the experiences of her family's everyday lives. Susan's insistence on learning to dye fabric and spin her own materials demonstrates her desire to participate in these traditions and to uncover past generations' unique forms of knowledge – knowledge that is under threat due to modern production and commercialization of textiles. Through her work, she has both revealed and participated in a gendered archive that is deeply meaningful to her personally and artistically.

Storytelling and Identity

This genealogy work is important for Susan because it provides knowledge about family members, and that knowledge helps establish connection with them. She says, "It really disappoints me [if] all you know ... is your great-grandmother's name. Or your ... great-grandfather, what did he do? Usually when people do genealogy they learn names, but they don't learn much else" (10-I). Susan wants more than a family name – she looks for the *stories* she knows are concealed in her family tree. Poetry and textiles allow her to form an imaginative connection with those family members, because in her creative projects she can "imagine what their life must have been ... [and] it helps me ... to ... kind of know where I come from" (10-I). She now considers herself the "family repository" (10-I), since her siblings are not as interested in family history, so she has become the bearer of the family archive. Susan doesn't simply store this genealogical material; she actively incorporates it into her writing and into the objects she treasures. In this way, she weaves her family history into her storytelling, an endeavour that she thinks about frequently since attending the workshops.

Not surprisingly, many of our collective metaphors about storytelling have close ties to textiles. As I noted earlier, the etymological and generative links between "text" and "textile" have a long history. We write about the thread of a story, or perhaps talk about how a story unravels, as Shields and Anderson highlight. Discussing an exhibition called "The Fabric of Myth," Byatt (2008) notes several more as she thinks about an essay by Kathryn Sullivan Kruger, including

> words that connect weaving with storytelling: text, texture and textile, the fabric of society, words for disintegration – fraying, frazzling, unravelling, woolgathering, loose ends. A storyteller or a listener can lose the thread ... The processes of cloth-making are knitted and knotted into our brains, though our houses no longer have spindles or looms. (n.p.)

Susan has directly employed the work of weaving and creating textiles into her poetic storytelling, but she also relies on the metaphors of this work in describing how the writing workshops challenged her foundational ideas of storytelling. A story doesn't have to start at the "beginning," she tells Jennifer; "you can start in the middle. You don't have to start at the first days I was born ... you could really pick up the thread of your life at any point and then write forwards or backwards from there" (50-II). She finds that she isn't wedded to a chronological notion of storytelling; instead, there are different threads that can be followed, and some, as Byatt notes (n.p.), can fray into oblivion while others can be integral stitches that keep the structure of the piece strong. The red currants, in one sense, had for a long period of time been tangled into a painful knot, but one that can finally be unravelled and rewoven into her larger story.

Yet storytelling for Susan remains both an essential activity and a complicated aspect of identity. As mentioned, and in keeping with the "positivity effect" that researchers on ageing have identified (Carstensen & Mikels, 2005), she doesn't "deliberately write about the ... bad stuff in my life. It tends to be the good stuff" (13f.-I). It also points to another thorny aspect of her relationship with her mother, whom she describes as a great storyteller, one who would captivate audiences. Her mother began telling stories to entertain her young children but soon became known for telling them to neighbours and friends who would visit the family home. There is now an element of competition to storytelling for Susan, such that she says, "I don't think I'm that good a storyteller. I just compare myself to other storytellers I've known" (2-II), like her mother. Weaving and poetry are two activities that allow her different media to explore her own individual approaches to storytelling. For example, she tells stories in everyday conversation, but notes that "I would say for me, the process is better on the page and that's partly because it's a place where I can [um] change things ...; it's a place where I can do my editing kind of as I go, whereas, if you start editing an oral presentation it really sounds awful" (3-II). Written storytelling lets her shape and rethink ideas in ways that oral storytelling doesn't (see de Medeiros, 2011).

The workshops have encouraged her to do more memoir-writing lately, and she has begun dealing with more difficult topics, such as saying good-bye to her camp. She and her husband had built it, and they enjoyed many years there watching their son grow up before they had to sell it because of health issues and accessibility problems related to the camp's location. Prior to writing about the camp, she had been mainly focussing on fiction in her personal writing practice. The workshops, however, have inspired her joy of writing memoir – even if it can be challenging to deal with the emotional implications. As she later thinks, the workshops encouraged her to "cover [...] ground that I really don't think about a lot ... leaving that camp behind ... it's kind of like an unresolved thinking process in my head because I don't want to think about it a lot; it just makes me sad" (2-II). Yet, the written submission sparked by the workshops and the interviews allowed her to explore "how hard it is to leave ... those camps behind [and how] they're an important part in the ... fabric of my life" (1-II). Once again, she takes the opportunity to sort through some of the snarls and knots of her story; the workshops have created a collaborative, safe space in which to untangle and process some of those knots through her writing.

Laurel Richardson (1994) thinks of writing as "a way of finding out about yourself and your topic ... Writing is also a way of 'knowing' – a method of discovery and analysis. By writing in different ways, we discover new aspects of our topic and our relationship to it" (p. 515). Though referring primarily to researchers, Richardson's point finds an echo in Jerome Bruner and Susan Weisser's (1991) observation that "autobiography turns life into text ... It is only by textualization that one can 'know' one's life" (p. 136). This emphasis upon writing as a form of discovery and knowledge, which the chapters in Part 3 will each say more about, certainly applies to the work that Susan does as a writer and poet. Her preference for written storytelling provides her with a way to gain new knowledge of past events of her life and of how she has shaped her identity along the way.

Writing as a practice involves "embedding those bits of memories into individual poems" (10-I) and stories as Susan gradually re-evaluates her texistence. Much like the work of gathering plants, dyeing fibre, and spinning wool, storytelling for Susan is an embodied practice. She prefers to write her poems and manuscripts by hand before eventually transcribing them on the computer. The craft of producing a product – be it yarn or fabric – is an essential part of the process and is very much akin to storytelling. This facet of embodiment remains a vital part of her stories: "I think about my own body and how often I tell stories about it ... you do have the ... tales of your life ... on your body" (2-I). Seeing stories as embodied, living entities prompts her to remain open to reinterpreting some of her past experiences after much time has gone by. For example, she views events that happened in her twenties much differently now that she is retired. "There was a time I wouldn't write about early boyfriends," she says to Jennifer, "and now I've written thoroughly about them" (13-I).

Her willingness to delve into these memories when prompted to do so during the workshops highlights her sense of narrative openness. Her story is far from over. As she says, "I'm very aware that I only have a certain number of years left and I ... [have] all these ideas" (22-I). Moreover, she constantly immerses herself in new learning opportunities, frequently taking new writing and art courses and contributing to two writing groups. The writing groups offer circles of supportive people with whom she feels comfortable sharing and receiving feedback on her work. The process of being critiqued entails trusting the other members of the groups to be constructive and learning from their insights. As Shields and Anderson (2001) observed in their own project involving women writers, trust plays an important role in allowing a person to open up their stories and share them with others. They note, too, that creating these supportive environments encourages people to reflect on their experiences and apply their insights to future situations (p. 16).

Reflection has therefore played an important role in Susan's life. She writes often – fiction, poetry, blog posts – and her writing frequently engages with organic themes of nature, growing food, and family. While she hasn't much written about painful events, like the deaths of her parents or selling her family camp, the writing workshops have helped with this issue, to a degree. She mentions that she actually wrote about her mother's accidental death at the workshops, and that "it was kind of surprising to me because I also read it out with the group and it's unusual for me to write about the worst things that have happened to me" (13-I). There is no fixed timeline for grief, but she has slowly started working through her vulnerability and sense of loss by exploring her emotions in writing. As evidenced in her written submission about the camp, she ends up highlighting the positive memories of family time spent there, focussing on feelings of serenity, connection with nature, and her relationship with her growing son.

The Poetics of Genealogy

All of Susan's artistic and literary activities highlight Randall's (2001) observation that "from a narrative perspective … the personal is inseparable from the poetical" (p. 38). Susan's work as an artist is fundamentally tied to how she thinks about her life and how she conceptualizes her identity. Randall further draws attention to Jerome Bruner's (1999) comment that "a life is a work of art, probably the greatest one we produce" (p. 7). However, our stories – our life-novels, if you will – possess no definite end point for when they are finished, which means that we can continually work on them, adding pieces and refining aspects, throughout our lives. It's a process that Susan knows is an integral part of being an artist. For example, she paints watercolours and acrylics and has sold a painting through a charity auction at a local restaurant while intending to submit more in the future. She is happy with the experience, but notes, "I'm quite proud of that … I'm getting better and … as I get older I hope I'll get better and better" (17-I). Improvement – getting better and cultivating one's skills – forms a necessary component of making art, be it a painting or telling one's story.

Her artwork – both literary and visual forms – offers a concrete example of her desire for interpersonal relationships. She longs to connect with others and to leave things for others to see and engage with, like her blog, where she posts regularly and makes contact with people from all around the world. She states, "I'm very motivated by what other people think" (20-I). This motivation in part has become an accountability measure, because she wants to continue providing content for her readers. But it also indicates how much her writing reaches beyond her own sense of self to connect with others. This intersubjective dimension emphasizes how "our lifestories are shaped by and entwined with the lifestories of other individuals, whether in our families and our friendships or in our intimate relationships" (Kenyon & Randall, 2001, p. 7). Literature scholar Hanna Meretoja (2014) puts it this way:

> Narrative conceptions of identity and subjectivity emphasize their social character: we become who we are in social contexts as we experience, act, speak, perceive and apprehend the world with others, and narratives – including the larger socio-cultural narrative frameworks in which they are embedded – play a constitutive role in shaping how we interpret our experiences and (inter)act in the world with others. (p. 7)

Meretoja's point focuses on how story-making is a dynamic process that necessarily involves other people. Our stories, and thus our identities, are influenced by a range of factors, including other people's stories about who we are and the larger sociocultural stories that constantly circulate around us. To return to the metaphor of textiles, our stories are all woven together in profound ways, our narrative worlds intricately entwined, such that it is sometimes difficult to separate the stitching of whose story is whose. Susan incorporates this dynamic understanding of storytelling in her interactions with her readers, and she directly responds to their thoughts and ideas on her blog.

Susan expresses this desire for intersubjective storytelling in other ways as well. Throughout all of her artistic and genealogical work runs the longing to leave a narrative legacy to others. Just as she feels the textures and weights of the stories from family members such as her mother, grandmother, and aunt, so too does she want to pass along her stories, ideas, and thoughts to someone else's narrative. As Randall and McKim (2008) suggest:

> This passion for genealogy which many of us develop naturally with age is fueled in part by the desire to bequeath a feeling for our heritage to those who come after us, lest they fail to appreciate the complex layers of history that lie beneath them and the nests of stories into which they have been born. (p. 277)

Genealogy, then, is a multifaceted process of locating one's own roots as well as looking forward to help others identify their own backgrounds and narrative circumstances. Genealogy, which reaches into the past, is in a real sense tied to generativity, which reaches out to the future. Part of what Susan wants her legacy to be involves imparting lessons to her son, to continue the storytelling genealogy she has inherited: "I try and get him to think about things as being part of a larger fabric … that we're … involved in" (26-II). A major part of her impetus for writing stems from her desire to leave something, some piece of herself, for others to discover. At the same time, she contributes to a larger human narrative:

> We're all gone … after a certain length of time and what's left of us except this wonderful great big story of humanity? All this information that somehow gets carried on and every one of us has something to contribute … It's almost like a living thing that … goes through time and … there's a bit of you in there and there's a bit of me. (43-II)

Susan here offers a beautiful vision of a grand human story in which everyone plays an important part. At its centre lies her acknowledgment of the limits of individual mortality, but death does not mean that her story must die. Instead, she invokes a more capacious sense of human temporality in which she participates with a multitude of others. It's a reflection that has profound implications for her own relationship to the loss of her parents, wherein the red currants come to symbolize how painful events can be rewoven into a new story of familial love and care.

Taken in conjunction with Susan's interest in family history, we could call this view *genealogical time* – our individual stories are all knitted into a larger story of humanity as family. She once again connects this idea of storytelling and time to the metaphor of textiles: "ordinary lives can be of importance … not just for … study [but to] add to the … historical fabric" (42-II). Jens Brockmeier (2002) also understands memory and personal identity as being "inextricably interwoven with the countless texts and contexts of culture" in which such memory "is part of an infinite intertext that stretches out not only into the present but also the past" (p. 457). Randall and McKim (2008) further see the motivation to be part of a larger cosmic or historical fabric as a significant element of positive ageing. They write of a person's "need … to leave a legacy, to harvest the wisdom that has been silently amassing inside us across the years, and … to mix it in with the soil of the world, for the benefit of others' growth as well" (p. 276). Susan desires to pass on objects in the form of stories and textiles that have been meaningful to her and that will hopefully be significant for others.

Susan notes that while she may be retired, she finds herself as busy as ever, becoming engrossed in her writing and art to the point where she dislikes interruptions such as appointments or grocery shopping. Her writing, spinning, and genealogical work provide her with a rich source of learning and value, and these activities motivate her to be mindful of the different stages of her life and her relationships with family and friends. She is also, as I say, continually trying out new storytelling tools, such as a blog that allows her to make virtual connections with people around the world. At the same time, she frequently returns to the work of textile-making[3] as a tangible reminder of her relationships with the women in her family. The physical touch of the material and the process of artistic making help her to reflect on the complicated emotions, expectations, and insights that are embedded in the several threads of her texistence.

3 *Editors' note*: An activity supplemented by perishable objects held in suspension in a freezer until the time is right for them to colour the woven threads.

12 Mahogany Table: Bringing Things Together

MATTE ROBINSON AND BRANDI ESTEY-BURTT

What is really going on in things, what is really happening, is always "to come." Every time you try to stabilise the meaning of a thing, try to fix it in its missionary position, the thing itself, if there is anything at all to it, slips away.

–John D. Caputo (1997, p. 31)

In this concluding chapter of Part 2, we turn to a gentleman who has done much of our work for us. And he has done it by implicitly weaving together a number of the themes that we've been considering in the book – about the larger stories that we live within and the master narratives that live within us, about shadow stories and family stories and possible selves, about genealogy and generativity, about sense-making, symbol-making, and myth-making, about our landscape of consciousness and our horizon of self-understanding, about autobiographical reasoning and post-formal thought, and, overall, the incredible complexity, the poetics, of narrative identity in later life. Each of the things considered in previous chapters emerged as significant in the pieces of writing that our participants submitted or in their interviews with Jennifer, or both. However, "David," as we call him, had already chosen a cherished object and made it the focus of his meditation on its symbolic value in his life in an eleven-page essay complete with endnotes that he composed prior to the second interview. The family table, from its origins in the building materials and the craftsman who made it, through its role as gathering place to its travels and its uncertain future as a material object, is transformed in this searching piece of prose into a powerful symbol of gathering. The table is the linchpin of the text, which was born of the writing workshop, and the essay now functions as a newly created text-thing that can be reproduced and disseminated to future generations who may never see or experience the table itself as an object.

Through his memories and reflections in this essay, David connects the family's memories and genealogy to the origins of humanity, to the original gathering that forms the first communities of the first people. Matte has already highlighted in Chapter 3 the deep etymological connection between the word "thing" and a sense of gathering – the first sense of the word, now archaic, remains "a meeting" (*Oxford English Dictionary*), and thus a thing was an event, bound less by matter than by time and location. David's written submission, entitled "Our table, a time for gathering," links the table via the unconventional appositive to *a time* and not to an object, and he makes full use of the "excess" of the table-object, its thingness, to expand his meditation to the scale of the cosmos: "the Universe's emergence through deep time has carried a spiritual dimension," and the emergence of that dimension is inseparable from – is identical to – the emergence of human beings, "co-creators" through the process of gathering (p. 2).[1] The table as symbol (which is how we first encountered it; it is safe to say that few, if not none, of our readers or our research team have been in the table's physical presence) operates on these many scales at once. David is co-creator of this symbol, along with the craftsman who fashioned the table, but chiefly also with the table itself, which did the job of gathering friends and family to it and which also exceeded this role such that it would so occupy his thoughts during the workshops. The symbol he has made out of the table gathers, in the manner in which symbols gather, thoughts of gathering – in the manner in which people gather around a table, a fire, or some other thing. The moment when gathering first occurs is the moment when humanity first arises as co-creation.

David's submitted essay, or story, focuses on that moment of the first gathering-spot, which was probably a fire and not a table, he reasons, "sometime between 2.5 million and 30,000 years ago" (p. 2). Though the table has largely replaced the fire as the locus of gathering in this written piece, the fact of gathering, he speculates, probably brings about the fact of language. As Matte has traced in Chapter 3, thingness likely did emerge, in a primordial way, along with language as the narrating

1 *Editors' note*: This seems a classic, even extreme, example of what psychologist of ageing Jeffrey Webster would call a "time expansive" orientation on one's life and one's world (Webster 2011, p. 436). In a sense, it also illustrates Lars Tornstam's (1997) controversial concept of "gerotranscendence," which he calls "the contemplative dimension of aging," one aspect of which is an increasing blurring of the boundaries, in an older person's mind, between the past, present, and future, or, to put the point in more narrative terms, between one's story as an individual and the story of the universe, of the cosmos. (For more on the experience of time in later life, see McFadden & Atchley, 2001; for more on "contemplative aging," see Sherman, 2010.)

human mind grew up alongside the things that humans co-created with their environments; in other words, humans are always already technological, narrating beings. David uses the process of imaginatively recreating the emergence of the first human consciousness to rediscover the intimacy – and spirituality – that once characterized life on Earth (p. 3), "the grand liturgy of the universe itself" (p. 3), he says, borrowing from creation spirituality theologian Thomas Berry (see, e.g., 1987). The birth of humanity is also the birth of ritual, and ritual joins the here and now with the totality of the universe – ritual, thing, and gathering all emerge at once to co-produce the human and the universe.

The Table's Shadow

These meditations in his story lead to a recognition that Indigenous peoples in Canada "maintain this tradition of recognition of intimacy with a transcendent power" (p. 3). Is this a suggestion that Indigenous people of Canada maintain an unbroken tradition dating back to ancient, primordial times? His experience as a lawyer with the government discussing treaty rights appears to have deeply affected him, seems to have confirmed for him that gathering is somehow the beginning of spiritual and thus for him human existence. The "sharing of stories" came out of those first meetings, he reasons (p. 4). The spiritual consideration of gathering, through ritual and symbol, to a single place or moment or thing contrasts with the temporal movements of peoples, occupations, and settlements that form the other main thread running through both the interviews and his written story. Apart from the force that gathers is a force that scatters, brings into conflict, requires thoughtful consideration and reconciliation. These shadows of gathering are also gathered together under the symbol of the human thing.

Before we can get to the bottom of these far-reaching meditations, the text of his writing interrupts its own flow to focus on the deeply personal and speak directly, in the second person (as if in a letter), to his children, the intended immediate audience of this text. He prompts them to recall certain important, character-defining moments that happened around the table over the years: "You will remember ..." (p. 6). Though the piece is written from a distinctly Christian faith, there is an ecumenical openness to other faiths. For instance, Tibetan Buddhism sits at the table in the form of a singing bowl that they have brought back from their travels. There is the recognition that the family's heritage was Jamaican and Jewish, that their ancestors had travelled to Jamaica likely to escape pogroms and over time been made to convert to Christianity. The Sephardic Jews of Portugal began emigrating to Jamaica as early as the 1490s, the decade of the so-called discovery of the "New World," but his own genealogical researches on his family suggest that his ancestors from the Iberian peninsula were later immigrants who had already been forced to lose most of their faith and had left to join the large community of Sephardic Jews in then-British Jamaica (6-I).

His meditation on the table is also a complex and multidimensional meditation on colonial relationships, on the strife and oppression that prompts human movements and migrations, on the miracle that any group can come together at all in fellowship. At the same time, it points to narrative fractures and fragments that arise when people turn against one another in violence and oppression. Who would he and his family be had they not been forced to convert or to move a continent away? Two significant contrasts appear in the figures of the First Nations people he will meet with after his move to Canada, who offer the possibility of an unbroken tradition that is nevertheless colonized and imposed upon by the very government he represents, and the craftsman who made the table, who though displaced nevertheless retains noticeable ties to Africa.

As a work of craft, the table is bound up with its Jamaican craftsman, who is named in the text of the story and whose African heritage contrasts with the Christianized Jewish heritage of David, who shared the same island with him. There is profound respect for the craftsman, who brings a relationship to the materials of the wood that David considers as an extra human sense, "an inner feeling for the nature of the wood he was so carefully crafting into our table" (p. 8). The family, together with the craftsman, chose three "different kinds of African mahogany" (p. 8) for the table, and in the mind of David the table and its craftsman share a mystical bond in that connection to Africa, the birthplace of the first human gatherings: "I remember one of the pieces of wood was particularly aromatic and caused him to sneeze a lot – an allergic-like reaction. Was it that the tree-spirit was reminding [him] of his deep roots in the land from which the boards came?" (p. 8). This animistic way of thinking places the agency with the thing, the table, whose inherent properties (spirit) draw out an involuntary physical relationship in the maker's body, though both material and maker are displaced from their place of origin. Through the shared African heritage of wood and woodworker, David seems to believe that the table itself, produced by hand and without "fancy electric tools" (p. 8), helps connect first the craftsman and then those who gather at the table itself to the rich heritage of human gatherings dating back to the dawn of time. Though his own family history, stories, and traditions have been changed by oppression and forced conversion, through the making of the table he is able to bypass the intervening millennia and reconnect to the original gathering that must have taken place amongst a group of human ancestors somewhere in Africa.

David's tendency to single out African and Indigenous North American cultures as somehow more authentically connected with *things*, with the materials from which things are crafted, is a romanticizing one, and it calls attention to his relative silence about his own cultural heritage. There is some anxiety about the privilege afforded to a white, Christian family that has the power and resources to leave Jamaica in 1976. There is on the one hand an identification with the island and its "sociological background, the nature of the island of Jamaica, how it was formed, what traumas it went through, and, and we are products of that" (5-II), and on the other an unexplored sense of *not* having such direct access to the culture or things that are enjoyed by members of North America's First Nations or the African craftsman who built the table.

The craftsman is also a "wonderful storyteller" (p. 7), who is still in possession of the tales of Anansi brought over from Africa. David does not seem to have any delightful stories from his own cultural ancestry, but a member of his family does the illustrations for a book about Anansi, with text written by a white, knighted British Jamaican and produced as a charity project for underprivileged children and reprinted in 2014, again as a fundraiser. All this information is included in the rich text that David was inspired by the workshops to compose.

The text about the table thus serves to educate his children about the complexities of Jamaica, part of his desire "peel off the layers of Jamaica and say something significant as far as I can see it for [his children] to understand who they are" (17-II): the family left Jamaica in 1976, when the children were still young, and before he dies David wants to give them the narrative tools to understand their Jamaican heritage, uneasy as he might himself be about his place in it.

What is left (mostly) unsaid is that, despite identifying with the dominant, privileged cultures first in Jamaica and then in Canada, an erasure has happened somewhere in his own family history, cutting one thread of tradition and replacing it with an oppressor's. The table is the thing he has built to make anew the connection to the primordially human gathering with things, to build a family and a community around gatherings for meals. Through the symbolic table, and the text-thing that is his meditation on it, he can connect his family, the microcosm, with the original act that was the co-creation of the human and the divine; though the gaps in his own family history can likely never be filled in, the table represents an attempt to reconnect to the wellspring.

The Table as (Spiritual) Thing

> It wasn't Moses leaving, leading the people out of slavery, but we too packed up and left Jamaica. (6-I)

In her book *Material Spirituality in Modernist Women's Writing*, Elizabeth Anderson (2020) seeks a middle way between Bill Brown's emphasis on the "excess" of things and the work of anthropologists such as Arjun Appaduari (1988), who uses the social life of things to describe identity formation:

> My work hovers between these two views. I am interested in the relationship between subjects and objects, that is, where the boundaries between the two erode, where material objects provoke intersubjectivity, and the ethical and aesthetic implications of the meeting, meshing and differences of subjects and objects. Yet I am also concerned with how material things (natural, handcrafted or manufactured) remain irreducibly other, and where this radical alterity may be an instantiation of the sacred. (p. 11)

Bill Brown's thing theory served as an apt departure point for Matte's chapter in Part 2 of this book, on sea-glass and the "excess" of the thing, a mystery from which springs the possibility of new narratives, metaphors, and combinations of subjectivities. Anderson's reformulation of the "irreducible otherness" as a potential means to the sacred – as Leonard Cohen (1992) put it, "there's a crack in every*thing* / that's how the light gets in" (emphasis ours) – speaks particularly well for this table, whose role as gatherer of people, communities, and stories mirrors the role of the literary symbol that it has become in its owner's meditation.

In closing this part of the book, we ask in what ways the "excess" of the thing opens up new possibilities for telling one's own story: it is a means to the sacred, but to what other hermeneutics of our own life narratives might it also speak? We argue that writing about cherished objects can shift the significance of those objects away from the things themselves – things that clutter up our lives in the end – and towards a level of abstraction that can nevertheless be passed on to future generations and enrich our life narratives. In a very real sense David's meditation on the table is a process of saying goodbye to the physical table and replacing it with the idea of the table, the table as generator of stories but also as gatherer of meaning. It is a different kind of *thing* after having undergone this process, which takes the form of mourning the physical thing while also celebrating the thing's abstract value. It is a celebration of life through the ritual discarding of the physical shell of life.

Rather than recalling Moses leading his people, the move from Jamaica to Canada suggests Noah's journey, and the table acts as a kind of ark, not in the sense of a vessel but as a container, such as the Ark of the Covenant or even the ark that carried Moses to safety, of something about the family's history and connection to the sacred. The table's dimensions are listed carefully in David's essay, just as Noah's ark's measurements are specified: "It measures 79" x 47.5" and 2.5" thick. The base on which it rests is also heavy, two blocks measuring 27" x 26" between which is a bar 38" x 8". These are also 2.5" thick; it is solid and well-made, but its heaviness and bulk make transport a real problem ... Its future is therefore uncertain" (p. 8). While now a potential problem because of its sheer physicality, that heavy table had previously acted as an anchor for the family, joining them together in mutual presence and companionship. David describes to Jennifer the first time that they sat at the table in explicitly religious terms:

> So we decided that the first meal on this table would be a eucharistic celebration ... [with] close friends and family and it was a wonderful experience reminiscent to a degree of the Seder meal that the Jewish celebrate at Passover. (6-I)

This first meal combines the Jewish and Christian elements of David's family history into a harmonious whole, in which different religious traditions were honoured together. At this moment, several human beings take time out of busy routines to come together as a family, nourish each other, and renew their relationships. The presence of others has a sacred connotation: it is a gift to be both given and received. As he puts it, "it has a sense of community, it has a feel of openness and sharing" (6-I). He goes on to connect "gathering at a table [with] these folks ... and then this development of a kind of spirituality that there is something larger than us here" (8-I).

This memory of their first meal at the table functions as a cornerstone for David, in which his family and the table become permanently fused in an experience of ritual. It is one to which he often returns, sometimes as a point of comparison to his life in the present. Perhaps this is why he laments the busyness of contemporary life and the fact that his children seem rarely to pause or unite within a physical space. All adults now, they are spread across the globe with their own families – "So, so far away" (4-I), he wistfully remarks. At the same time, though he senses that things, that life, must change, he laments the "hectic busy rush" (9-I) in which family gatherings now seem to occur only at Christmas or special occasions a couple of times a year. There seem to be few opportunities for presence anymore, and this fact causes him some regret. There is thus something about preservation and loss in this text: he feels the urgent need to write about his family's Jamaican heritage for the kids, and the table gathers unto itself both its physical components and ties to the storyteller-craftsman who provided the deeper cultural connection to African Jamaica and its symbolic components as "a time for gathering."

But first and foremost, the text about the table is a preservation of the essence[2] or thingness of the table itself, even if the actual physical object has an uncertain future. Any table of a suitable size can fulfil the necessary function of tablehood, but this particular table's story, which includes the story of its components, its African-Jamaican storyteller craftsman, and the family's meetings and gatherings around it – as well as the way such meetings and gatherings connect the family to the larger ritual and sacrament of gathering for meals, which they share with the first human gathered around the first human-produced fire, the very first things – is the family's story and, by extension into the macrocosm, the story of humanity and the emergence of the first sacred thing.

The table is, in many respects, his romanticized vision of gathering, his own familial version of what happens in other cultures and groups. Discussing Canada's Indigenous peoples, he values in his essay how many Indigenous communities prioritize the transmission of knowledge and spirituality to the next generation: "So again you see … this is a kind of spirituality that has been handed down to them from generation on … generation and so again, I see that as … reflected or resonated in our tradition of giving thanks at … the meal" (p. 9). Once again, however, he hesitates to explore the complex dimensions of either his relationship to Canada's Indigenous people or his own role in his Jamaican heritage, a reticence perhaps tinged with ambivalence, not unlike Hermann, perhaps, and his heritage as a German (see Chapter 7, this volume).

Playing on Brown's "Secret Life of Things," Elizabeth Anderson (2020) writes of the "spiritual life of things" in modernist texts, the consideration of which reveals "not only how these texts represent things (mimesis) but also how they participate in world building (poesis)" (p. 7). David's table was built with the intention of its having a spiritual life, originally also having matching benches to suggest "monastic simplicity" (p. 8). The family's first meal together at the table was a mass, at which the discussion of Jesus's communal meals also recalls the Seder (pp. 8f.). David had recently gone on a pilgrimage, his first, at the time of this table's coming into being; he had walked the Camino de Santiago pilgrimage in Spain, and in the future would take many Camino journeys. But the solid, beautiful table was created only a few years before they would leave for Canada, and there remain many details as yet uncovered, stories yet untold, about that parting that threw the table's future into uncertainty.

2 *Editors' note*: With apologies to Clive in his Afterword.

After the family's move to Canada, the table has to be "deconstructed" to fit into the smaller kitchen of their new home. It must be cut down to a more appropriate size that will correspond with the dimensions of their much different life in another country. The table is no longer an ark carrying a single family into a new life together but an object vulnerable to being cut and recut to new shapes. David realizes that, on a practical level, it is a massive object that cannot easily be carried around or managed by his son, who is now in possession of it. In this sense, he is grieving a loss of connection with his family, but he is also grieving the table as a material object that has played a tremendously important role in his life. He has formed a unique sense of kinship with the table, which is more than simply a passive object.

"Things act and interact," write Miguel Astor-Aguilera and Graham Harvey (2018, p. 2). Astor-Aguilera and Harvey discuss how understandings of things and their relational aspects are changing in light of new studies in animism. Different forms of animism emphasize how the spiritual and interactive aspects become entwined in things so that they are not merely viewed as inert objects. Animism – including Indigenous, pagan, and some Christian practices – highlights how things can be agents and underscores how humans can have significant spiritual and emotional bonds with that which is other-than-human. These insights are becoming increasingly important as human communities seek more respectful relationships to the more-than-human world in response to issues such as climate change, mass extinction, and exploitative economic policies. Yet, these perceptions of things as spiritual agents applies not just to non-human animals, but to a range of things that play key parts in people's lives.

The thingness of the table therefore emerges as a multidimensional concept layering symbolism, spirituality, and relationality together. It's no wonder David is having difficulty letting it go – it has functioned as more than an aid for his family gatherings and instead become a thing with which he has formed a significant personal and spiritual bond. His emotional investment in this relationship means that his feelings of bereavement are very much legitimate responses to a situation of loss. This table has been with him for decades, throughout the growth of his children and through one very difficult move to a far-away country.

A major problem for David, however, now lies in reconceiving the symbolic and spiritual aspects of the table to reflect his family's new diasporic reality. Visits to his children in Australia offer new opportunities to have meals and embrace different objects and practices such as the singing bowl. But he also is in the process of reflecting on other possibilities for connecting to his family and to a shared heritage, one that can cross the vast distances between them in a way the table simply cannot. The workshops appear to have offered him another such tentative way forward, helping him to understand his own story and adding to his narrative resilience.

The Workshops

The workshops and the act of writing that they inspired him to do have encouraged David to see new possibilities for reflection. He frequently points out how his professional career, as someone involved in the Canadian legal system, made him something of an over-preparer. The workshops' spontaneous exercises encouraged him to try new ways of expressing himself and not worry as much about perfection in the resulting story. Moreover, they helped him take ownership of his own story and invest himself in the process of structuring, revising, and editing it as he sees fit. As he frequently mentions, he does not plan to publish this story – it is for him and for his family alone. Perhaps this is also why it is never finished for him – writing is a process that does not necessarily have an end point. He can go back to his letter, to the story he is telling his children, and add details, add memories. At one point, he even thinks that he will encourage his children to add their own memories or perspectives on events so that *their* children can hear those views. Talk about generative narration, and narrative openness! The process becomes an open invitation to unfold, embracing new reflections and incorporating the voices of others. It also helps him reappraise his identity as one that is perhaps more open to uncertainty and spontaneity than he had thought, given the extent to which his professional identity shaped his sense of self.

In other words, the story itself can potentially function in similar ways to that of the table. It provides a point of connection among family members, through which they can renew their relationships to each other and to their own family history. As the writer, David gives of his own presence and time to stitch the various memories and reflections together. Yet he also invites collaboration by asking his family members to add their own versions of memories to the essay once they get it. They, like the craftsman who built the original table, can participate and share in the co-creation of this new family object. Though it was written in part to address his sense of loss at the table and physical gathering, the letter and the stories it contains offer him an opportunity to rethink connection in a digital, frantically busy age. Connection does not *just* occur at the table – it can be forged and enacted in multiple ways, ways that David and his family are still figuring out.

David's anxieties about the table and today's pace of life echo sociologist Sinikka Elliott's ongoing work on how food, family gathering, and the kitchen table become romanticized (see, e.g., Bowen et al., 2019). David's concerns about how dispersed his family is as well as how little they are able to sit down at their own meals due to their work and activity schedules are common. For Elliott, they demonstrate a shared feeling that families are fragile in the midst of significant societal changes. These are valid worries, she notes, but they risk focussing on gathering in the kitchen as symbol of moral good that places much pressure on families. The danger lies in moralizing a symbol to the point of nostalgia and ignoring the social realities that burden many families today – and burdened them in the past. Nor does it account for the inequalities that structure who can sit at the table in the first place. Those who are working several jobs to pay the bills or those who live in food deserts often do not have the luxury of sitting at the table together to share nourishing food, stories, and rituals. In other words, the table can never be a neutral object, nor can any lament for it be untethered from sociological matters.

To some extent, David realizes this aspect, even as he wants the table to provide a structure for his own memories and his own hopes for connection. The table in its bulk and its tactility has offered a comforting touchpoint for his own spiritual and genealogical identity. How does one do this work of identity-making without the mooring of this particular object, especially in later life? If the table no longer holds his family and his spiritual convictions about gathering together, what will help stitch the resulting fracture in his life story?

The chapters in Part 1 of this book explored one pivotally important means of doing identity-work in later life, namely narrative reflection. And they noted the largely narrative challenges that can face older adults, including perceptions of ageing as inevitable deterioration in terms of physical health: the powerful "narrative of decline" (Gullette, 2004) that shapes our society's views on what ageing is. Moreover, a person's story becomes entangled with that narrative when it is assumed that there is, in fact, little possibility for real growth in later life. Happily, recent research in gerontology – certainly in narrative gerontology (see, e.g., de Medeiros, 2013) – contests such a narrative, positing instead that ageing can be an exciting process of discovery and the opening up of new opportunities, for meaning, spirituality, and wisdom (Randall & McKim, 2008). Having a strong story – or narrative resilience – emerges as one key element for this more positive understanding.

Though in the interviews David demonstrates a profound reflectivity about his life, he points out that actually writing down his thoughts and shaping them into a coherent entity is an entirely different activity. He starts asking new questions and going in unique directions: "I started wandering off into the question of why do we gather? Why don't we just go off in the corner and eat? Or by ourselves?" (1-II). Writing solicits a different kind of attention to the subject of one's life. Like other artistic activities such as drawing or painting, the writer must rethink the elements that are often taken for granted and – like drawing – learn to see people, memories, and events in a new light.

This process of defamiliarization via writing requires David to choose which memories to focus on and which details to include, all the while considering his audience – his family. His son's asking him to share his memories shows him that there are other viable ways to pass along his knowledge and reflections to his children than just gathering around the table. David thinks of his own father who, after being diagnosed with a terminal illness, was unable to write about his experiences in local Jamaican politics. Having also experienced the deaths of two friends, David is considering his own mortality and what he will leave of himself for his family. Now, "the table story is ... a chapter in ... what is going to be quite a long letter to my children and grandchildren" (2-II). It can be shared amongst all of them, while only person at a time can retain possession of the table.

Through this letter, the table transforms into an altogether different object: a digital one. Digital objects are decidedly more portable, as well as more instantaneously shared, but there are both positive elements and drawbacks to such portability. They raise important questions about the symbolism of all types of objects: for example, do digital objects function in ways similar to those of material ones? What impacts do they have on virtual and other relationships? In one research study, digital objects were perceived to possess fewer lasting symbolic connotations (Petrelli & Whittaker, 2010), yet digital objects such as photos, videos, art, communications, and more are being increasingly preserved by families. In other words, digital objects are becoming more and more important parts of our lived environments. Researchers Daniela Petrelli and Steve Whittaker suggest that family members are asked to become "digital curator[s]" (p. 155). At the moment, David seems to be debating the role of digital objects as a one-to-one replacement for the physical object that has meant so much to him. It's another subject of ambivalence for him, but for now his letter provides a unique mode of connection to his family that the table can no longer give.

Despite his misgivings about the table, David discovers a level of intentionality to writing his story that he finds exciting as well as challenging. The activity also offers an opportunity for growth, wherein he can continue to work at his writing and improve; he remarks to Jennifer that "the writing process is a constantly changing, hopefully improving business" (4-II). He may be thinking about mortality as part of the impetus for his story, but life has not stopped in the meantime. Rather, it is still full of possibilities, even for new-found confidence in his writing and reading skills (8f-II).

Writing also possesses spiritual possibilities, in a way becoming a kind of pilgrimage into the self. David's fundamental question about why human beings gather instead of eating alone is, for Rowan Williams (2007), a highly spiritual one. At its centre, the question of how we gather for a meal asks how we are to relate to our neighbours as individuals. Williams, a theologian and the former archbishop of Canterbury, understands this type of query as an open-ended invitation that seeks a relationship rooted in sharing and presence instead of an attempt to control others. Discussing the early desert Christian monastics, Williams notes the "compromises that the presence of other human beings entails" (p. 12), but he observes that the "literature associated with the early generations of desert ascetics" grapples with "how humanity is to be understood – about life, death, and neighbors" as well as the interior spiritual life of prayer. In other words, their writing formed a significant part of their spiritual experiences and how they dealt with the challenges of life, mortality, and relationships.

For someone like David, who often meditates on his own spiritual experiences and path and seems to operate at a somewhat advanced "stage of faith" (Fowler, 1981), writing has become an important tool of interpreting and understanding himself and his history. Like Williams, David invokes the necessity of coming to terms with uncertainty by linking the spontaneity of writing to a broader sense of unpredictability in life. His is clearly no "security narrative" but a "growth narrative" instead (Bauer & Park, 2010). Nor does he exemplify the "positivity effect" (Carstensen & Mikels, 2005) that gerontologists have identified at work in many older adults. Rather, he is notably open to the questions and ambiguities with which life presents him. In talking to Jennifer, for instance, he says that "I like the uncertainty because I think … that's part of the reality of our life journey. I mean you … can't detail this thing … called life down … many have tried, I think, most of them have failed" (36-II). Part of his own spiritual journey has involved reckoning with the instability of life as well its implications for how he meets with other people along that path. It is not necessarily an easy activity, as demonstrated by his conflicting feelings about the busyness of life, the future of the table, and the scattering of his family across the globe. It is, however, a noteworthy pursuit that does not have a definite end point. David plans to revisit his letter, adding and subtracting pieces and memories; it is a never-finished process subject to perpetual reinterpretation and new perspectives on his past and his future.

David's feelings about his life journey mirror his thoughts on his own family history dating back to Spain and Portugal. This history is one of continuous change and migration, in terms of religious identity as well as geographical location. It is a pattern of transformation that he thinks about in his own spiritual practices, such as when he walked the Camino. That particular endeavour melds the physical activity of walking with spiritual contemplation. Like writing, the Camino is an exercise in uncertainty and exploration; it creates a space for wonder as well as an opportunity to confront the uncomfortable aspects of one's life. Lee Hoinacki (1996), a former Dominican priest and political scientist, writes of this curious conjunction of pain and exhaustion with an intensity of joyful feeling (p. 15). Immersing oneself in this intensity becomes an important element of appreciating the beauty of the journey. Hoinacki and David both share a gratitude for those human pilgrims who have helped shape the path they too have walked. The Camino becomes another way for David to explore his place in a much longer story of family – and human – change.

Thanks to prompts from the workshops, David's written story becomes a meeting point for all of his interests in spirituality, genealogy, and human history. The materials for his table had been carefully chosen – as noted above, it comprised three different types of mahogany, all of which could be traced back to Africa, the birthplace of humanity – but so too is his story carefully composed from raw materials. Words are shaped into new form like the wood, and memories and details are sanded and cut into a new kind of object as he goes beyond "just basic memory" (28-II) to parse the central issues of his life. Just like gathering at the table, writing requires a sense of presence (10-II), and the workshops have helped him "view myself more carefully, perhaps more objectively" (35-II). The letter itself provides a link to the important objects, traditions, and rituals of the past while opening a productive gateway to a new, more virtual form of gathering via the Internet and digital objects. David hasn't yet addressed some of his more painful moments – the trauma of leaving Jamaica, for example, the very sort of troubling experience that "demands more storytelling work" (McAdams, 2008, p. 253). But perhaps those issues will be worked through in future iterations of his letter, or even in more personal, written meditations.

PART THREE

Pathways of Practice

13 Things to Know about Life-Writing Groups: Some Variables Involved

WILLIAM L. RANDALL

There is little of greater importance to each of us than gaining a perspective on our own life story, to find, clarify, and deepen meaning in the accumulated experience of a lifetime.

–James Birren & Donna Deutchman (1991, p. 1)

Writing Our Life Stories

Through these inquiries into our participants' worlds, we've seen how the things that people refer to, and write about, as significant in their lives – a packet of love letters in the case of Joy, a quilt in that of Amelie, a torn page for Harriet, some currants in a freezer for Susan, a ring for Hermann, a beer stein for Joan, a table for David, or "tens of thousands" of pieces of glass for Mary and Bob – can serve as windows onto just how intricate and intriguing their stories really are. It is time, then, to tap back into some of the concepts we introduced in Part 1, especially Chapter 2, and, taking a more practical tack, consider how older adults can explore their storyworlds more deeply by participating in groups that help them write about their lives. With that in mind, let me introduce my friend Viviane Edwards.

Two months prior to beginning this chapter, I helped Viviane celebrate her eightieth birthday. To mark the occasion, some twenty of us toasted her with budget champagne at a lovely little garden party organized to recognize yet another year that the group she launched and leads has been going on. A retired professor, she had emailed me some nine years before asking if we could meet at my favourite coffee shop so that she could run by me an idea she'd recently been toying with. In turn, a short time before that, she had attended a one-day event put on by me and my colleague Beth McKim entitled "Reading and Writing Our Lives: A

Workshop on the Poetics of Growing Old." "I was so inspired by that day," she said to me eagerly once we were seated with our drinks, "that I want to start a group like that for other older adults my age who, like me, want to write some of our stories. It could be a lot of fun."

Thus began "Writing Our Life Stories," or WOLS as its members fondly call it. Now heading into its tenth year (during COVID, using Zoom to hold its meetings), WOLS brings together twenty or more older adults ranging in age from sixty to ninety for two-hour sessions twice a month each fall and winter to read aloud to one another the stories they've written in the intervening weeks. Often, the stories they write and read concern comical or unusual situations that they're eager to get down on paper before their memory of them dims. Since the audience they have in mind is typically their children and grandchildren, it's a way of engaging in *transmissive* reminiscence, one of the types that I outlined in Chapter 2. It's a means of passing on information about what their life was like in the past, and some of the life lessons they've learned, the hard-won wisdom they've gained – what John Kotre (1984) calls *generative transference* (pp. 30f.). But as a number of them confessed to me the afternoon of the party, it's something they do for themselves as well. It's a way of revisiting events that are somehow central to their sense of self – their turning-point stories or signature stories, for instance, or memories that are especially self-defining. It's a way of pulling themselves together in memory and imagination, of engaging in the identity work, the "storywork" (Randall, 2010), that is vital to our continuing development in later life. It's what psychologists call *integrative* reminiscence, one variation on which, as per Erin's thoughts on Harriet, is conceivably *feminist* reminiscence.

Every autumn, I invite Viviane to bring along a couple of group members with her to my course on narrative gerontology, where naturally reminiscence is among the many topics that are on the docket for discussion. I ask them to tell my students what it's like to be part of such a group and why they think it has gone on so long. The last time they came, Viviane brought with her a collection of stories that had been written by a number of the members and that she had self-published in a book called *Remembered* (Edwards, 2018). Literally, the stories have been transformed into a thing, one that more than a few WOLS members may view someday as having "cherished" status. She also distributed around the room copies of a two-page statement that she had taken the time to prepare in order to explain what WOLS is and isn't. Here are a few excerpts from it:

> When people ask me what "Writing Our Lives" is all about, the best answer I can give is: "We get together, we read our stories, and we celebrate who we are and what we were." ... Unlike a "Writer's Group," which usually is intended

> to support people who hope to publish and to improve the quality of their writing, this group is for anyone who has something to say to future generations ... What WOLS provides is a secure environment for reading what you have written, an opportunity to be inspired by what you hear others read, an opportunity to share your thoughts with others, and a constant reminder that the time to write is NOW. *"Too soon our tomorrows are yesterdays"* ... For some people reading is the impetus that forces them to write. They will always be applauded. Their writing skills are never questioned. We consider the story that is read *a gift to the group.* (emphasis Viviane's)

The group that Viviane so faithfully facilitates (she speaks of it as a personal mission almost) is but one of the two growing trends that I wrote about at the start of Chapter 1 and that constitute the context to which the book is addressed. Narrative scholar Robert Atkinson (2006) cites evidence of this trend in a full-page article in *The New York Times* in 2000 heralding how "thousands" of American adults are "getting together to look back at their lives and share their stories" (p. 86). It's impossible, of course, to access accurate statistics since, like the members of WOLS, so many of these thousands are getting together in a comparatively informal, ad hoc manner. Furthermore, if such statistics were available they would likely be tipped in favour of women over men, in keeping with the gender differences in narrative activity and narrative complexity that I noted back in Chapter 2. That's certainly the case with WOLS, as it was with the workshops that our participants attended, where there were four women for every man. It's a pattern that others have noted as well. "It may ... be that writing an autobiography," posits one source cautiously, "is a typically more feminine activity than it is a masculine one" (O'Neill et al., 2011, p. 155). If so, and as I hinted back in Chapter 2, this pattern implies that women in general may be more narratively resilient than men, which in turn could play some part in why, as statistics routinely show, they live longer.

Such gender imbalances aside for the moment, the proliferation of life-writing groups period is a trend that's worth noting, I submit, for the validation it implicitly lends to a narrative perspective on ageing. And it's a testament to the need that many older adults in general experience to engage in some sort of "life story work" (Kunz & Soltys, 2007; Soltys & Kunz, 2007), and the potential of that engagement to enrich the inner resources that they bring to the challenges of later life. This third part of our book, then, is where the rubber meets the road as far as narrative gerontology is concerned.

My aim in this chapter is scarcely to survey the many different types of life-writing groups that exist out there. Given the "thousands" of older adults involved in them at any given time, that would require writing another whole book. But I would at least like to consider some of the broad variables that are at work in how such groups operate. Doing so will provide some context for appreciating the workshops that were central to the research on which this book is based – workshops that I participated in myself, as did Jennifer and Clive – and which, in the chapter to follow, their facilitator, Deborah Carr, will be describing. It will provide context, too, for the conversation featured in the chapter after that between Anthazia, also a life-writing leader, and Shelley, a life-transition professional who works mainly with older clients, about the soulful, on-the-ground connection – in a strange way, the *convergence,* as Matte hinted back in Chapter 3 – between our stories and our things. In short, it will provide context for pathways of front-line practice with older adults that are rooted in a narrative perspective on the complexities of biographical ageing.

From Thinking to Talking to Writing

Let me begin by saying a bit about why writing about our life – as opposed to merely talking or thinking about it – is especially important in terms of the kind of storywork just referred to. This is a huge topic, of course, with many larger ones lurking in the background, topics there is neither time nor space to do more than nod towards here. Among these is the question of the relationship between orality and literacy in general, a question that cuts across the fields of philosophy, psychology, linguistics, and anthropology (Olson & Torrance, 1991). Nor is there space – or need really – to sketch the scope of scholarly inquiry concerning the history, theory, and analysis of autobiographical literature per se, or beyond that, and embracing it, of "life writing" overall, a category that includes biography. These limits acknowledged, there are nonetheless layers of awareness and depths of insight that, it may be argued, only become accessible to us when we express our thoughts and feelings through the written word, through some sort of overt autobiographical activity. Talking out our thoughts and feelings with a counsellor or confidant, for instance, can be an important step in gaining distance on issues that we might otherwise mull over obsessively in our minds. It can afford us an affectionate detachment, a measure of irony, on what is happening in our lives (Randall, 2013). However, writing our thoughts and feelings out of ourselves and onto the page or the screen adds an additional degree of concentration and intention that can fix them even more clearly in our minds and help us drill down even deeper into what is most important for us. "All writing," the author Joan Didion has said, "is an attempt to find out what matters." But more than fix them better in our minds, it can open them out for us on an emotional level to where we have a more dynamic, more interactive relationship with them overall. To adapt a comment made by Hermann more than once in his interviews with Jennifer, "I don't know what I think – or feel – until I see what I say." That interactive relationship paves the way, not just for clarity of thought, but potentially for personal transformation, for healing (Anderson & MacCurdy, 2000), by widening our landscape of consciousness, our horizon of self-understanding. It can change the relationship that we have to our life, our self, as a whole.

The idea that healing and life-writing are linked has inspired the research of psychologists such as James Pennebaker (1990, pp. 46–48). Pennebaker and his colleagues at Southern Methodist University have demonstrated, for instance, that having students write in their journals about traumatic experiences in their past has the effect of providing them with distance on the pain. It helps them, as narrative therapists might say, to externalize the problem, and thus experience a greater degree of narrative agency towards it. It opens up a space where they can play with multiple perspectives on the original experience, entertain alternative interpretations, and not be (narratively) foreclosed on one reading alone. As a consequence, so Pennebaker and company claim, it can even strengthen their immune system (Pennebaker & Seagal, 1999), something that I submit can conceivably occur whenever we help people tell and write their stories in ways that make them stronger (Wingard & Lester, 2001).

Journalling in general, several have proposed, can have a similarly life-changing effect on us, permitting us a profounder, more soulful relationship with our innermost self. Among many volumes to have appeared on this subject, Tristine Rainer's *The New Diary*, published in 1978, was instrumental for me personally in heightening my awareness of the healing that is possible through the discipline of writing each day in a journal. Kate Thompson (2011) writes persuasively, as well, about the power of therapeutic journal writing. In his book *At A Journal Workshop,* Jungian psychologist Ira Progoff (1975) makes a number of particularly provocative claims about the profound personal growth – the "philosophic deepening" (p. 12) – that people can experience when they participate in the "intensive journal" workshops that he has pioneered.

Among the novel activities that are part of Progoff's process are keeping a "daily log" of our life's events (pp. 86–97), as well as a "life history log ... in which we gather all the facts of the past of our lives" (p. 132). Included as well is "listing the steppingstones" in our life's path, or in other words, our turning-point events or nuclear episodes, or memories that are especially self-defining. Then there is, as he puts it, "moving back and forward in our life history," which he refers to as "time-stretching" (pp. 140–152), plus engaging in a "dialogue" with our dreams, with our bodies, and with events, persons, and situations in our lives – ultimately, with our "inner wisdom" (pp. 269–284). By submitting ourselves to such activities, he proposes, we can establish "a new quality of relationship … to the events of the past" (p. 11). We can "enter the inner movement of our whole life history and connect ourselves to it from within" (p. 13). In words reminiscent of McAdams's definition of a lifestory, "we see *an inner myth* that has been guiding our lives unknown to ourselves" (p. 11; emphasis mine). And in keeping with what has been said previously in this book about the increasing need as we age for a measure of narrative resilience, "we can each develop interior capacities strong enough to be relied upon in meeting the trials of life" (p. 15), can "strengthen … the inner muscles of [the] psyche" (p. 55).

Such strengthening, and the storywork that gives rise to it, comes at the cost, though, of stirring up our inner worlds, as we hinted back in Chapter 2 had occurred with participants in this study. It can mean disturbing our "narrative habitus" (Frank, 2010, p. 49), thus causing a measure of dis-ease or distress, of narrative disorientation. Through journaling, in other words, we embark on a journey of restorying that can be both exciting and unsettling. We may uncover a counter-story that has been quietly taking place beneath the surface, as we saw in the case of Harriet. She had inklings of such a counter-story – a larger story, as it were – as she mused with Jennifer on the transformative potential that was latent in the tragic tale of her lost possible violinist self. And she began to see how "the roads not taken earlier in our life are not necessarily dead ends" (Progoff, 1975, p. 138) but "may have gone underground … incubating beneath the surface of events" until such time, as she showed with the creation of her retreat centre later in life, that they "may now be taken, both more appropriately and more successfully" (p. 138). Here is Progoff's metaphorical description of the process he envisions going on:

> Under the pressure of events, our lives become hard packed like soil that has not been tilled for many years. They pile up and are pressed tightly together inside of us, leaving no room in between for the fresh air of consciousness to enter, nor for something new to grow … As we work in our Journal, however, we gradually break into this hardness … The solid clumps of past experience are broken up so that air and sunlight can enter. New awarenesses come in and have a fertilizing effect. Soon the soil becomes soft enough for new shoots to grow in. (pp. 99f.)

Arthur Frank (2010) enshrines a similar process of stirring up and thus rendering more fertile the soil of our lives in the last word of the title of his book *Letting Stories Breathe.* In Progoff's case, however, the process is no solitary enterprise. It happens within a group. In a passage that anticipates the notion of "wisdom environment," which I'll come back to later, here is how he describes what can occur and how it can feel:

> For many persons the experience at a Journal Workshop is like entering a sanctuary, for it provides a protected situation safe from the outer pressures of the world in which an individual can quietly reappraise his relation to his life ... The presence of other persons in the workshop, each exploring the individuality of his own life history, builds an atmosphere that supports and strengthens his inward work ... Being with many others while each is delving into the uniqueness of his own life, has the effect of reinforcing our intuitive sense of the integrity and validity of each individual existence. A Journal Workshop thus serves as a retreat in the traditional spiritual sense of the term. (1975, p. 14)

The kinds of claims Progoff is making in passages such as these are intriguing, and even inspiring. They suggest that journaling can indeed assist us in developing what narrative researchers Bauer and Park (2010) have called "eudaimonic resilience," which "involves an explicit concern for making meaning and growth" (pp. 71f.). It can be a means, as yet another source puts it, of "writing ourselves into being" (Sinats et al., 2005). Although Progoff's vision overall may sound somewhat mystical in tone, it nonetheless permits us a measure of insight into the intimate, inner process – part psychological, part spiritual – that we open ourselves to undergoing when we shift from musing upon events within the privacy of our own minds to exploring them intensively and extensively through writing, in the context of a group.

Comparing Life-Writing Endeavours

For the sake of argument, the broad variables according to which life-writing groups can be compared include context, structure, intention, duration, and strategies. Though these variables inevitably overlap, I'll discuss them, briefly, one at a time.

By context, I mean, for instance, where the group meets. Is it in a church, a synagogue, a spiritual institution of some sort or other? If so, this could colour the narrative environment within which people write about their lives, not to mention signal something about why they are writing in the first place, whether it be, say, to compose their spiritual autobiography (Wakefield, 1990) or to deepen their awareness of God. Alternatively, is it in a local seniors' centre, a palliative care unit in a hospital, a psychiatric ward, a nursing home, a community clinic of some kind, a school, or perhaps even a prison? Different contexts mean different attendees with different needs and different agendas, and will lead, no doubt, to different outcomes too.

By structure, I mean the degree of organization that is entailed. With WOLS, comparatively little structure is evident, or at least not an especially complicated structure. While technically Viviane is the facilitator, there is little "facilitation" as such. People write stories about their lives and then meet monthly to read aloud – some of them at least – what they have written. Everyone claps, and then they go home. Other sorts of life-writing groups, however, can involve considerably more structure, with step-by-step manuals offering would-be facilitators training and tools, plus ethics to adhere to, protocols to follow, do's to be done, and don'ts to avoid.

By intention, I mean the central aim of the group. Naturally, any one group can achieve a number of aims at once. While some will be in the foreground, others will be in the background, less intentional than incidental, as it were. One such intention is intervention. A life-writing program implemented by Dutch gerontologists Ernst Bohlmeijer and Gerben Westerhof (2013) entitled (in English) *The Stories We Live By: One's Autobiography as a Source of Wisdom* combines life review therapy with elements of narrative therapy, for example, to help middle-aged and older adults suffering from depression. As its title suggests, it has been designed with a narrative model of human development deliberately in mind. As is the case with narrative therapy per se (White & Epston, 1990), mental health issues are deemed to arise, in other words, when people's life stories "become chaotic, contaminated, problem-saturated" or, in some way, narratively foreclosed (Bohlmeijer et al., 2011). The goal is thus to promote within participants a greater sense of mastery, meaning, and agency and to pry them out of stalled or stagnant stories by helping them integrate into their overall life narratives the "negative life-events" that they are reminiscing obsessively about. The goal is to critique the dysfunctional life-scripts and limiting narrative templates – including the narrative of decline regarding ageing per se – by which they have unwittingly been living. The goal, in short, is to open their stories up again and get them moving. The intention is intervention; its aim, therapeutic at heart. A similar intention is implied, of course, by Gillie Bolton, Victoria Field, and Kate Thompson in their book *Writing Works*, composed as a resource for professionals like themselves who put on workshops in "therapeutic writing" (Bolton et al., 2006). Along the same lines, Geri Chavis (2011) has published a parallel resource entitled *Poetry and Story Therapy: The Healing Power of Creative Expression.*

In contrast to these avowedly "therapeutic" approaches, one highly popular life-writing program has been pioneered by veteran gerontologist Jim Birren (Birren & Deutchman, 1991). Entitled "Guided Autobiography," or GAB, for short, its aim is to get people together in groups of eight to twelve individuals for ten weekly sessions of two hours each to write about their lives with the aid of broad life themes – education, health, love, faith, and so on – that steer their reflections and discussions from one session to the next. The very first one, in fact, is designed to get them thinking about their life as a whole. Called "The Major Branching Points in Your Life," a variation of it was employed by Deborah in the workshops she did as part of our project. Between sessions, participants are asked to write a maximum of two pages about their lives in relation to the theme in question and, the following week, to read what they have written to the others.

The intention of GAB – which, true to the pattern just noted, attracts three times more women than men (O'Neill et al., 2011, p. 155) – is not to address issues of mental or emotional health in the way that the Dutch group does. It is "not designed to be used as formal therapy" (Birren & Deutchman, 1991, p. 3). Instead, it is intended to assist members in the process of *reviewing* their lives, the goal being psychosocial more than psychotherapeutic in nature. The goal is to "explor[e] the fabric of life" and, in so doing, achieve a greater sense of "ego integrity" (Erikson et al., p. 37), something signalled by the positive outcomes that GAB participants regularly report. Among these are a "sense of increased personal power and importance," "recognition of past adaptive strategies and application to current needs and problems," "reconciliation with the past and resolution of past resentments and negative feelings," and "greater sense of meaning in life," plus, as an added bonus given that some participants might be suffering from social isolation, "friendships with other group members" (Birren & Deutchman, 1991, pp. 4, 6). While individuals within the group may derive a small-*t* therapeutic benefit from their participation, by for instance shoring up their sense of "retrospective self-continuity" (Bluck & Liao, 2013, p. 10), and with it their sense of self-esteem, therapy as such is not the group's reason for being.

Another intention that can guide the formation of a life-writing group is to help members refine their skills at writing – writing about their lives, to be sure. But it's the writing as much as the life that is the focus. A memoir-writing group would be a prime example. The goal is to coach members in composing and perhaps eventually publishing their autobiographies. To use a distinction proposed by narrative gerontologist Kate de Medeiros (2011), the goal is to write one's story as a whole (to the extent this is possible!), not just isolated episodes from different parts of one's life. The latter she calls "self-stories" and the former "life stories," a distinction that parallels one mentioned in Chapter 2 between recounting "small stories" from one's life and engaging in "big story reflection" (Spector-Mersel, 2017).

One long-standing program focussing mainly on self stories was begun in Galveston, Texas, under the leadership of Kate and her PhD supervisor at the time, gerontologist Tom Cole. Initially titled "Share Your Lifestory" (de Medeiros & Lagay, 2000), it has widened its reach considerably and become known as the Pentimento Project (Sierpina, 2007). During its regular meetings, usually eight in number and no more than two hours long, between twelve and sixteen participants are given various prompts to engage them in timed writing activities that get the creative juices flowing. They are then asked to take whatever story they may have started and develop it further before they meet again. At the next session, they share aloud with the whole group the more extended, more finely crafted piece that they have each composed in the interim. Once a participant is finished reading their piece, the others respond to it with their observations and suggestions. They could recommend, for instance, that the writer play a bit more with a particular metaphor that might be running through it, or try out different techniques for going deeper into the experience in question, thereby peeling off another layer of the onion in terms of their knowledge of themselves.

Such techniques include writing about the experience not just in a straightforward, first-person manner but in the third person, thus permitting a degree of distance and perspective on what it's about (de Medeiros, 2007). Members are also invited to write about life events in the form of a poem, a journal entry, or a letter to a deceased relative who possibly played a pivotal role in the original experience. Deliberately using a range of literary genres to write about the same event can elicit different emotions concerning that event. It can tease out different interpretations of it, in the process widening the writer's "horizon of self-understanding" (Berman, 1994, p. 180). This is akin to what Ruth Ray (2000) has in mind when discussing the unique brand of wisdom that she believes is evident in the life-writing groups of which she, too, was a member: not wisdom understood as a compendium of life lessons that we pass along to our offspring, but as a dynamic, open-ended orientation towards our lives overall, and to the stories we have spun around them. In her words, "'wise' people watch themselves tell life stories, learn from others' stories, and intervene in their own narrative processes to allow for change by admitting new stories and interpretations into their repertoire" (p. 29). People become wiser, if you will, when their ways of talking and listening to one another within a group setting transform the narrative environment among them, subtly but surely, into a "wisdom environment" (Randall & Kenyon, 2001, pp. 169–171). In general, then, group members experience therapeutic benefit from thus broadening their narrative horizons but, once again, the group is not meant to be therapy per se.

By the same token, the Pentimento Project is not Creative Writing 101, a context where the emphasis is often on the writing first and foremost, not the writers themselves nor their personal growth. Such growth may happen all the same, of course, but if so it is a by-product of the process, not its main aim. And the classroom environment can at times be critical and defensive in tone – in stark contrast to WOLS where, as Viviane says, members' "writing skills are never questioned," where they "will always be applauded," and where the ultimate goal is to feel good and have fun. In other words, it's a setting in which, implicitly, social-emotional development is given priority over social-cognitive development (Bauer & McAdams, 2004), hedonic well-being over eudaimonic well-being (Bauer & Park, 2010). In the Pentimento Project as well, even if tensions sometimes surface as members offer their comments on the pieces that they've each composed and read, "the sharing is bigger than the writing" (Cole, 2002). A sense of closeness and community thus frequently develops among them. Indeed, in some cases "participants will remain in the groups for long periods of time, often years" (Sierpina, 2007, p. 84).

This leads to the variable of duration, which is understandably a factor in terms of (among other things) the experience that members have of social cohesion. Groups differ widely on this point. Many of the members of WOLS, like those of the Pentimento Project, have been connected to one another for nearly five years. A feeling of "family" almost has emerged among them. I could sense it in the air the afternoon of the garden party! Something similar has been reported with those who participate in GAB (Birren & Svensson, 2006). With respect to the process that the individuals we focussed on in Part 2 were part of, the three full-day sessions (9 a.m. to 4 p.m.) were spaced one month apart. Despite being together longer at any one go, and despite the chatting they did at their table groups or over lunch, there was not much chance therefore for a long-lasting sense of community, and thus a wisdom environment, to develop among them. (Such an environment, I would offer, was more likely to emerge amid the interviews that Jennifer conducted with them individually.) If there had been, it might well have made the whole experience that much more powerful for all those involved. This, though, returns us to the topic of intention.

The intention behind these workshops had less to do with combatting social isolation, let alone guiding people through a theme-by-theme review of their lives, nor even with coaching them to become better writers. The intention – our intention as academics at least – had to do with testing a specific hypothesis. This is not uncommon among researchers investigating the impact of life-writing activities with regard to different aims, whether to improve memory function (de Medeiros et al., 2007; de Medeiros et al., 2011; Hartman-Stein, 2011), awaken creative talents, stimulate life-long learning, slow down cognitive decline, or even hasten the healing of wounds (Koschwanez et al., 2013). In our case, the hypothesis was that taking people progressively more extensively into their stories (regardless of the quality of their writing) would assist them with tackling the developmental tasks of later life that I referred to in Chapter 2 – the primarily *narrative* tasks, that is – thereby rendering them more narratively resilient. In short, it would assist them, as Jim Birren himself would say, in "strengthening the fabric of life" (Birren & Deutchman, 1991, pp. 1–22).

In terms of strategies, as we've started (I hope) to appreciate, there is hardly a limit to those that can be employed to trigger the "autobiographical drive" (Cohen, 2005, p. 23), depending upon the intentions informing the group in question, the constraints (physical, logistical, and so forth) imposed by the context within which it meets, and the creative talents of the facilitators themselves. I've already alluded to a number of those that a given life-writing group could incorporate. One is getting people to tell a story from their lives that comes to mind when they look closely at their hands, which links to what was said back in Chapter 2 about our bodies having stories too. As Anthazia will explain in Chapter 15, another strategy involves having people ponder the significance that a particular object in their lives might have for them, and writing the story or stories that are associated with it. Gillie Bolton (2006) labels this activity "writing from objects." Indeed, as our explorations in this book have so far shown, there is no end of objects, cherished or not, from which such stories can spring.

Another strategy, which Deborah made use of during the workshops, employs the prompt "a story I was told ..." This strategy has the potential to tap into the whole issue of family stories that I touched upon in Chapter 2, and of cultural stories too, stories that for better or worse have wormed their way under our skin (Stone, 2008, p. 6) and become narrative resources for storying our lives, stories we may never have acknowledged nor critiqued. Still another strategy, as we've seen with "Princess" in Chapter 10, is the "Once upon a time ..." prompt, which she passionately picked up on, a simple but ingenious way to invite individuals to step back from their lives, engage in a brand of "big story reflection," and put words to the underlying myth by which they've been living, or as the case may be, might yearn to live.

The entire topic of life-writing strategies is especially germane, of course, in connection with the workshops that Deborah designed and delivered as part of this project. I say this because it was precisely upon our participants' experiences of such strategies that they reflected during Jennifer's interviews with them – interviews in which the things that they made mention of happened to catch our attention and thus drove us to write this book in the first place. In the following chapter and in a moving, autobiographical manner, Deborah will tell her own story of these workshops, beginning with an account of her experience facilitating a life-writing group in disaster-torn Haiti. Pulling in strategies from this and other such events that she has led, she generated a delightful array of questions, cues, and prompts, as well as journaling exercises, to stir up the compost heap of participants' memories (Randall, 2007) and entice them to write their way deeper into their own unique lives.

14 Writing Things about Our Lives: Exploring, Examining, and Embracing Our Stories

DEBORAH CARR

All that we are is story. From the moment we are born to the time we continue on our spirit journey, we are involved in the creation of the story of our time here. It is what we arrive with. It is all we leave behind. We are not the things we accumulate. We are not the things we deem important. We are story. All of us. What comes to matter then is the creation of the best possible story we can while we're here; you, me, us, together. When we can do that and we take the time to share those stories with each other, we get bigger inside, we see each other, we recognize our kinship – we change the world, one story at a time.

– Richard Wagamese (2012)

From Haiti to St. Thomas

The room was dim, cramped, and quiet. Dust motes swam through the diffused light from the open doorway. Beyond the rectangle of light, a semicircle of second-hand sandals and dust-covered flip-flops, scuffed shoes, and frayed sneakers – some clearly too big or too small for the feet within them – shuffled on the dirt floor. To be here, the dozen or so Haitian farmers, field workers, midwives, mothers, and market vendors wearing them had walked for hours from the small mountain villages of Gwabari, Grand Savanne, Mombin Crouchu, Vinbal. They'd come to learn how to write their stories.

A critic of the project thought this was trivial training for people struggling with a subsistence life. I wasn't sure she was wrong. As I looked around the room, I worried that North American writing methods wouldn't translate well to a foreign culture, especially one so rooted in struggle, oppression, and poverty.

Language provided another complication. Formal Haitian education was delivered in French, the language of oppression. Haitians learned lessons through memorization rather than comprehension, leaving little freedom for creative expression. To encourage them to value their own thoughts and heritage, it was essential to conduct the workshops in Kreyole, their native tongue, a musical dialect with hints of French.

In the hours to follow, using a translator, I led them through various writing exercises and listened to stories that revealed Haitian life. They wrote about places and people meaningful to them, about fears they'd overcome, and dreams they'd held hidden. They wrote the language of their ancestors, and it was both creative and healing.

A work-weary farmer with calloused hands wrote of taking his rest beneath a lone mango tree in his field, regaining his strength in the gift of its shade. I fought back tears. A young man wearing oversized shoes wrote that when the full moon shone bright, he felt he could walk to the ends of the earth. I believed he could. A diminutive woman, wearing the black of a mourner, described the misery of women working in fields, hauling rocks and sand and water, washing the dirty clothes of others to feed their children. I felt the anger and sorrow of injustice.

When they wrote about dreams, they put words to a vision that became more real and more possible when it was written on the page and then voiced aloud. An idea birthed in the heart made its way to the mind, then out the arm to spill upon the page, where it became words to be spoken aloud, stories to be heard and received. "Stories," writes Daniel Taylor (2001), "not only help us make sense of our present and past experience, they also allow us to imagine possibilities for ourselves in the future" (p. 27). They began to see themselves not just as characters in an ongoing story, but as characters with choices. This seemed to give them a greater sense of agency – *narrative* agency – in a world where they often felt powerless to change their circumstances.

One man commented, "Many times things are there, but they are hidden. For example, when you learn how to write stories like this, you can also do the story of your locale or city or town, and you can show an NGO [non-government organization] this and perhaps find help for how to do things." The participants also realized that they had a responsibility to bear witness to the time and place in which they lived. As one of the women expressed it, "Thank you for helping us write the knowledge that we have and to value it, because we have just used the ideas of other people and we know the stories of other countries, but I feel that we haven't left an image of ourselves for the people who come after us."

The realization that their thoughts and stories were both revealing and worth writing filled them with a sense of significance, and when we were finished, I asked them if they thought this training would have value in their lives. One woman summed it up well: "May we go home and write our stories so that our children's children will know who we were and what we did on this earth." Writing had given them a means of leaving something of themselves behind in a world that was in constant flux, and where death was a familiar companion. It was this experience that convinced me that understanding our past, finding the meaning in our lived experiences, can give us strength and resilience to meet the future. And it was the memory of this that I brought to the St. Thomas University (STU) workshop series.

Far from the concrete walls, glassless windows, and dirt floor of the Haitian community centre, the STU workshops took place in the chapel of Holy Cross House, a room with tall, paned windows and a lofty, beamed ceiling. The key to delivering a successful workshop, I've learned, lies in creating a safe and sacred place for the explorations, a wisdom environment, of sorts (see Chapter 2). Attention must be paid to the small details that contribute to helping people feel welcomed, respected, and at ease. The chapel setting afforded us padded chairs, adequate spacing at tables to ensure privacy when writing, quiet surroundings, plenty of natural light, and a casual, relaxed atmosphere.

We did not use full names in the group, nor did we discuss careers or our places or roles in society, other than what may have emerged in the process of sharing the writing, or in personal conversations, for I've found that it's important for participants to feel they're on a level playing field. They worked and shared in small groups, although there were also chances for them to read in front of the whole group if they so desired. Reading aloud was always voluntary so no one felt pressured to share their writing. I asked everyone to respect the sanctity of stories and maintain confidentiality within the group.

In addition to the writing techniques that were part of the instruction I provided, participants also learned passive listening etiquette. For instance, when someone read aloud, others were to keep their eyes down or closed, listening only to the words, and allow the reader to remain the focus. When one person shares their writing, it often stimulates memories in the listener, who then wants to share their own experience, taking the focus off the reader. It's hard to do, but I asked that opinions or feedback be withheld during first readings and offered later only if expressly requested. In this way, we learn to accept the words as they are and to honour the honesty of the writing. This is critical to learning how to receive our stories with all their flaws and mistakes.

The three workshops took place from 9 a.m. to 4 p.m. on successive Saturdays one month apart in the winter and spring of 2015. In the planning and designing, I intentionally sequenced them as "Exploring Our Stories," "Examining Our Stories," and "Embracing Our Stories." In the remainder of this chapter, I'll provide a sense of how each of them unfolded, drawing on examples from other workshops, including the ones in Haiti, that I've had the privilege to lead.

Exploring Our Stories: Workshop One

During this first session, we discussed the role that storytelling plays within the trajectory of a life – why stories matter, how we learn from them, and how they help us better understand our experiences. I provided instruction on basic journal writing techniques designed to uncover hidden memories. We also reflected upon the various roles we play in life and learned about the difference between descriptive writing and reflective writing. This would help provide a framework for the more in-depth work I'd be getting participants to do in the sessions to follow.

One of my favourite warm-up activities is an acrostics exercise in which a participant assigns a characteristic or attribute to each letter of their name, then chooses one attribute to self-identify with for the rest of the day. Jennifer, or Jenn as she's often called, used the adjectives Joyful, Energetic, Nice, and Neat to describe herself to the others at her table group. I've always found this an effective ice-breaker that not only sparks camaraderie and laughter, but also gives each person a degree of anonymity until tablemates get to know one another better and build mutual trust. Past participants have told me it had a positive effect on them by encouraging and highlighting that particular characteristic. As I call on them during the day using their "name," it serves as a reminder for them to be "Happy" or "Courageous" or "Spontaneous."

Following the icebreaker, I showed a short, three-minute video by Nova Scotia author and filmmaker Shandi Mitchell (2006), which explores the questions a daughter wants to ask her father. Entitled *Tell Me*, the film features Shandi's soft voice-over narration as she asks her father question after question. "Tell me … what is your favourite time of day?" "Were you ever afraid?" "What makes you cry?" The responses are silent images of her father's expressions, sometimes a long shot, sometimes up close and intensely intimate. Sometimes he is fully clothed, sometimes naked from the waist up. The starkness of the minimalist treatment, the vulnerability of the ageing man, the manner in which the film's message pierces the very heart of our relationships – we desire the intimacy of knowing and being known, but often don't know the questions to ask or the answers to give – moved me to tears the first time I saw it. It perfectly captured my relationship with my own father and my fears that he might die before I really have a chance to know who he is. It captured my frustration that the questions I really want to ask so often remain unspoken.

The first time I showed the film to a class of participants aged fifty to eighty-five years, I asked if they could relate to it in some way. There was a long silence. Some shuffled uncomfortably. Some looked down at their hands and others doodled on their notepads. I waited. Finally, a woman said that the man's nakedness bothered her. "How so?" I asked. "There was no hiding," she replied. "Why do we want to hide, do you think?" Someone else piped up: "As parents, I suppose we get in the habit of hiding our emotions or the truth from our children to protect them, or because we think they're too young or immature to understand. So, hiding becomes the norm." Good point, I thought.

I know my own parents hid much from me as a child. And I certainly hid a lot of my activities from them. They still hide certain situations from me. Once, on our way home from a vacation in Portugal, my husband and I had to stay overnight in Toronto due to a delayed flight. I called my mother to let her know. "Oh," she said. She paused. "I'm having surgery in the morning for a broken shoulder," she said. Her voice wavered and I knew she was scared. "Do you think you can get to the hospital before I go in?" She'd fallen four days before while walking my dog and had broken her arm and shoulder in five places. It was on a Friday, so the ER personnel had immobilized her arm and sent her home with painkillers until a surgery could be scheduled the following week. Fortunately, I arrived at the hospital just in time to see her for a few minutes before they administered the anaesthesia. Afterwards, I blasted my dad. He shrugged, "She wouldn't let me call you." She hadn't wanted me to know until I was back in Canada, as it "might ruin our vacation."

There are also the stories that perhaps *should* remain hidden, left untold. During one workshop I led, for instance, a woman wrote about reading her mother's journals after her death. In them the mother had expressed feelings about her daughter that were tremendously hurtful. "I never knew she felt that way about me," the woman said. It's hard to fathom that kind of pain. And yet, we often reach a place as we age where we wish for the relief of being known for who we truly are, but don't know how to have these conversations. To say, "I'm this kind of person!" is unconvincing, superficial. We want to be known by and through our actions and choices.

With my memories in mind of the Haitians who saw writing as a means to leave something of themselves behind, I hoped this film would press home upon the participants this unspoken desire, and to assure them that their experiences are of value to their children and grandchildren. If the latter don't appear to be interested, chances are they haven't yet recognized their own need to know. The more we can express about who we are, I believe, the greater the gift. So, understanding our own stories is not only of benefit to ourselves, it's a gift to others, particularly those we brought into the world. My message to the participants, then, was this: You are important. Your stories are important. They're gifts of intimacy, and even though questions remain unspoken, the stories you tell provide clues to the answers. What is more, and as was mentioned in Chapter 2, those stores are always embodied. In the eloquent words of Carolyn Myss (1996), "we are all living history books. Our bodies contain our histories, every chapter, line, and verse of every event and relationship in our lives. As our lives unfold, our biological health becomes a living, breathing biographical statement that conveys our strengths, weaknesses, hopes, and fears" (p. 40).

Following the film, the workshop exercises were structured with increasing complexity. I started with easy free-writing exercises (using pen and paper) to give confidence, as well as the occasional glitter of a diamond unearthed, the tip of a memory worth excavating. I hoped to encourage them to a practice of journaling regularly in this fashion – not so much in the format of a daily diary, but daily exploration. The process of journaling and of working with the images and memories that emerge in doing so can lead us to become more conscious and aware of our life lessons and turning points, of those "nuclear episodes" that McAdams (1996, p. 140) talks about. Pursuing this as a practice might create in us a greater awareness of the underlying significance of events. What is the purpose of our living – our pain and our triumph – if we cannot share the lessons we've learned, or if we do not share how living changes us, makes us stronger or wiser?

Free-writing, also called stream-of-consciousness writing, begins with a supplied phrase, and then the writer simply follows wherever their mind takes them, writing steadily without stopping, for ten minutes. The aim is to write what comes to mind, keep the pen moving, and not stop to think. The value of this exercise, beyond being an excellent warm-up, is that it trains the writer to get their first thoughts on the page, without editing or overthinking, which sends a subliminal message that our thoughts are worthy of writing down. Beyond building confidence, free-writing prepares the mind for the real work, the deep "storywork" (Randall, 2010), which will come later. Often, during the final few minutes, the writer will have worked through all the chaff and idle thoughts to reach something concrete and surprising: a memory, an association, a situation that can be explored further in other writings.

I personally use free-writing as a means of exploring ideas, digging for the truth of an experience, or settling myself into more focussed writing. It helps me write my way to the centre, to clear through the clutter that generally occupies my mind. It's one of the most valuable tools in the writer's toolbox. Julia Cameron (1995) calls the practice "morning pages"; Natalie Goldberg (1986) calls it "writing first thoughts" (pp. 8–10); Tristine Rainer (1978), "free-intuitive writing" (pp. 61–68). Whatever it's called, it's an effective means of giving voice to our subconscious and giving buried images permission to rise.

Once, on a whim, during a workshop in a lovely artist's studio overlooking the Bay of Fundy, I asked participants to write about the kitchen sink. One of them, a beautiful young woman in her mid-twenties, stared at her page when I called out the ten-minute mark. She was visibly upset, but when I asked if anyone wanted to read their work, she lifted her eyes and took a deep breath. She'd begun writing around "everything but the kitchen sink." Near the end, however, she found herself comparing her marriage to a sink piled with dirty dishes in need of a deep cleaning that she felt too tired to undertake. The kitchen sink gave her a side entrance through which she was able to examine some of the problems she was facing.

People who are new to this practice will sometimes find it challenging to keep the pen moving, but after two or three exercises they generally loosen up and are writing more freely, and with confidence. After a half an hour, they seem surprised that they've accumulated quite a few pages of words. In regular practice, this helps access our intuitive inner consciousness and override the resident editor in our head. It's an effective way to warm up and to combat our fear of writer's block. It's actually fun and revealing, rather like following a maze. Follow the words, and seek the truth, because truth is where the energy lies.

After this, we moved into a more focussed writing, which I call "Topic Writing." The method is the same; however, a single word is given as a topic and the writers write down all their associations with it. If they start to wander onto another subject, they circle back to the topic word. This trains the mind to be more focussed, but it also opens the door to rich memory and symbolism. For example, writing on the word "Hands" frequently brings up visual memories of a grandmother's or grandfather's hands and the work that they perform. "Bread" enlivens the sense of smell, touch, and taste, and is a reminder of home. Writing on "Mountain" can raise a number of metaphors as the mountain becomes an obstacle, a challenge, a symbol of strength or endurance, a new viewpoint or perspective. Or the writer may find themselves circling around the topic from various angles, like searching for an earring in the grass, until the glint of a hidden memory sparkles forth.

One of the Haitian groups I worked with produced only a few stilted lines during the free-writing exercises. Since the very concept of free-writing seemed hard for them to grasp, I decided to do the exercise as a group. I asked them to tell me everything they knew about mangoes. They looked at me blankly. The mango was such a commonplace thing in their lives that they struggled to "know" what they knew. I asked about shape, colour, size, smell, and soon synergy took over and everyone was contributing something new and different. They shared "mango" stories and memories in what turned out to be a rich cultural learning lesson for me. The common mango had become an open door for them to share with me something of their day-to-day life, and also took down the barriers that had prevented them from writing freely. As I've seen repeatedly in small groups that are open and willing to share, synergy happens. One person strikes the match that sparks another's flame, and we quickly realize how our writing can become both an act of collaboration and an act of love.

Another technique is list-making. Lists are easy ways to generate topics that the memoirist can later explore more fully. A list can be made of places worked, lived in, or travelled, of jobs held, childhood friends, fears, pets, family vacations, or the significant turning points in our lives. The linear thought required of us helps us to categorize experiences or topics, and gives us a structure, and a wealth of themed topics to explore later in depth, using one of the other techniques. It can also reveal patterns that might prove significant.

During this first session, I asked participants to make a list of the roles they play in life, starting with the general and moving towards the specific. I provided them with examples to get them started: mother, father, daughter, son, aunt, student, mentor, artist, manager, nurse, caregiver, cook, gardener, listener, dog-walker, bed-maker. The exercise helps them realize the integral part that they play in the lives of those around them – how their stories intertwine – as well as revealing to them the many skills and talents they possess and the service they provide to others.

Participants often express surprise at the length of their lists. During a previous workshop I'd conducted, one person commented that she never realized how valuable she was until she reviewed her list. In this group, one of the participants – who had earlier divulged that he didn't want anyone to really know him and didn't like to write about himself – noted that the majority of roles on his list were from his youth and adolescence. We can often learn as much from what is left out as from what is included. Did he see himself as disconnected from others in his adult years? Did he feel a lack of purpose, disengaged and unneeded? Or was he more drawn to dwell in the past rather than the present? Once the list was complete, participants were asked to pick one role in particular and do a free-write around it to see what emotional responses or connections emerged.

After lunch, we moved into more descriptive writing, where the writer focuses on creating word pictures using specific nouns, adjectives, and strong verbs. This is more thoughtful writing and reflects the writer's own unique perceptions and language, how they see the world. It is a practice in specificity and concrete images. A robin instead of a bird. A brittle paring knife instead of a knife. Descriptive writing exercises help us to expand our perception and enrich our appreciation of a given subject, allow us to explore word choices and similes that work (or don't), and encourage our own examination of the subject matter in question. We begin to take ownership of that subject or experience and thus begin to shape it for our purpose. I like what Tristine Rainer (1978) says about such writing: "When I describe an experience, I no longer feel controlled by it, but responsible for it in the overall context of my life. I affirm my own existence and validate my vision of the world. In describing my experience, I am recording not what happened or what exists, but how I perceive it. In doing so, I define myself" (p. 61).

For the first such exercise, I asked them to write a character sketch of someone they knew well. There are many different ways to think about people, including their physical description, character traits, likes and dislikes, curious mannerisms, hobbies, habits, values, and influence. What we write about people says as much about us, and what matters to us, as it does about them. We don't always closely examine our relationships with others, and such an exercise allows us the opportunity to do so; to take stock of what we know and what we don't, what we notice and what we overlook.

The second exercise, divided into two parts, was a description of place. Places, real and imagined, literal or metaphorical, are useful and can generate powerful and revealing writing. We often use place as a metaphor for a more general feeling about our lives. An example for this might be "home" as a place of sanctuary, or a meadow as a place where we feel possibility, openness, and vibrant life.

In the first part, I simply asked them to write about a place where they experienced comfort and safety. I instructed them to close their eyes and recall all the details about it, using all their senses, for our senses can carry us into the past to connect with memory, and how we recreate sights, smells, and colours generates a specific feeling. A gentleman who had served in the Second World War, for instance, wrote about being holed up with his unit in a monastery in Cyprus, trying to get some much-needed rest. Afterwards, they discovered that enemy rebels were there as well, resting in another area, at the same time. His unit bombed the monastery a few days later. I felt this was an extraordinary story with much potential, and I told him I hoped he would explore it more fully.

The second part of the exercise focussed more on the emotional connection to place. I asked them to write, "If fear were a place ..." This generated some exemplary writing. One participant, a self-declared "writer," wrote a moving piece describing the fear she felt while in the line-up to make an overdue payment at the bank. She described the red velvet ropes holding people in line, and her own "holding back" of funds so that she could buy groceries. Another woman wrote about dark basements and spiders. As she read her piece aloud afterwards, her eyes were as big and round as her glasses. "My own writing makes me too afraid to continue," she said with a little smile.

The third and final descriptive exercise was to write about a lesson learned, which is a simple way to introduce story structure. Whenever we consider a lesson learned, it involves a student and a teacher, a particular setting, a desire, a challenge, a choice, and a result. It's a situation where obstacles are encountered, growth occurs, and change happens. These are the intrinsic elements of a story. In most circumstances, the teacher is elder to the student – often a parent or grandparent. This was a nice note on which to end, as it brought us all back full circle to the beginning of the day and the message that when we share ourselves – our skills and talents and stories – with another person, we're infusing our lives with value and purpose. Life is about learning, in other words, and sharing what we learn with others.

Often, as the workshops I lead progress, participants observe a pattern emerging in their writing that may have connections to their present situation. For example, during a previous workshop, one woman had selected "baker" from her list of roles to explore more fully because she loved food and baking. Later, she wrote a place description of the renovation of her childhood kitchen, and a memory of her mother standing in it saying, "I'm married to this place." As the day progressed, her writing kept coming back to her relationship with food and her mother, and her mother's relationship to the kitchen. When her own writing led her to shed tears, she confessed that the anniversary of her mother's death was only days away.

This is what I love about this process ... a network of patterns and connections lie below the surface of our lives just waiting for us to notice them. Once we do, and we tug one of those connections to the surface, up comes another, and they become a string of memories, like a strand of pearls fed through our fingers, each one asking to be touched and appreciated, then finally leading to the clasp, the piece that pulls it all together.

For homework before the second workshop, I asked the participants to select one story from the writing class, or from subsequent journaling they might do, to work with for the coming two sessions. They were instructed to do research on it and to gather additional details, including photographs, mementoes, journals, and the like, to assist them to write settings and character sketches of others involved in the story. As they all left the room that day, and I packed up my materials, I felt elated. In one short day, I'd seen them progress through the excavation of memory to the rich, emotional reliving of detail.

Examining Our Stories: Workshop Two

The second workshop, one month later, was devoted to understanding the nature of story. What makes a story? What are the elements and framework? What are story layers? How do we determine themes and focussing statements? My aim was to give them the tools to dissect an experience and tease out the narrative arc – the desire, the obstacles, the resolution – and thus to find the meaning in the story.

Meaning is intrinsic to storytelling. A tree is just a tree, until a connection is made through experience. Perhaps I plant a tree in memory of my father. Tree and father become intertwined. Maybe the tree was reduced in price at the nursery because no one wanted it and I brought it home to nurture it. It becomes a symbol of mothering, of caring for what has been neglected. Perhaps on my daily walk, the hemlock tree is a turning place, the point where I turn towards home again. It has meaning. When I describe this tree and its attributes, its species – birch, pine, spruce, maple – I connect it to personal knowledge. And when I write about it, I have a chance to enliven the reader's own experience of trees and help them make similar connections, or perhaps see things differently.

The writer Rust Hills (1977) says that every good story contains a moment after which things can never be the same again. It's a moment of profound change for the characters and reader alike. The act of writing about our lives also moves us towards change, towards "restorying" our lives to some degree (Kenyon & Randall, 1997). Every story works through a series of complications and resolutions. The narrative arc advances the characters (and the reader) through these changes in situation, including key turning points and moments of tension and choice. Why did characters choose or react the way they did? How did they change as a result of that choice?

Writing from a point of hindsight (Freeman, 2010) allows us to see how a positive or painful story impacted lives, strengthened resolve, or affected a subsequent direction. Distance allows us to determine meaning. Ultimately, the goal is to understand the significance of the lived experience and how it shaped who we are. Such understanding places us in a better position to embrace the story for the value it brings to our lives and relationships.

First-time story writers – and there were a number of them in these workshops – often struggle with this shift in thinking, as it drops below the surface of the visible actions and searches out the underlying motivations taking place. Sometimes more information is needed to develop the segments, but this is essential in determining the significance of story. This kind of analysis also helps the writer deepen their story. While we most often think of an experience as simply a series of actions, the story actually has multiple layers. As Jon Franklin (2007) explains, "All stories have three layers. The top layer is what actually happens – the narrative. The next layer is how these events make the main character feel. If the writer succeeds in getting the reader to suspend disbelief and see through the character's eyes, then a connection has been made. The third layer is the rhythm of the piece and evokes the story's universal theme. Good wins, love endures, wisdom prevails" (p. 110).

So, this session was about identifying the setting and characters, the desire and complications, the struggles and the resolution. It's a different way to think about the things that happen to us and, as opposed to the journaling process where the work is spontaneous, internal, and reflective, this process is intentional, external, and analytical. It allows us to gain some distance and see ourselves as a character in our story and to objectively question why we did what we did. "An autobiographic story is not just an account of events," writes Tristine Rainer (1998), "it is the charting of your emotional, moral, and psychological course, which gives meaning to those events" (p. 38).

During the workshop we discussed various ways to start and end stories, and we considered different points of view that we can take on them, or different sorts of narrative positioning that we can adopt. Each participant learned how to develop a focussing statement that defined the desire-complication-resolution arc of their story, and tried writing from a different perspective to see how this might help to deepen their understanding of the events. They plotted the flow and structure of their story, identifying its conflict points and resolution so that they could understand how they changed in the course of the story. And they tried to determine the story's underlying theme as well.

It was clear to me that the session was unearthing lots of memories and reflection. As I made my way around the room, speaking with participants, one man who had been writing what seemed to be an iconic adventure story when he was a young man abroad told me that when he got back home, his wife had left him. He went on to remarry, but had been estranged from his daughter for sixty years. When he spoke of seeing something that she'd written about him on Facebook, he wiped his eyes. He'd gone beyond the story he wanted to tell. I touched his shoulder. "It appears this story was far from over. How do you see it ending?" I asked. He shook his head. Another woman – Mary, whom Matte discussed in Chapter 5 – talked about an annual community yard sale that had been going on in her neighbourhood for thirty-two years, how she was now aware of all the relationships between neighbours and all their stories of "things." She was excited because she could see so many possibilities for stories *within* the story.

As we wrapped up at the end of the day, the participants were to spend the coming month shaping and rewriting their stories, choosing a perspective and structure, and giving consideration to symbolism or metaphor, to the layers and overall flow of the story. My hope was that it would help them craft what Bill likes to call "a good, strong story" (Randall, 2013, pp. 5f.).

Embracing Our Stories: Workshop Three

At the start of the final session, which took place on a sunny Saturday in April, participants had the chance to discuss any problems they'd encountered or observations they'd made during the previous months, and then read out loud their completed stories, or have them read by another. The rest of the day was then devoted to taking a wider view of life and applying some of the lessons learned about narrative structure and flow to their personal "life-lines." I hoped the exercises would help them uncover common themes and threads throughout their lives, or give them a basic outline to follow. Within this structure, they could then begin to fill in the stories and explore the underlying desires and motivations that may have driven and shaped their lives to date.

Many of us, I believe, grew up understanding important life lessons and story structure through the fairy tales that we heard as children (see, e.g., Randall et al., 2022). So, I reviewed with them the basic narrative arc of desire, complication, and resolution by working through the familiar story of Cinderella: her desire to escape her life of drudgery and to go to the ball, the obstacles of the stepmother and stepsisters, the unexpected appearance of the fairy godmother who gives her the chance that changes everything. She meets the prince, then at the climax, the stroke of midnight, realizes she must either leave or else reveal who she really is. Fearful of the consequences, she chooses to run, losing her slipper in the process, which leads to the resolution as the prince searches for the girl who can wear the slipper, and eventually finds his way to her. The shoe fits, she produces its mate, they marry, and they live happily ever after. She has overcome her obstacles and achieved her desire.

This served as a lead-in to the exercise entitled "Once Upon a Time" that "Princess" made much use of (see Chapter 10) and that I first discovered in Rainer's (1998) book *Your Life as Story*, whereby we consider our life story as a fairy tale. Rainer explains its effectiveness: "People have an instinct for what story is – beginning, middle and conclusions – and when writing a fairy tale, they intuitively use the essential ingredients in the right order" (p. 42). I like the exercise because it helps focus the complexity of a long life and also allows the participant to assume the third-person perspective, if they choose, or to apply elements of fiction to the process.

Another exercise from the same book, "The Story You Were Told," explores the paradox (or similarity) between the way we were taught to see ourselves in the world and how we really came to see and understand ourselves over time. It asks three questions:

1. What story did the world you grew up in tell you about who you should or could become? (The word "world" meaning environment, family/friends, society, class, and/or culture of your formative years.) In other words, what message did you receive about who you were and who you might become?
2. What story did you tell yourself about who you should become?
3. What story has life told you about who you really are?

It's a more difficult exercise, for it asks us to pinpoint what we understood about ourselves as children, whether we believed this or not, and what "truth" we have learned or had confirmed about ourselves as adults. This reflection can reveal crucial, and sometimes painful, growth or career curves, but it can also help participants understand some of the choices that they made along the way. It was a particularly meaningful exercise for me, personally, and one that helped me reconcile some of my own choices ...

At eighty-seven, my mother still has a love of pretty dolls and keeps a number of them around the house as decoration, a leftover from her own childhood dream to have a daughter. I often teased her that if I'd been a boy or a homely baby, she'd probably have sent me back. She temporarily left her career as a secretary when I was born, delighted that she finally had her little girl. As a child, I remember dresses, ankle socks, and patent leather shoes. She did my straight hair in spikey rollers every Saturday night so it would be curly for church on Sunday and bemoaned the Band-Aids on my perpetually scraped knees.

My Barbies were less interesting to me, though, than my books or my bike. For a school project when I was ten, I made a newspaper, complete with photographs, stories of murder and mayhem, cartoons, advertisements, and classifieds. One of the photos was of myself, at perhaps four years old, in a frilly dress, typing on my mother's old Underwood. The story I wrote was entitled "The World's Youngest Author."

And yet by high school I understood my career choices were either secretary, nurse, or teacher. I chose the easier role of secretary, which afforded me an immediate salary, enabling me to move out on my own, which I did the year after I graduated. But there was always this other side: the girl with the scraped knees who loved to write stories. Each time I pursued something with even the barest hint of danger or adventure, my mother protested that I might get hurt. She often lamented, "Where is that little girl with the curls?"

As I mention in my brief bio in Appendix 1, I left my chosen career in office work in mid-life. I've since learned to respect my femininity but also to give expression to my tomboy side. I'm as comfortable in my long, loose, flowing skirts as in my T-shirts and jeans. I enjoy physical and mental challenges. I rarely hike on level paths, preferring the rewards of a climb. I'm a writer with a curious mind and a love for the environment. But a curious mind without the structure of scientific inquiry often flounders. I regret not furthering my education and pursuing the sciences, and sometimes wonder about the path not taken.

This exercise, though, gave me a spine to work with; it helped me identify the backbone of the choices I've made, the directions I've taken, and provided me a map for tracing any one of the connecting ribs to its conclusion. It also gave me the strength to stand tall and accept the choices I've made, and reflect how each one carries multiple storylines, multiple points of conflict. It helped me identify the points of struggle between who I was expected to be and who I really was. As I walked among the participants, their heads bowed to their work, I hoped it would afford them something similar.

One participant in another senior workshop I've led was a retired Vietnamese professor, a brilliant man who worried about his memory and his structured academic thinking. He hoped the class would help him generate memories and incorporate more creativity in his writing. This exercise generated a story that he had worked on at home but was reluctant to read aloud, so I read it for him. That day, each one of us in the room learned that the story we were told about Vietnam's fight for independence from France was not the same one experienced by a young boy, hiding in trenches and caves from soldiers and bombs. As conflict raged around him, he reluctantly studied the language of the aggressor. His father told him that French did not belong to the soldiers, but to "a people who had much to offer the world." His adeptness with the language eventually aided his immigration to Canada. His memory provided compelling detail, and his academic skills gave us concise historical context that helped us see the bigger picture that preceded the American intervention. That day, we all walked away changed.

By late afternoon of this third and last session, we'd worked long and hard with words. So, for the final exercise, I wanted them to break out their artistic aptitudes and sketch a life storyline for themselves, although it was less about talent and more about seeing the span of their life creatively through metaphor.

We supplied everyone with sheets of paper, coloured pencils, and markers and asked that they sketch their life story as a picture, providing some examples to get them thinking: a river, a tree, a mountain, a circus, anything that helped them envision the major twists, turns, and milestones of their life. The result, I hoped, would give them a map to guide their writing when they returned home.

One woman sketched her life as a river with tributaries; another as a quilt where some blocks lined up, others did not. Along the lines of the "major branching points" prompt used in Guided Autobiography (see Chapter 13), another participant chose a tree with many branches. Another opted for a snakes-and-ladders game, another a series of worlds spilling into one another, and another – Hermann – a maze (see Chapter 7). One woman drew herself in the form of a goddess almost. Her splayed fingers on one hand represented phases of life. On the other hand she assigned broad themes to these phases: for childhood, play; for her teens, rebellion; and so on, until later life, which she saw as creativity. All of the participants were creative with the images they sketched. I particularly appreciated the woman who drew a cross-section of landscape including hills, a pond, trees, a rising sun, the sky, and beneath it all, multi-hued layers of soil. I smiled. She was going deep.

When we reach a deeper understanding of our story, as workshops like these can help us do, we can begin to see that it may not be over yet, that there may be more chapters still to write, that our story is still open, that there is "a lot more to it" (Berman, 1994, p. 180). And maybe we can admit that we have much to offer and contribute through our lived wisdom. It was, I think, a fitting end to the whole series.

15 Stories and Things: A Chat with Two Professionals

ANTHAZIA KADIR AND SHELLEY SWIFT

I watch old people look around their houses and wonder what to take [to the nursing home] and watch how every object becomes a container and synthesizes an entire lifetime, becomes a reservoir of memories.

– Barabara Myerhoff (cited in Kaminsky, 1992, p. 310)

This touching comment is by the anthropologist Barbara Myerhoff (1992), author of *Remembered Lives: The Work of Ritual, Storytelling, and Growing Older*, a book linked to her Oscar-winning documentary about field research with a community of Jewish older adults in Venice, California. Myerhoff captures many of our own sentiments during the two-hour conversation that we enjoyed one afternoon in February 2020 (just before COVID closed things down!) when, as part of working on this book, Matte, Denise, and Bill interviewed us about the boots-on-the-ground work that each of us does with older adults.

For Anthazia, not unlike Deborah, that work involves leading life-writing workshops with people of all ages, though mostly those in the second half of life. One workshop in particular deserves mention here, for in it stories and things are tightly entwined. It's one she's facilitated in numerous communities throughout the Maritimes, with newcomers to Canada primarily in mind. Its title is "Arrivals and Departures: Objects, Memories, and Transitions," and the stories participants told as part of it have been published in the literary journal *Fiddlehead* (Kadir, 2018). As for Shelley, her work as a Certified Relocation and Transition Specialist (or CRTS) involves meeting with her clients, most of them older adults or the adult children thereof, to assist them, often over a number of sessions, in the process of downsizing to smaller quarters, such as an apartment, retirement home, or nursing home. As you can imagine, it's a process fraught with complicated feelings, insofar as many of the objects to be sorted through are, in Myerhoff's words, "reservoirs of memories."

Using a bit of editorial licence, we'd like to draw on our own words – mostly from the transcript of the interview itself, but also from the notes that each of us jotted down to prepare ourselves for it – to provide a flavour for the wide-open territory that the five of us ended up exploring that delightful afternoon. It was territory where, again and again, the topic of stories converged repeatedly with the theme of things. Thankfully, though, Matte and Bill sent us a few questions in advance to help ensure that our explorations didn't take us all over the map, for there were no end of rabbit holes to wander down!

Question 1: What do things, or objects, mean to your clients, or to participants in your workshops? Why?

SHELLEY: That was the hardest question, a loaded question. Objects that are especially meaningful represent snapshots in people's lives. Sometimes they're happy, sometimes they're not. Sometimes they represent an event – that trip you took to the Louvre, for example – and sometimes they represent a person – the sister you made the trip with – and sometimes both at once. Generally, though, I tend to distinguish between the heart value that objects have for us and the monetary value. Of course, the "meaning" and "value" of things are in the eyes of the beholder. For many of my clients, their things are their legacy almost, while for some, they have a monetary value only and are, well, just things, just stuff. That said, I've seen the value that people assign to things change with circumstances, as I think we'll be talking about later when we get to the third question. But overall, when I think of what objects mean to my clients, what comes to mind first is obligation, responsibility, and burden. I don't like to use that word, "burden," because it's such a negative word, but it's there, okay?

The downsizing business is about making choices, and about dispersing things. This means there's always the fear of making the wrong decision, because some decisions have to be made in a very short time frame. That's a huge burden on people, especially if they are an only child or they're the one sibling who's here and the others are elsewhere across the country, and they've been given the task of dealing with mom and dad's estate, so that would be the burden part. But it's very real for people and it doesn't necessarily mean it's related only to the expensive stuff. It's all the little things that have meaning for a family too, that are encased in those four walls of someone's home. So, unfortunately, "burden" is the word that we talk about a lot in my industry.

ANTHAZIA: Building on what Shelley is saying, but coming at it from another perspective, people can feel a sort of burden, I think, when they're going into a workshop in which they're "writing from objects" (Bolton, 2006), knowing that they're going to write about an object that is dear to them. I've had some workshops, in fact, where the same person comes in with two objects! What I've witnessed often is that it's as if the object itself represents a person in their lives. It's like they're seeing their grandmother or their grandfather in front of them having a conversation, so objects can be very much attached to relationships. Because of that attachment, the burden a person feels can be one of guilt out of not wanting to let go. I remember doing an activity in a workshop in Saskatchewan once where we were actually speaking to the object, which was weird, but it's amazing what can come out of that. It's the relationship, it's the attachment, that holds some sort of meaning. In my experience, people sign up for these workshops because they are at a point in their life where they're trying to make sense of things; it's like a turning point in their life. So, when they bring an object, they're expecting that writing about it should do something for them. It's like a passage to healing or something.

I've had teenagers in the immigrant community, for example, who started school in another country and who bring their workbooks with them to the workshop because they symbolize some attachment to a teacher, or to some other important relationship back home. So, if you see the tears are coming, or there's silence while they're staring at the object, that's where the workshop goes to another whole level. In ways like this, I've seen time and again how objects become sort of a passage to healing amid the ebb and flow of life. And often it's not really the object but the relationship that the object represents. The object becomes a person that stands beside them through the journeys in their life, offering comfort as they figure out what they are and who they are.

SHELLEY: That is just so parallel to what I do. When you start, you've got all these things and all these decisions that have to be made, all this prioritizing that has to be done. But then you have this one particular item, maybe they'd forgotten all about it, that suddenly elicits a memory for them and makes their eyes light up. And, although they maybe can't describe it at the time, there's obviously a lot of emotion attached to it, and a story or two that they can tell about it. Of course, my clients can have hundreds of such things, which they have to go through and decide which is most valuable. One client, for example, had spent a lifetime surrounded by family and things and by generations of traditions, and she became the caretaker of the family history. And at the beginning it was as if *everything* was cherished.

But I can see a certain object ending up in your workshop as the person tries to make sense of why it's so significant for them. In fact, I should recruit some of my clients to attend your workshops! Because in your area, the paring down has happened. They have already put aside what they're going to hold on to and what they are coming into that workshop with, whether it be, say, their grandmother's dress or a pair of earrings.

MATTE: I'm struck by the contrast between your situation, Anthazia, where your participants bring one object that's already been pre-selected, and yours, Shelley, where you go into clients' homes and find all kinds of objects that need sorting through.

SHELLEY: Yes, that's right. One of my clients would say, "Okay, this is an overwhelming situation, so let's just shake it down." And that's kind of what we do in the downsizing business, and that "shaking down" gives us a smaller sampling of what's meaningful, but it has to be done in a very short period of time, so it's very stressful, which again is where the burden comes in. Decisions have to be made because you can't keep everything, but if you have time to go through it, it's an amazing process. I've always wanted to do post-interviews to follow up with them, maybe every year or so, to see if they have any regrets, for example. Also, because in working with clients, it's become clear to me that, say, I can cherish a particular item at this particular period of time, but as time passes and as my life changes and my situation changes, its cherishableness – assuming that's a word! – may change as well. All of a sudden it may become not a burden but a responsibility that I'm not capable of dealing with because, right here right now, there's something else in my life that is more immediate and more valuable to me. So, as to how you cherish things, there's like a scale to it.

ANTHAZIA: That's interesting because last November I was in Halifax doing a workshop and a woman brought along her wedding photo. Although she was divorced from her husband, she was still holding on to this photo. At the end of the workshop, after writing about it, she said to me, Anthazia, I'm done with this. I've written about it, deconstructed it, or done whatever I had to do, and he's out of my life, so it's going in the trash. Its meaning had shifted for her because she was now at a time where, if she remarries and moves on, she doesn't really need this in her life. So, there is the holding-on part but there's also the letting-go part. Even though they have pared down and come to the workshop with this one thing, at the end they can say, I don't really need this. And when you're writing from objects, that shift can happen in just a few hours. With her, I think the decision was always there; it was just waiting for the right time for her to sit with it and contemplate. In all our busyness, we don't find the time to really sit and think about why we are hanging on to these things.

SHELLEY: I agree. If my clients have the time and if I have the right questions to probe them, well, then, you can see so much on someone's face and they get emotional; they don't know where they're going with it. I see that on my clients' faces all the time, when something has to be set aside and dealt with later. They just need a little bit more time to think about it.

MATTE: In the case of both of you, it's like you're creating a space between people and their things that isn't really there in their daily life. They've got this cherished object, or whatever it is sitting in the hallway on a special shelf, but what you're doing is causing them to open up a very reflective, very self-conscious space that changes their relationship to that object, because they're having to pay attention to it.

ANTHAZIA: Change, yes, but also coming to grips with what is there, because I'm a firm believer that your decisions are in you but just need that prompt, like an object can be, for you to really look in the mirror and say, well, it's there and I need to deal with it. Sometimes, though, when there isn't an object, a memory can be used as one, whether a memory of an event or a memory of an object. In a sense, a memory itself becomes an object.

DENISE: That's interesting, Anthazia. I have maybe a strange question for you: when you ask people to bring in an object, I would expect that they'd bring something that had a happy memory associated with it. But from what we've been discussing, it seems that people can bring what you might call *difficult* objects too. Is that something you purposely ask of them, or do you just leave it open?

ANTHAZIA: Yes, I do. It's a workshop in which we're dealing with objects and memories, so I leave it open. In my workshop "Arrivals and Departures," with newcomers to Canada, for instance, we explore how the memory connects with the object – whether it has happy memories associated with it or not – and then we look at how understanding that connection can help them make the transition to their new life in Canada.

SHELLEY: I'd like to pick up on that point, as well as Denise's comment about "difficult objects," and share a story that I think illustrates the role of objects, and the memories associated with them, in managing transition in later life.

This one client I worked with – we were two years together – had the luxury of time, so we just picked away at things. There were many days where we would just talk, and nothing really got accomplished in a practical sense. But she was processing and processing, and she had the responsibility of two uncles, her mother, her husband, and a good friend. She really was the collector of their things. Her uncle had served in the war, and he had amazing memorabilia. He was actually in the prisoner-of-war camp that they made the movie *The Great Escape* about. In fact, he was there during the escape itself. He had journals of sketches of the bunks and the camp and it was really amazing, all this history, and she took great pride in and responsibility for these things of her uncle in terms of where they were going to go. Are they going to stay in the family or go into a museum? Anyway, there was this one item that for some reason really got to me – a little shaving brush, which I thought was really cool and I would send pictures of it to my husband, who has a military background. He would say, Shelley, I've never seen one of those before; the museum at Gagetown (a local military base) would love to have it. But she just backed right up and said, no, it's going in the garbage. And I thought, wow, what a response! It took me off guard, for this wasn't just the first few months that we were working together; this was well into our relationship and we had built up a very trusting rapport. Still, although I knew there had to be some meaning behind her saying this, I let it go at the time. And in fact, she actually did throw it in the garbage, which really saddened me because I felt there was something going on in her concerning it.

When we finally talked about the matter, she said it was simply too personal to give away, this shaving brush of her uncle, a man whom she truly cherished. However, as she explained her reasoning to me – her "autobiographical reasoning," I guess you'd call it – the brush had been owned by a bombardier [her uncle] in a plane that killed and destroyed. It shaved a rough face into a clean face, so meticulous and smooth. Meaning that it was in stark contrast to her uncle's actual job, which was bombing people and causing such incredible devastation. That's what it symbolized to her. She knew the person, she knew the history, and she knew the devastation, and somehow, she wove all of that together. She's not someone who just reacts, she's a thinker, so obviously it had prompted this thought process for her and therefore it had to go. That was, like, my biggest "wow" moment. I don't understand it myself but that's the connection she made with that brush ... the destruction and the devastation and this horrible time in our history.

ANTHAZIA: Yes, it's something bigger; it's where the personal becomes political. Difficult objects can also be cherished, but it might not be until you can really sit with them that you can say, it's going in the garbage. So "cherished" and "difficult" can go together. If people have experienced, say, a traumatic loss or an ambiguous loss of some sort, whatever it might be, then maybe they hang on longer to the things that remind them of it? In which case, it's almost like going to surgery, isn't it? Finding healing within yourself by using that object to pull apart and take away what you don't need. You need the object to write and to make sense of what is happening, but you don't need it after that. It's like coming to a sense of peace within yourself.

Question 2: Do you have any stories about the metaphorical, symbolic, emotional, or even spiritual significance that certain things have had in your clients/participants' lives?

SHELLEY: You know the story, Matte, that you and Brandi wrote about the chap with the table [Chapter 12]? Well, I have much the same sort of story. There was nothing else in this one client's home. Even the dinnerware and china and crystal weren't as important as the table itself. Which surprised me: sixty years in a home and it's just the table at the end! The house was cleared out, it was empty, and the last thing in it was the table. Oh, my gosh, I have goose bumps now just thinking about it! If you could have seen pictures of the home, it was a full basement, and all the bedrooms full, but the last thing that we sold was the table. And that took a lot of back and forth, figuring out where the right home for it was, because it was too big to fit in her new home. If it's passed on to someone who will cherish it like you did, then it's not so hard to let it go.

Fortunately, the table ended up going to a family that mirrored her own family, her younger family, that is. But it was the stories around that table that remained. Every time she and I would visit, sitting at it, there'd be another story, about how it was purchased, for example, or about "all the dinner parties we had, for my husband's work colleagues, for family holidays, neighbourhood parties, with so many people sometimes – once there were twenty-seven! – that we had to put a card table at the end of it and bring up extra chairs from the basement ..." It was symbolic of so, so many memories, and of her sense of being a woman who stayed home for her family, supporting her husband, and that gave her such great pride. You know, there's a generation of people that really did have dinner parties and created that sort of environment. They all had pianos and were musical, they had cocktail parties with singing, and the décor, and the attention to detail, and they valued relationships. And so, for this client, and it can happen for many others too, it really came down to that table.

ANTHAZIA: Yeah, the objects people bring to a workshop – I haven't seen anyone bring a table yet; I'd be amazed if that happened! – but it's the relationships, right? It's not really the table per se, it's what happened, the life experiences that happened around it, and what that symbolizes for the person holding on to it. And I think life writing can help us get at that. Do you mind if I read a little here from the notes I prepared for this question?

> Life-writing asks us to be real with ourselves. The writing process can move very quickly from learning and being interested in the technical aspects of writing to becoming a pouring-out exercise, an emptying of oneself. Life-writing as a genre affords us the freedom to remember and to feast on our lives, to investigate what Ta-Nehisi Coates (2015) describes as "the cold hard truths of our life" (p. 38). What objects do in this metaphorical process of emptying oneself is take us beyond the boundaries we have set out for ourselves and invite a sense of vulnerability necessary for the writing to be real or to come alive.

I remember facilitating a series of workshops entitled "The Suitcase Stories" for the museum downtown, right here in Fredericton. During the workshop, a participant – we'll call him Fernando – brought a hat that he had tucked away for some time. As I was guiding the warm-up sessions, he revealed that he was able to link his father's hat to the strong, determined, resilient person that he himself had become, a person with the kind of personality to withstand the horrible experiences he had to endure through his life journeys, like being exiled from his country and having to leave his profession and having to live in different places around the world. In being invited to write about what the hat represents, Fernando is pushed to remember the times he shared with his father, whose funeral, by the way, he never got to attend. During our conversations, I sensed that Fernando had a going-back-in-time moment, but more so, he was able to reach within the depths of his soul and make connections with the truth(s) of who he is, that truth, that spiritual connection – some call it a gut feeling or a nudge – that often fades into the background of our lives because we're too busy to listen to it. For this participant, it was when he took a moment to sit with himself and connect with his father's hat that he was able to experience an awakening through deep contemplation and connection. Fernando began to see writing as an avenue that, in the words of Louise DeSalvo (1999), "permits the construction of a cohesive, elaborate, thoughtful, personal narrative in the way that simply speaking about our experiences doesn't" (p. 41).

BILL: It strikes me, Anthazia, that this kind of working with memories and using things to help you face what are perhaps difficult parts of your life is a classic way of engaging in what psychologists of ageing call "integrative reminiscence." It's a type of reminiscence where you integrate the good, the bad, and the ugly of your life, and it's associated with maturity in later life, with the achievement of some kind of wisdom or insight or transcendence even. It's the pulling-yourself-together, as it were, that is so important. And you're helping people do that in a very rich way in these workshops, where people can sometimes be brought to tears – not sad tears necessarily, but rich tears almost. And, Shelley, in your own way, you're doing something similar.

SHELLEY: Yes, it's coming full circle – or 360, as it were – with moments in your life, and "integrated" is a good word for it.

MATTE: We've talked about how a thing can signify a relationship. This got me thinking about the relationship, and in a sense the responsibility, that we can have to a thing itself. Because our lives are bound by death, things tend to last longer than individual lives, especially well-made things. Forget about disposable razors; I'm talking about a well-made razor, or a well-made bag or tool or whatever, something that can and should be passed on. What I'm talking about is integrating enough of what the thing means to me so that I'm able to say, okay, I really don't need to hang onto this anymore. I'm done with it. Then my responsibility – to that thing – is to find another place where it can go.

SHELLEY: Yes, a huge part of letting go is knowing that someone else will, maybe not cherish it, but find it useful and appreciate it. You don't know how many times my clients have said that it's not a monetary thing, it's not about selling it, it's about wanting it to go to a home, or a person, that will appreciate it like they have done. Then they can let it go. That's my responsibility as well to my clients. It's all about finding the right home for things and then they can let them go.

There was this one lady I worked with very briefly. She was very meticulous and very decisive with things, and there was this beautiful old milk pitcher in her kitchen. I said to her, this is gorgeous. She said, oh, that was my grandmother's. And then I saw her body language change and this faraway look in her eyes as she stared out into her backyard. She said, I just remember my grandmother and the sweetened milk she used to make in it and pour on our pancakes, and that is such a beautiful memory. She wasn't looking at me, but I was watching her, and I said, so would you like to keep this? She said, no, that's okay. I can let it go. It wasn't one of her most cherished things but there was this beautiful memory attached to it. Once she shared the story of that memory, though, it's like it gave the object more meaning and, at the same time, enabled her to let go of it. And so I said, well, I know someone who would really appreciate this, who would absolutely love it, and she said, perfect. So, I feel that that's my responsibility: to ensure that their cherished items make it to a new home, and then it's easier for people to let them go. That's why the charities around are really nice. People pick charities that resonate with them and then it's easier to let something go, if they know that it's going to, say, the homeless shelter, or whatever. It's sort of like your responsibility too, Anthazia, which is to guide people through the workshop process and allow them a safe space. That's one of the things that I like to do, that I need to do, for my clients.

ANTHAZIA: Jumping off of that, I remember this lady at a workshop in Halifax who had these beads on her wrist. She told me: I didn't bring any object. I don't have any object. So, I said, well, is there a story behind those beads? She's, like, they're just beads, but I wear them all the time. I asked, why? She said, oh, they were my mother's. Is your mother with you? No, she said. And then I suggested she begin writing, and from that, she started telling us all these stories about her mother. And she said, yeah, probably that's the reason I always wear them, right? So sometimes, it's knowing, yet not knowing, that there's a story there; that there's a connection that, deep down, you care about. But maybe you can't just put your finger on it, so the telling of that story releases whatever was inside. By the way, I find that participants use the word "care" a lot: if I can find somebody to care for the thing, then I can let it go.

MATTE: Yes, on that point I was thinking of one object that I have that I got after completing my PhD. I looked into buying a robe for Convocation, but I thought $1,200 bucks, no way, for a piece of clothing that I'm going to wear only once a year. But then somebody who was retiring from the university announced that he wanted to give a robe away, with a fancy hat and everything, and I said, oh, give it to me. I'll take it! And I went to try and find the man and thank him, but he didn't actually want me to know anything about him, nor did he want me to know the story of himself and his career. So, I got the sense that he just wanted this thing to be useful, to go to somebody who should have it and would take care of it.

SHELLEY: It wasn't about him anymore, right? But, yeah, there's people that, once you see them let go, it's like they experience this relief from the burden that we talked about before. You can just watch their body language. Like, I'm sitting there right next to them while we're doing these things, and once they make the decision, it's great. I give people options, right? That's my job, to give them options as to where their things can go, and they can decide whenever they're ready.

ANTHAZIA: Sometimes, four hours in a workshop is not enough time for people to make that sort of decision, so I find myself occasionally having phone conversations with them afterwards, because even though they want to let go of an object and give it to, say, the second-hand shop, it's not time yet.

BILL: When you both talk about letting go, I'm wondering if maybe that's not an important part of so-called successful ageing, which is a term I actually don't like. But, particularly as we near death, which you might say is the ultimate in letting go, if we're not ready to let go of stuff in our lives, then there's work that we should maybe have done a lot earlier. I'm reminded here, for example, of what the old miser said to his minister when told he wouldn't be able to take his possessions with him when he died: "Well sir," he replied, "if I can't take it with me, then I ain't a-goin'!" But in the workshops and in the phone conversations, Anthazia, you're helping people to engage in that important task of letting go of things, and in the task of making sense of them that precedes it. So, I wonder sometimes if there's almost like a small-*s* spiritual dimension to what's going on in these workshops …

ANTHAZIA: I think it has a lot to do with it, but of course how do we define "spirituality"? Everybody will have their own definition. For me, it is thinking about something that is bigger than ourselves. When you work with seniors, it's often something that's higher than them that they're depending on, and then it goes back also to the authenticity, the truth, that lives within them. And it doesn't necessarily have to be "a spiritual being" like a god, but it's that inner nudge or soul-searching that is meeting them in the flesh, so to speak, and it's becoming one with that, or communing with that, that is helping them to let go. I've seen people nearing death who have regrets and it's hard for them, even without an object, to just sit and have conversations with you as their time approaches to leave this world. It's hard *because* of those regrets, which they haven't really had an opportunity to talk about it. And that's my concern with social media, and how everything is so quick, and it's google this or google that, and we're not giving ourselves time to process our lives in preparation for that final phase. So, yes, going back to your question, I think it has a lot to do with spirituality.

BILL: Is it a fair question, I wonder, to ask you both to think about the concept of regret? If so, do you have any wisdom or any stories to share from your respective work about the role that regret plays as people think about their lives and about the value of certain objects to them?

SHELLEY: Well, I think it's the *fear* of regret … it's not so much the regret itself as it is, you're afraid that you're *going* to regret. Part of that fear, too, is that if it – the thing – is gone, then eventually the memory will be gone. Forever. And when you're in the position of getting rid of something that was valuable to someone else, for instance, you may feel *guilty* that, although what you're getting rid of was cherished by your mother, it's not cherished nearly as much by you. And that can be hard to live with.

ANTHAZIA: I think, for you, "fear" is a good word, but in writing, people experience redemption, for want of a better word. The redemption comes with, okay, I'm in this workshop, I'm having conversation with others in the room, and there's somebody here to guide me through the process, so if I have regrets – about, say, things that I've done or not done – then I'm in a safe space to think about them and work them through. The foreshadowing or fear of regret is something, to be sure, but with writing, I think, there is a way to redeem yourself from that pain.

MATTE: I wonder what kind of conversation we're going to be having after a generation has grown up on Google and disposable things and they're thinking about downsizing? Do you think we are looking at a changing relationship with objects on a cultural scale, or will there always be cherished objects in the sense that we have them now?

SHELLEY: That's a really good question.

ANTHAZIA: That's a very good question.

SHELLEY: I always think things will come around again. You know, we have a minimalist movement out there nowadays where we're told that you don't need all this stuff around you. You need clean lines, only two books on the shelf, that kind of thing. I personally don't live like that, though, and I don't want to live like that. My things around me represent my life, and I like that, and I'm afraid that twenty or thirty years down the road we won't have any of these beautiful historical things that were handmade so amazingly by craftsmen who were often in our families, and that worries me. I'm afraid we're going to have a huge regret because, as a society, when we let these things go because of a trend – and I mean there are extremes, of course: there's hoarding at one end and minimalism at the other. But I tend to think there's going to be a great deal of regret. Of course, maybe that's just me and maybe I want there to be a regret, because I *do* value things. I do value the historical significance of things, and I would just hate to see them gone. Because we can't get it back when it's gone. That's what people deal with as well. They can't get it back once it's gone.

ANTHAZIA: I think there's a generation coming along that doesn't have an attachment to physical things. They don't know what that relationship is, because of all the gadgets they have, where everything is instantaneous. I have a sixteen-year-old at home, for example, who asks me, "Why are there all these books in the house? Why can't you just google stuff? Look, mom, I'll teach you how to use Google!" But I like the smell of pages, and you can't get that from a device.

SHELLEY: And is that good or bad? Is that us putting our values on them?

ANTHAZIA: Who knows? Time will tell. Time will tell.

Question 3: In dealing with cherished objects, have you ever observed a participant/client making a new observation about a particular thing/object – either because they are looking at it in a new way for an exercise in the workshop or because a decision has to be made about discarding it (or not)? Do you have any stories that come to mind as you think about this question?

SHELLEY: I have a little story. One of my clients had all these Christmas decorations of her mother's, and among them there was this blue ceramic angel. It was old and dilapidated, but I thought it was beautiful. It was in a box, circa 1950s maybe, and the plastic was ripped. But I thought, oh, I can fix it up for her. Well, she didn't really care about it; there were other things that were more meaningful to her. So, I took it anyway and cleaned it up and made the box look really pretty, and I gave it to her just before Christmas. Sometimes I make those decisions. I could be right or wrong, but it's not hurting anybody. So, I gave it to her and she looked at it again and – it was like one of those moments, maybe because it was the holiday season – she started telling me how her mother was an educator, a teacher, and for years and years, she put these pageants on at Christmas time. And that angel was the one consistent thing that was always at the top of the tree during them. It was the one thing that represented her mother's commitment to education and to her career, and being a single mom who struggled, who didn't have a lot of money, who got her education and did really, really well in her field. I mean, she told me that the people at her mom's funeral were past premiers of the province and lieutenant-governors. So, all of a sudden, this Christmas angel, which was going to be gone … I gave her an opportunity to rethink its value. In her new place, in fact, she had it sitting nicely in the box on her piano. So, I just get a sense sometimes that there's something more to things. She would never get rid of it now. It's a cherished item for her, for certain.

BILL: If you take that same kind of personalized approach with other clients, where you think, hey, with this object, there's something more going on and I'm going to help my client revisit it, like this woman did, that lends a whole other layer of wonderfulness to the kind of work you do.

SHELLEY: Honestly, I find something in everybody's home that, during the chaos and the moving and all that stuff, I hear little tidbits about, or they'll mention something about it, but because of time and everything else that has to be done, it kind of gets dismissed. So here's another story for you …

With one client, there was this horseshoe hanging in the garage – remember how people used to do that? – that went back to, like, 1820. I mean, the family heritage in this province is huge. Which, by the way, makes me want to use a word like "stewardship" instead of "obligation," because it's about maintaining part of your family history, your community history even, in the hopes that it will carry on. Rather than "obligation," which makes it sound like a burden, "stewardship" suggests that you want to carry on, that there is value to it. In any case, with this horseshoe, I actually cleaned it up, framed it, and put it in a nice little shadow box, just the horseshoe all by itself. She can't put it over her door in her new apartment, of course, but it's on the wall just inside the door. And, well, the tears were coming on with that one! It's hit or miss, right? But with every one of my clients, I try to find something of theirs that I bring back to them as sort of a house-warming gift.

There was another client where I did that. She had this little clay pot sitting on the wall just inside the back door, and she always had fresh flowers in it from her garden. So, after working with her all through the spring and summer, I kept it and I put some dried lavender in it from my own garden, and I gave it to her at Christmas. It's that kind of connection, something that was attached to the home. If it's not the table or the pictures, then it's something that represents the house, or a memory of the house, something they can bring with them. People are incredibly resilient, I find, when they face a major life-change like this, but they need some sense of continuity in the midst of it, and this sort of thing can help. It's nothing ever that big or burdensome, of course, and nothing that's ever really been of value, or at least of monetary value. So, anyway, that's what I do try to do for everybody.

BILL: Do you think others in your line of work do this too?

SHELLEY: I don't know; you'd have to ask them. But I'm very fortunate that I can do this. Very fortunate.

ANTHAZIA: We were talking earlier about memories as objects. Well, I had a lady who came to one of my workshops but didn't bring anything with her. However, she was talking about the Caspian Sea and swimming in it as a child with her father, and all the wonderful memories she had of it, and then about going back and seeing it littered with plastic and garbage. And so, from that wonderful memory she is now building a career as an environmentalist. Her attachment as a little girl to the sea and to her father has now changed into her building a career, wanting to clean up not only the Caspian Sea but her own environment where she's living in Halifax. It's interesting, then, how one thing can lead to another and another and another. And that's just one example.

There was this other woman some years ago in a month-long creative writing course for seniors – this would have been in Mississauga, Ontario – who talked about her husband, and how she had kept all of his and her journals about being in Japan, and the war, the Hiroshima bombings. She never thought she could become an author, but she said to me at one point, "Can I take all of this and make something out of it?" So, we sat over lunch and talked and, well, it's like that opened the floodgates. She's still writing, at eighty-five! It's amazing what can come out of these workshops.

BILL: Then there's the woman I recall you telling me about one time who takes the memories that she has thought about, sparked by certain objects in your workshops, and she ends up producing a very important thing, a new thing, that book that she's now extremely proud of, and rightly so, but that represents the integrating and valuing and raising up of key things in her life.

ANATHAZIA: Yes, and then she went on to write a second book mentioning our meeting and about what that has done for her. I've often continued relationships with some of the participants in my workshops, and it's amazing what they do after that – the ripple effect of my involvement with them, I guess you could say.

DENISE: It strikes me, Anthazia, that this process can't be done in just a couple of hours. But with you, Shelley, although you often have time constraints, you tend to have quite long relationships with your clients, and a lot of follow-up with them.

BILL: Yes, and what strikes me, too, is that you each are agents of both transition and transformation. I mean, Shelley, you use the word "transition" in the name of your company – Gentle Pace Transitions. But the transitions and the transformations are closely linked, aren't they?

SHELLEY: Yes, they are. In fact, I'm inspired now to go back and have conversations with my clients – that post-interview sort of thing that I talked about before. I mean, I'm very close to probably seven of my clients and we've actually moved on a bit from our time together around the whole downsizing process. I really would like to go back, as there are a few questions in my head right now because of what we've just been discussing, and visit with them again one or two years later to see, you know, what they're feeling and thinking about these cherished items once they've gone through the transition process and are settled in their new place, because there's another step or phase in that process. I love what you do, Anthazia, it seems just to be the perfect extension of what I do with a lot of my clients. It's therapeutic, right?

ANTHAZIA: Yes, it is.

SHELLEY: And with some of them, it's not done the day they move into their new home. It's definitely not done, that transition. There's a lot of follow-up afterwards, and there's a lot – like with your phone calls and emails, Anthazia – a lot of hanging on. They don't need me there, but they want me there. "Oh, Shelley," they'll call me up, "I wonder if you could come by and hang this picture …" I know they don't want to bother me, because they know I'm busy, but still they'll get me there on a sort of pretext, if you like, and it's really, for them and for me too, about continuing that relationship. And it is just such a gift!

ANTHAZIA: And it turns sometimes into beautiful friendships. You become part of their family almost.

SHELLEY: Yes, you do. Especially with the seniors, the ones who are alone. And then their extended family who don't live here, they will call you, because they trust you, and ask, you know, "Is she okay?" Granted, family dynamics can be challenging sometimes in my line of work. Family can be supportive, for sure, but sometimes it's like "You don't need that, mom.

Why do you want to keep that?!" Which I guess I can understand. They're in a hurry and their lives are busy, but they don't allow their parents the time to reminisce and think about things and make the decision on their own, when in fact they're more than capable of doing so. Thankfully, though, that sort of situation is the exception more than the rule, and the sweet connection you can develop with family members, well, I embrace that, because it fills my cup – as a person, not as a business owner. That just fills my cup.

ANTHAZIA: With the immigrants I've worked with here in Fredericton, some of them have reached out to me with situations that I don't have a clue how to solve. I'm not a policymaker, I'm not a politician. But they can say things to you that they can't say to somebody else. They just need me to listen, not to solve anything, just listen. That's all they need.

BILL: I don't think I realized it until this afternoon, but the work that you two people do is so closely linked. And it's amazing the personal relationships that you develop. It's not at all just about doing a job.

SHELLEY: No, it's not. I always say that anybody can go into a person's house and help them pack up and move and disperse stuff. Anybody can do that, but when I come into your life it's, it's so much more, just so much more. I don't mean to be tooting my own horn here, but I've been doing this for four years and I truly believe that it's a gift to do it. I'm sure you do as well, Anthazia, with your workshops.

ANTHAZIA: Yes, it doesn't feel like work. I'll do this for free! And when I'm in the classroom as a teacher, this is how I teach. What I do in the classroom is just an extension of what I do in my workshops. I have a standardized curriculum, yes, but how do I want to implement it? It's through storytelling.

SHELLEY: Exactly. And what you're doing is you're guiding them. I have never told a client what to do with anything. I give them the options, we talk them through, and they make their decisions. It's the same with you, Anthazia, isn't it? You're not telling them what to write, you're coaching them. You're a writing life coach.

ANTHAZIA: Yeah!

Question 4: Do you have any thoughts on the sort of reasoning or reminiscence that your clients/participants engage in when reflecting on the place or meaning of certain things/objects in their own lives?

SHELLEY: The nature of your relationship to items changes, or can change, based on circumstances, and where you are in your life. Take, for example, your husband's razor. Its value can change dramatically for you from the time when he's alive to the day after his death. Or, depending on the thing and the relationship, it could be the other way around – like, three months from now maybe not so much.

ANTHAZIA: I agree with you. It depends on the circumstances, and what activities you're involved in, so it's always kind of in flux. In fact, I had a few thoughts on this question that I wrote down …

> Storytelling, or story-making, pushes us to think not only about the past but to engage in a sort of foreshadowing towards the future. Sometimes there are participants that come to my workshop who are not wanting to remember but wanting to write. Not to begin in that place of reminiscence because it is too painful, because they had so much fun there, and knowing that, in reality, they may never have that fun again can be painful.

What I find can happen with reminiscence is that if participants are encouraged to go into places of deep remorse or nostalgia, then they end up coming out of the workshop saying, "It was good for me. I needed that to make connections as to why my life has turned out the way it did." I mean, maybe they were beating their head against a wall trying to figure out why, or they were papering over something, or holding onto one thing or another. Again, that's what you might call "autobiographical reasoning," right?

SHELLEY: I think your example earlier of the wedding photo is perfect here, Anthazia. I mean, ten years prior, that could have been that woman's most cherished possession, right? And then her situation changes. The cherishableness – there's that word again – is time-specific, and an object can lose its sentimental significance over time. Or the other way around, as we've talked about already. Some things are just things, in other words, until suddenly they're not anymore! It's as if the passage of time itself helps us to decide what we cherish, or not.

ANTHAZIA: And, yes, sometimes just a few hours, like in a workshop, can cause that change to come about.

Question 5: How has your work in the downsizing industry or in facilitating writing workshops affected or changed your relationship to or your experience of things in your own life, and why?

SHELLEY: I realize that I don't hang onto many things, don't keep many things. I'm certainly not a hoarder, although I've had a few clients who were. For them, it's like *everything* is meaningful! For me, though, I'm more of a *symbolic* keeper. My grandmother, for instance, had this one thing that, when she died, I was desperate to have. It was a doughnut cutter and, well, it reminded me of all the doughnuts she had made for her family over the years, and all the cooking she did. When Dad asked if I wanted anything of hers, I was so afraid someone else would want it too. But they didn't. Of the thirteen grandchildren, I was the only one. Whenever it comes up in conversation, even thirty years later, my cousins and siblings will say, "Oh, you're so lucky to have it!" To me, that thing is the personification of my gram; it personifies my sense of her, my relationship with her. Happy memories …

If circumstances were to change, however – like, for example, when my parents pass away – I don't know how much I would keep. An item can be cherished because, say, the original owner cherished it. Maybe we could call that "deferred cherishableness." There's a new term for you! But, so far, I haven't lost my closest family members. Maybe that will change everything … Up until six or eight months ago, when he began paring things down, my husband was one to hang onto a lot, because he was afraid to have regrets. As I say, that weighs on people. Fear of regret is a big burden.

ANTHAZIA: I know that, after facilitating all these workshops, I've stopped holding on to stuff in the way I used to do. Like you, Shelley, I've stopped being a hoarder. And moving has helped of course, because I've moved around a lot in my life, so every move I make, it's, okay, I haven't used such-and-such for a year, so it's going! It's become easier, for example, for me to let go of my high school notebooks, something which after thirty-plus years I really have no use for anymore. Now, I keep things that I have a connection with, or that I can have, you know, sort of a conversation with to help me through difficult times. Like, my grandmother's dress is something I would never give away. The smell of her is in my closet. I need that, and her earrings. I mean, I lay with her as she was dying. And my grandfather's walking stick – which I don't have because I couldn't get it on the plane, but it's back home in British Guyana where my mom and dad are – that's something I definitely wouldn't get rid of. So I guess you could say I've been brought to a point of really reflecting on my own life and on what I want to keep and what I want to give away.

But still, this whole decluttering process is a work in progress, isn't it? Like when it comes to, say, hand-written letters sent to me back in the 90s. Hopefully, some day, I can create something out of them, a collage maybe, but for now I'm hanging onto them.

SHELLEY: I agree with you a hundred per cent. And I've been like this for a while. I need, like, a token thing that represents someone meaningful in my life. Once again, with my grandmother, who sold her doughnuts at the market, the only thing I wanted was that doughnut cutter. I remember, as a kid, going up to the farm while she was making them on Mondays and Tuesdays and she would let me help her. She included me, even though she was crazy-busy and this was her livelihood. I remember making those doughnuts next to her in that hot lard and I cry, you know. That was just the one little thing that was so meaningful. I was so afraid that someone was going to take it. I don't need a lot of things of my grandmother's; I didn't need this and I didn't need that, but just that one thing. Because I remember, I still cherish it today, you're darned right I do! I mean, she had a whole other side to her where she loved to act and things like that. My sister has the book, like a couple of her play books, and that was meaningful for her to have those.

As far as my other grandmother is concerned, I have a little ceramic cow that was sitting in her kitchen, and I was visiting her one day and I said, "Oh, my gosh grandma, I just love that. I don't know why, but that cow reminds me of you." And she said, "You take that," and I said, "No, I'm not." In any event, I ended up getting it long before she died. So, going back to my comment about being a symbol keeper, I don't need a lot. I just need that symbol. If I don't have something to remember, I'm afraid I might forget. So it's just that little trigger. Not a house full, because that becomes a burden, mentally. If everything you looked at was a memory, good or bad, that takes up a lot of brain space. It'd be exhausting. No, it's about travelling light.

ANTHAZIA: Yes, travelling light ...

So then, that's the gist of the conversation that the two of us had with Matte, Denise, and Bill. In very much a meandering manner, with one comment leading to another and another and another, we ended up covering a broad range of themes – and certainly emotions – that the "industries" we each work in involve, both for us and for our "clients." Among them, to name just a few, are guilt and regret, fear and relief, relationship and redemption, attachment and integration, transition and transformation, hoarding and healing. And we talked as well about heart value versus monetary value and stewardship versus obligation, about difficult objects and about degrees of cherishableness. But we could have covered many themes more if we had had the time, maybe a whole conference worth of it! Two hours was not enough. We didn't touch at all, for instance, on the fact that both of us are women, as are the majority of our participants or clients. As earlier chapters in this book have pondered, when you factor in gender as a dimension of the relationships people have with things, is it possible that women are more sentimental, and more narrative-y, all around? If so, why? Or is it more complicated than that? In any case, the one theme that stood out for us with stunning clarity is that things and stories are very, very closely linked, which of course makes for lots of common ground between what we each do for a living. With so many life-transition professionals like Shelley in Canada alone, and life-writing groups like those that Anthazia leads springing up at an ever-growing rate, we can only assume that appreciation for this link – and all that it implies for what people value and for how they live, and story, their lives – can only increase.

Afterword: Changing Things Changing Us: Further Reflections on the Role of Cherished Objects in the Stories of Our Lives

CLIVE BALDWIN

> The world, the human world, is bound together not by protons and electrons, but by stories. Nothing has meaning in itself; all the objects in the world would be shards of bare mute blankness, spinning wildly out of orbit, if we didn't bind them together with stories.
>
> – Brian Morton (1999, p. 185)

When I volunteered to write this Afterword, I thought it would be quite straightforward to do. After all, my task was to summarize some themes, draw some connections, and suggest some possible directions in which further research might usefully go, the same tasks as I have done multiple times before for multiple projects. I was wrong. The more I read and reread the various chapters, both as they were being developed between members and within the CIRN group as a whole and the versions that finally emerged, the more I realized that the task was not at all going to be the straightforward one I had imagined, or perhaps had hoped for. Just as my colleagues had crawled inside of our interviewees' transcripts and stories in carrying out their narrative inquiries, I, too, was compelled to crawl inside the resultant chapters, not only to do justice to their work but also to understand the nuances, connections, possibilities, dynamics, and depths at work in our participants' worlds, and in our interpretations of them in turn. At the same time, in identifying key issues and considerations I do not want this piece to be viewed as a substitute for reading the rest of the book. You will not find here a Coles Notes version of my colleagues' efforts. Rather, my intention here is to take up certain themes and ideas that run through what they have written and let them lead me in some reflections upon: (1) the nature of cherished objects, (2) how material things become cherished objects, and (3) the work they do or are called upon to do and, along the way, the relationship between cherished objects and our sense of self and belonging, our sense of narrative identity.

The Nature of Cherished Objects

The word "cherish" means multiple things. On the one hand, to cherish an object means to hold or treat it dear, to have a sense of attachment to it, an attachment that is often, but not necessarily, emotional in nature. On the other hand, to cherish can mean to care for, protect, or nurture; often this is used to refer to another person or a sentient creature. To cherish can also mean to keep in one's mind, as in a cherished memory. While the focus of this book has been cherished *objects*, it is, I think, important to recognize in the interviews and stories in which these objects feature that participants' cherished objects might fall under more than one meaning of the word.

In Joan's story of her grandfather and being given her grandfather's beer stein by a neighbour who intuited that it might be important should someone ever come looking, she is clearly attached to the stein. This tangible object seems to function at least in part as *reminiscentium* of her grandfather, and thus she expresses emotional attachment to it (more on the work that cherished objects do later). Now, of course, such *reminiscentia* are cared for and protected in that we tend not to want such cherished objects damaged, lost, or destroyed. And in this case the object is clearly linked to cherished memories, quite self-defining ones in fact – even though the object appeared late in the story of Joan and her grandfather and was not directly linked to any discrete memory of time, place, or event involving him.

For Bob and Mary, on the other hand, sea glass appears to be slightly different. There seems to be less of an emotional attachment to any particular piece of sea glass – so any given piece is not necessarily *reminiscentium* or linked to specific cherished memories. However, there is a sense in which sea glass is cared for in a way that is in excess of protecting. I want to suggest that the couple care for sea glass in a more nurturing way than perhaps we normally think of people taking care of an object.

In Chapter 3, Matte alludes to Aristotle's four causes of things: matter, form, agency, and end. In fashioning matter into form with the intention of creating jewellery, the couple, I suggest, are nurturing the sea glass. They are transforming it, enhancing its beauty (or at least allowing it to be displayed). They care for the glass enough to want to find ways that it can become more of an actant, a non-human actor that changes the world – becoming *reminiscentia* for others. It can also be seen as nurturing the couple – acting on them and their family in engendering gathering, collaboration, and new ways of seeing things. Similarly, we see Susan nurturing the currants that her mother had picked in transforming them into dye for yarn in order to create something new to write about. As sea glass and currants are transformed by human agency, humans are transformed by the agency of non-humans. (Again, see below where I reflect upon another theme hinted at by Matte, that of actor-network theory).

In the stories that our participants shared or wrote, and that my colleagues have been reflecting on in this book, one form of cherished object does not seem to be represented – the object to which there is a non-emotional attachment. I think here of objects that are cherished for what they are rather than for what they represent, what place they have in our lives, what work they do. Among my books I have one of which I am particularly fond – I would say that I cherish it. I came across it on the AbeBooks website's list of weird books. I had not heard of it before, nor has it any place particularly in my story, but I treasure it as something that is beautiful and mysterious. My copy is not a first edition, it is not signed by the author, it was not a gift (save to myself) nor do I know the authors, so it has no relational import, and I cannot read the text as it is in a language devised by the author and which no one has ever been able to decipher, so it is not informative, does not transport one into another storyworld, and cannot be connected to other ideas or texts by what it says. Nonetheless, I do cherish it. Not being useful, it does fulfil William Blake's alternative to usefulness – it is stunningly beautiful. The script, the illustrations, the paper on which it is printed, the binding, and the dust cover make it something special that I am pleased and proud to have in my life. I cherish it because it is the *Codex Seriphianus.* It is what it is, no more, no less. This is perhaps the "thinginess" to which Matte refers in Chapter 3 – but I see this essentialist thinginess in these stories less than he.

How Do Objects Become *Cherished* Objects?

The second theme I want to discuss, which is linked to the first and linked, too, to the question raised by Matte in Chapter 3, is how do objects become *cherished* objects? In the stories of our participants, it does not seem to be "thinginess" that is the primary reason for an object to be cherished. However, the objects are cherished. So, what are the factors that spur on a person to invest emotion, time, effort, and so on in a particular object?

The answer to this question lies, I think, in both high-level abstraction and concrete everyday experience, each in some way informing the other. On the abstract level, it seems to me that we might learn much about how culture shapes individuals by studying their cherished objects. Here, I am thinking particularly about Pierre Bourdieu's two theories of taste/distinction and habitus.

Bourdieu's (1987) theory of "habitus" (pp. 172f.) – a term that, as Bill noted in Chapter 2, Arthur Frank (2010, p. 49) enlists to talk about *narrative* habitus – is that the cultural environment into which we are born and within which we grow up shapes our worldview by its conferring of cultural value. This cultural value may be accorded to the material or the immaterial. Through this we become subjects that reproduce the habitus through our choices in the cultural domain. One aspect of habitus is taste or distinction – our consumer choices and aesthetic preferences being shaped by the cultural values within which we have grown up. We have seen these influences documented in works such as Paul Willis's *Learning to Labour* (1977) where the lads' choices regarding their approach to and activities in school are framed by their working-class culture, which at some level allows them to intuit the class-based structural disadvantage of the schooling system but ultimately serves to reinforce the habitus of school and thus the capitalist system. Although these lads do not have cherished objects, that is, tangible material objects, they do cherish (not their word, nor Willis's) their friendships, belonging, and so forth. A more concrete example might be anti-social behaviour orders (ASBOs) introduced in the United Kingdom in 1998. ASBOs were civil court orders issued against someone due to their behaviour, restricting their behaviour in some way in order to reduce the threat, fear, intimidation, or disturbance caused by the behaviour. ASBOs might, for example, restrict hanging around stairwells in apartment buildings, forbid being in certain places at certain time, forbid swearing or drunkenness. Although ASBOs could be issued against anyone, they were seen primarily as a means of addressing perceived problems of youth delinquency, and the vast majority of ASBOs were issued against working-class youth. ASBOs became part of the culture of punishment (Brown, 2020) and, while relatively ineffective, were generally popular (Kelly, 2012), more perhaps "for what they symbolized or expressed rather than necessarily their instrumental value" (Brown, 2020, p. 94).

ASBOs became embedded in popular culture – people could purchase T-shirts and other ASBO merchandise, there were popular songs written, ASBOs appeared in autobiographical and fictional works, and so on (Kelly, 2012). Rooted in the notion of "naming and shaming," ASBOs sought to both prevent and deter anti-social behaviour. For some recipients, however, ASBOs became badges of honour (Solanki et al., 2006, p. 136): "The recipients were in effect inverting the shaming process and were using their ASBO as a tool to boast to their peers. These recipients of the ASBO were using it to express a message of deviance" (Brown, 2020, p. 96).

This might seem a long way from an individual's cherished object and, indeed, it is not a theme that has been explored in the chapters of this book and has been only sparsely considered in the literature, for example in Bhattacharyya and Pradhan's (2019) brief discussion on the cultural framing of cherishing. But I suggest that an analysis of how cherished objects differ across the larger narrative contexts of gender, race, ethnicity, class, religion, and so on holds promise for interesting research. Dyl and Wapner (1996) explore age and gender differences in the nature, meaning, and function of cherished objects between adolescents and children, but research on the relationship between cherished objects and other demographics might enrich our understanding of human relations with things, identity, self, and belonging, and how our seemingly individual, idiosyncratic selection of objects to cherish reflects wider social tropes, concerns, and constraints.

How Material Things Become Cherished Objects

When we turn to specifics – why this specific object came to be a cherished object to this particular person – I want to suggest three features here, *time*, *relationships*, and *narrative alignment*, and leave a fourth, the work such objects are called upon to do, for later.

Time

From reading the stories that our participants shared during the interviews and those that they wrote out, it seems evident to me that their cherished objects have a relationship with time. For some, such as David, the family table became a cherished object over a relatively lengthy period of time. The table was not a cherished object from the moment of its acquisition but became one due to accompanying multiple family members in their journeys. At a certain point in time, however, it became a non-human companion – I am tempted to say, a non-human member of the family – which ensured that it would continue accompanying family members on their journeys. Quite what that point was I cannot determine – and perhaps neither could David. But the point is that the table's persistence, its continued presence, attendance at family gatherings, faithful service, and so forth *earned* it a place among the family's cherished objects. Here I am aware that I am attributing agency to the table – an attribution that may seem wrong or misguided but one I will explore later on.

Other objects – like the currants in Susan's story – are similarly long-time occupants (in this case, of the freezer) until they emerge as cherished objects to be transformed into dye and appropriated into Susan's various writing projects. They had done their time as currants in the freezer and became enshrined in yarn and creative writing. As Shelley puts it in Chapter 15: "Some things are just things, in other words, until suddenly they're not anymore."

In contrast, there are some participants for whom objects become cherished almost immediately. I am thinking particularly of Harriet and Joan: the former serendipitously coming across the same textbook as was read from by her brother four decades before and she copying the page; the latter being presented with her grandfather's beer stein, rescued by a neighbour following the demolition of her grandfather's manor. These two objects appeared out of nowhere but seem immediately to have become cherished objects.

Yet other objects, illustrated here by Hermann's labyrinth ring, are selected to be or become cherished objects. There are objects that serve to represent something important. In Hermann's case, the ring represents his journeying through life, following or being presented with multiple pathways and having multiple centres, and his belief in unity amid multiplicity. For myself, in a personal memory box that I have, which is one of my own cherished objects that I say more about in my bio (Appendix 1), I have two wooden crosses. These I commissioned from a friend of mine with the intention of giving one to Anne-Marie, the woman I was very much in love with at the time, and keeping one for myself. And while that intention was never realized, these crosses were created to be cherished objects. Such objects encapsulate time and experience.

Relationships

A second feature of cherished objects – perhaps more obviously so – is how they reflect, represent, enhance, or create relationships (see Sherman and Dacher, 2005). Almost all the stories featured in this book – perhaps with the exception of Hermann's – point to the importance of relationships: David's gatherings around the family table; Harriet's relationship with her brother and mother, caught in a page of text; Joy's relationship with Scott captured in his letters to her; Joan's grandfather's beer stein; or Susan's currants picked by her mother. Even the sea glass of Bob and Mary's story, while not directly associated with any particular relationship, drew in their grandchildren.

That cherished objects are associated with important relationships should be of little surprise. Certainly, virtually all the items in my memory box are there because of the importance in one way or another of the relationship I had with the person or persons with whom they are associated. The other obvious point, which I raise for the sake of completeness, is that such objects are associated with persons with whom we had positive relationships. I have, for example, no desire whatsoever to place in my memory box the homeland security evidence bag into which my computer was placed after being confiscated by a US border control officer who had deliberately intimidated me and attempted to manipulate me and my words in pursuit of his narrative of wrongdoing when I had attempted to cross the border on a shopping trip. (I hasten to add that his suspicions were proven to be as unjustified as his behaviour.) I suspect others might feel the same about their own negative relationships.

The two possible exceptions to this association of cherished objects with positive important relationships are Hermann and Amelie. For these two participants, the cherished objects were cherished because they encapsulated some aspects of their lives rather than a relationship with others: Hermann's labyrinth ring, his journeying; Amelie's, her sense of identity. I will return to these two participants later, when I explore the work that cherished objects are called upon to do, and the relationship between cherished objects and self and belonging.

Narrative Alignment

The third feature I want to reflect upon is narrative alignment. In considering our participants' stories, it seems to me that the objects talked about become cherished objects at least in part because they align with an ongoing narrative. None of the objects discussed in the previous chapters, I would argue, seem to be the cause of narrative change. David's table became over time part of his and his family's narrative; Hermann and Amelie's objects served to embrace their existing self-narratives; Joy's letters, Susan's currants, Bob and Mary's collection of sea glass, Harriet's page of text, Joan's beer stein ... all found a place within an ongoing story. Objects become cherished objects because of what I'm calling their narrative alignment – whether that alignment be by choice or by chance.

While alignment might seem an obvious feature, I am puzzled by it. On the one hand, it seems natural, commonsensical, that alignment would facilitate becoming cherished. On the other, I can imagine easily that other objects might become cherished because they prompted change, opened up a new narrative path, inspired greater narrative openness, if you like. From my own experience, I am reminded of books that changed my thinking very significantly and that, consequently, I do hold dear – and while this may not be an exact example of what I am trying to get at, it serves as an opening to the possibility that others might have had their life changes provoked by objects that then become *cherished* objects – perhaps, to continue the book example, a particular copy of a sacred text and a person's subsequent conversion. Again, the nearest I have to this would be the Spring 1987 Teachers' Bulletin of the Urban Wildlife Group. While this was given to me by someone of whom I was very fond, that is not the reason for this object's having a place in my memory box (I have another cherished object that embodies my relationship with her). This bulletin opens up into a poster at the centre of which is a quote from Chief Seattle, and this gift, this object, changed my spiritual journey.

I do not have any answers to why it might be that among our participants we did not find any whose cherished objects were harbingers of change – but exploring this in future research would, I think, give us further insights into human and non-human agency and how objects participate in narrative production.

Decommissioning Cherished Objects

Before moving on to my fourth area of discussion – the work that cherished object do or are called upon to do – I want briefly to reflect on the "decommissioning" of cherished objects, a theme introduced in Chapter 15 in the story-rich chat that Matte, Denise, and Bill enjoyed with Shelley and Anthazia. To me it seems patently obvious that if objects can *become* cherished objects they can also *cease to be* cherished objects. This might appear somewhat unfeeling – as though the abandonment of a cherished object is also the abandonment of what that object represents, encapsulates, and so on – the "burden" to which both Shelley and Anthazia refer.

As part of the process of writing this chapter, I have returned repeatedly to my memory box and the objects therein. I continue to cherish most of these objects – indeed, I cannot imagine ever removing some of the objects. Others, however, I find now have less call upon me, or I on them. That is not to say that I wish to forget or abandon or discard them, but I do find myself wondering whether I now need them in my memory box. There are, in particular, two types of objects that are the subjects of my unsolicited discernment.

First are objects that are associated with experiences that are now so deeply part of me that I no longer need the object to do that work for me (see the next section on the work that cherished objects do). This is similar to the story recounted by Anthazia of the woman who came to a point of discarding her wedding photo because she no longer required it to do the work it had been doing – though in her case the object had become redundant through a different process.

Second are objects that have not stood the test of time; that is, objects that I have cherished but over the thirty-something years of placing objects in my memory box, things have changed, and whatever it was about them is no longer so important. In other words, cherished objects may be time and place specific and once those times and those places have receded the object too recedes. This is the experience to which Shelley refers in Chapter 15: "as time passes and as my life changes and my situation changes, [the item's] cherishableness – assuming that's a word! – may change as well." Returning to the example of the ASBO, I am able to understand how an ASBO might have the status of a cherished object in the late 1990s, but I find it difficult to imagine that those sixteen- and seventeen-year-olds for whom an ASBO was a badge of honour at the time still hold to it as such twenty-five years later. The interests, circumstances, desires, hopes, and allegiances of the now forty-plus-old ASBO recipients will be, I suggest, far different from those of yesteryear, and so a previously cherished object is no longer held to be so.

The decommissioning of cherished objects that I've described above is very much a passive decommissioning. One realizes in hindsight that these objects no longer fill our needs, substitute for our actions, or are required to do any work. However, as we've seen in Chapter 15, sometimes circumstances call for a more active approach to decommissioning. In effect, this is what Shelley does – helping people who need to make decommissioning choices as part of the process of downsizing. This active decommissioning involves, as Shelley suggests, a sort of scale of cherishableness and as such imposes some sense of burden on those having to make decommissioning choices. On reflection, I think it would have been an interesting question to ask of our participants, "What would it take for you to give up [cherished object]?" Such a question would help locate objects in wider discussions of values, desires, and histories.

The Work That Cherished Objects Do

My fourth area for discussion is the work that cherished objects do or are called upon to do. This stems from Matte's references to actor-network theory – a theory to which I more happily subscribe than does Matte (of which more later). In actor-network theory both humans and non-humans are attributed agency – the ability to make a difference in the world. Bruno Latour (2005) argues that non-human actants make a difference because of the impact they have on the world, and others make a difference because of the human work or agency that is delegated to them – the work they do and the work they are called upon to do. An example of the first would be the key fob described by Latour (1991), which, if large enough, will cause guests to change their behaviour from taking the key with them to leaving it at reception (see also Harman, 2009). Strangely enough, I had this experience prior to reading Latour's analysis, when I was working temporarily from a community college and was issued a key attached to a six-by-six-inch metal fob with sharp edges and of substantial weight; it was a key I never forgot to hand in when I left! An example of the second, delegated work would be the door closer (Latour, 1988) that is called on to shut doors for humans to save us from doing it ourselves.

So what might be the work that the participants here require their cherished objects to do and what work is delegated to them?

It is clear that the objects of which our participants made mention when sharing with Jennifer their stories work far harder than is required of simple *reminiscentia*. While some may play that role – for example, Joy's letters prompt memories of Scott or Harriet's page of text recalls memories of her brother – they are not limited in the way that *reminiscentia* are. Scott's letters do not simply prompt memory but act as a bridge to Joy's previous self – just as the letters between Marcea and Amy allowed them to travel "back through time to visit our younger selves" – allowing Joy not only to remember Scott and the times they spent together or corresponding but also to re-experience who she was at an earlier time, when she had not followed the path she did, when other paths were possible. I would suggest that, although not explored in Chapter 6, this is also the work of Amelie's map, transporting her to a different time and place, a previous storyworld in which today's storyworld was only imagined (if that) as but one possibility among many. Such objects act upon us in a way that promotes a heightened degree of autobiographical reasoning – a point raised by Jennifer in her reflections on Amelie's story – by bridging time and space. They thus facilitate connections between the present and the past, and generate a sense of historical continuity (Wapner et al., 1990) – or, as Bill noted back in Chapter 2, of both "chronological" and "retrospective self-continuity" (Bluck & Liao, 2013). Sometimes, as in the case of Susan's currants or Bob and Mary's sea glass, they also point to the future through being transformed by the participants.

Some participants mentioned that they took the workshops out of the desire to leave a legacy for future generations of their family. Certainly, the theme of legacy-leaving stood out for Jennifer and Marcea in their discussions of Amelie and Joy, respectively. In this connection, I am reminded of a story I came across in Sheldon Kopp's (1976) book *If You Meet the Buddha on the Road, Kill Him!*:

> When the great Rabbi Israel Baal Shem-Tov saw misfortune threatening the Jews, it was his custom to go into a certain part of the forest to meditate. There he would light a fire, say a special prayer, and the miracle would be accomplished and the misfortune averted.
>
> Later, when his disciple, the celebrated Magid of Mezritch, had occasion, for the same reason, to intercede with heaven, he would go to the same

> place in the forest and say, "Master of the Universe, listen! I do not know how to light the fire, but I am still able to say the prayer." And again, the miracle would be accomplished.
>
> Still later, Rabbi Moshe-Leib of Sasov, in order to save his people once more, would go into the forest and say, "I do not know how to light the fire. I do not know the prayer, but I know the place and this must be sufficient."
>
> Then it fell to Rabbi Israel of Rizhyn to overcome misfortune. Sitting in his armchair, his head in his hands, he spoke to God. "I am unable to light the fire and I do not know the prayer. I cannot even find the place in the forest. All I can do is to tell the story and this must be sufficient." And it was sufficient. (pp. 20f.)

This story teaches us that it is not the object or action that is all-important but the story. The cherished objects singled out by our participants are not simply *included* in their stories, but actually facilitate parts of those stories and are engaged in the production of those stories. As such, these cherished objects are sufficient to accomplish the miracle of averting the misfortune of one's life being of no consequence.

Objects are also called upon to undertake identity work – the work that is necessary to construct and maintain a viable and stable sense of who one is (see Kroger & Adair, 2008). In Chapter 3, Matte makes reference to actor-network theory in his discussion of human–non-human relations. In this discussion, I suspect that while Matte appreciates that humans and non-humans co-exist, he wants to hold more strongly to a form of essentialism, perhaps akin to Harman's (2009) critical realism, than I feel inclined to do. I am more convinced than he, I think, that objects are the objects they are because of their location in a network of other things, both human and non-human. If that network changes – and while many networks are incredibly stable, all networks are theoretically open to change – then so do the objects within that network. Objects are the objects they are due to the relationships they have. But I want to go one step further still and suggest that we are who we are due to the relationships we have, both with humans and non-humans – a network theory of identity. Provided that each actor in the network plays its part, it is possible to maintain a particular identity. Mike Michael (1996) explores just this phenomenon in his discussion of identity among the scientists involved in repopulating the scallops of St Brieuc Bay (see Calion, 1986, a now classic case study in actor-network theory).

In this view of identity, objects become non-human actors, helping to stabilize the network within which we are who we are. Their removal from this network would act to destabilize the network (maybe only a little, but the more central a role that an object plays in that network – a *cherished* object, for example – then the more that network is destabilized). This does not mean that people "fall apart" upon the loss of any single actor in their networked identity, though they may, but simply acknowledges the active part that non-humans play in who we are. Perhaps this might explain the burden Shelley says some people feel when they are faced with downsizing and making choices between things, that is, actors in their networked identity. Such choices are not simply about which objects we keep and which we discard but also about who we were and who we will become. Price et al. (2000) refer to this as a "de-selfing" process. Through the materiality of objects we can explore "the significant networks of forces, materials, and people – and therefore episodes and actors – that engage with and through objects" and "map the connections and transitions that occur over the life-course of an object" (Humphries & Smith, 2014, p. 477). These networks or maps are akin to Smith and Monforte's (2020) assemblages in which "there is not 'a knowing (human) subject who acts and a passive (nonhuman) object that is acted upon: everything is entangled'" (p. 5, citing Snaza et al., 2016, p. xvii) and by focussing on such assemblages we may highlight the reciprocal influences on our respective identities.

Other scholars have explored how people draw upon cherished objects for multiple purposes. Coleman and Wiles (2020) indicate how participants in their study used cherished objects to "to cope with times of challenge and change in the present, and in some cases, to cultivate a sense of being able to maintain aging in place" (p. 41); Bell and Spikins (2018) argue that people draw upon cherished objects to provide a sense of comfort and security in the absence of loved ones; and Howarth (2020) considers how objects can be used to "empower the voices of the cognitively disabled." Other such work is also performed by some of the cherished objects explored here. David's table creates a gathering place. Susan's currants are called into action to serve first as raw material for dyeing yarn and then as the subject of narration. Bob and Mary's sea glass is called upon to act as a focus of activity for them and their grandchildren. And all of these cherished objects have been dragooned into service in the production of this book.

Such is the work that objects are called on to perform. But what of the work they do silently, without being called upon, without acknowledgment? I am thinking here particularly of the association between cherished objects and well-being. Edmund Sherman (1991b) points to an association between such objects and mood and indicates a correlation between a lack of such objects and lower mood and life satisfaction

(Sherman & Newman, 1978), and Sherman and Dacher (2005) suggest that such objects can imbue a place with meaning. In addition, Wapner et al.'s (1990) study shows that in the context of the transition to long-term care, cherished objects may increase a person's sense of control, serve as anchor points that facilitate the exploration of the novel environment, and promote a sense of belonging.

Reviewing the chapters in this book, I think that there are echoes of this sort of work being undertaken by the participants' cherished objects. David's table certainly seems to operate as an anchor point as it is transported from one place to another, providing a sense of stability, continuity, and gathering for the family; Joan's beer stein prompts feelings of acknowledgment, affirmation, and vindication. And Harriet's page of text could be interpreted as restoring a sense of control over her relationship with her brother, with whom she had not had the opportunity to develop a positive relationship at the time.

Concluding Remarks

Although "conclusions" can be hard to come by in the world of narrative inquiry, I want to make one further observation before returning to my opening remarks. The observation is this: that we inevitably interpret the stories of others through the lens of our own life narratives. We see this most clearly in Bill's explicitness about how he relates to Hermann and the labyrinth ring, in Jennifer's disclosure regarding quilts occupying a significant space in her own story, and in Marcea's recounting of the importance of letters in her own life. And while less explicitly personal in style, I would suggest that Matte's discussion of Bob and Mary's sea glass and Matte and Brandi's treatment of David's table reflect a view of how to narrate the stories of others based on their own approach to narratives.

The interpretation of the stories of others raises two areas of concern: first, that of subjectivity, and second, the ethics of representation. I am less concerned, if indeed at all, about the subjectivity of our interpretations. If narration is indeed a meaning-making activity, then all narrations are to a greater or lesser extent subjective. The important thing is to acknowledge this and not to claim or, worse, impose our own narratives as definitive statements of how things really are. In proffering these interpretations, we are, hopefully, adding to the stock of potential meanings and the process of meaning-making. Others may take our interpretations and rework them as a part of their own meaning-making. We are all made richer by this process. This is the beauty, the open-endedness, of narrative inquiry.

I am far more concerned with the ethics of representation. All too often in academia authors present their narrations as highly robust interpretations based upon acceptable methods, data, and findings and upon location in the relevant literature. In actor-network theory, this would be seen as the establishment of a stable network. Indeed, we academics are encouraged to work this way – by our institutions, grant-making bodies, and publishers. The danger here is that *our* interpretations of participants' stories become *the* interpretations of those stories, or at least the dominant ones, edging out other interpretations, including those of participants themselves.

As far as I am aware, none of us involved in writing this book think of our interpretations in this way. Indeed, the very multivocality of narrative should steer us away from such thinking. I hope that we have done justice to the participants whose stories appear here, and that in some small way we have added value to them for other readers. Put simply, we have stood on holy ground, and have hopefully remembered to remove our hobnail boots.

Finally, I want to return to my comments at the outset regarding how I misjudged the task I had agreed to undertake. I do not regret the task; indeed, now that it is virtually complete, I recognize how I have benefited from thinking about the cherished objects of others. Academically, I have been forced to think through several issues around things and identity of which I had some inklings and, while I still have a good way to go on that journey, the opportunity presented to me here has been a welcome first step. Personally, I have visited and revisited the objects in my memory box in the course of working on this project and writing this chapter, and been prompted to reflect rather more deeply on them and their significance. As *reminiscentia*, they prompted memories that warmed me; as cherished objects they helped re-establish a sense of centredness and provided me with welcomed anchor points (Wapner et al., 1990). Revisiting these objects was also a process of revisiting myself, both past and present. At some point, I know, I will make choices about which of them to keep and which to let go – but not just yet.

Appendix 1: Some Things about Ourselves: Brief Bios of Our Lives

Given the personal-relational dimension of narrative inquiry (see Chapter 1), we'd like to offer here a bit more background as to who we each are and how we got involved in this adventure of exploring the ways that people story their worlds in later life. For, inevitably, our own narratives have played a pivotal role in every dimension of that endeavour, and certainly in writing our respective chapters in this book. They have been the lens through which we've looked at our participants' lives. What is more, our relationship with special objects in our own lives has sensitized us to the complexities of the relationships participants have with such objects in theirs. What follows (in the order in which our various contributions appear in the book) are hardly autobiographies per se, however, but simply quick sketches of our lives and careers as they relate to this project, with particular mention of those things that, for one reason or another, we hold especially dear.

Bill Randall

I've been teaching gerontology at St Thomas University (STU) since 1995. However, my interest in narrative goes back twenty years before that when I was training to become a minister with the United Church of Canada. In my final year of studies, I became fascinated with something called "narrative theology." Upon graduation, I spent ten years serving pastorates in Saskatchewan, Ontario, and New Brunswick: a full, intriguing chapter in my own story, to be sure, and one in which I practised narrative theology every single day. For I listened to the stories of more parishioners than I could possibly recall, between the lines of which they conveyed their convictions and questions in subtle but certain ways.

Wearied from such soul-stretching work, I shifted gears eventually and returned to university to pursue further studies, my dissertation amounting to the pulling together of scattered insights into the storied complexity of human life that I had gleaned from my decade as a pastor. I titled it *The Stories We Are: An Essay on Self-Creation* (2014). Through a string of delicious coincidences, publishing it led to meeting Gary Kenyon. The founder of STU's gerontology department, Gary had been working with scholars worldwide to develop a unique approach to the study of ageing known as "narrative gerontology." In 1995, he invited me to come to STU for one semester as a visiting chair in gerontology, an opportunity that resulted in our collaborating on a range of writing projects in this whole emerging area (e.g., Kenyon & Randall, 1997; Kenyon et al., 2011; Randall & Kenyon, 2001). It also led to my designing a course called "Narrative Gerontology," which I've taught each year since, and to other things besides.

In 2008, a group of us at STU obtained funding from the Social Sciences and Humanities Research Council of Canada (SSHRC) to establish the Centre for Interdisciplinary Research on Narrative (CIRN), then in 2011 another SSHRC grant to bring Clive Baldwin to STU as a Canada Research Chair in Narrative Studies. And the rest, as the saying goes, is history – a history that includes launching a series of conferences called "Narrative Matters," co-editing a journal entitled *Narrative Works* with STU colleague Elizabeth McKim, and co-authoring with her the book *Reading Our Lives* (2008), which lays out a conceptual framework for envisioning what we think of as "the poetics of growing old."

In keeping with my initial interest in narrative ideas, I've become increasingly curious about the spiritual dimensions of older people's storyworlds, and about how those worlds draw from the narrative resources (metaphors, symbols, and stories) of particular traditions. Above all, I've become committed to promoting the practice of "narrative care" with older adults in an assortment of settings, from therapy as such to simply listening, respectfully and compassionately, to the stories of their lives. Narrative care, I believe, can help them to cultivate "a good strong story" with which to meet the challenges of ageing (Randall 2013, pp. 13f.), to tackle the philosophic homework referred to before, and, overall, to *grow* old and not just get old – with meaning, resilience, and grace.

When I think about special objects in my own life, things I'd be careful to carry out with me if, God forbid, my house were burning down and I had mere minutes to escape, I think about my "happy tub" – a big, green, Rubbermaid bin into which I've tossed various cards or emails I've received across the years from students or colleagues or even total strangers: anyone kind enough to say nice words about things that I've written or done that have touched their lives in a positive way. Some day in the not-too-distant future when I'm feeling lonely or depressed and in need of some narrative care for myself, the plan is to pull this tub out, strew its contents hither and yon, paw through them at random, and hopefully experience a flash of affirmation that, all things considered, my living has not been in vain.

Matte Robinson

My grandmother had a big hand in raising me, living in our house and often taking care of my sister and me while my parents worked. When she was in her late eighties we found out that she had pulmonary fibrosis, and I had some thinking to do about what I'd been putting off asking her. Nana was both a great storyteller and a repository of generations' worth of family tales, including some she'd heard from her grandfather, dating back to the 1800s. I'd heard these stories all my life, and I wanted to be able to hear them again, in her voice, for many more years and to play them for any children I would have. I had a digital camera that could take video, and I wanted to ask her if I could film some of her favourite stories.

The problem was that she was, in her own words, "old-fashioned," in a British sort of way that I'm sure scarcely exists now. Not that she wasn't warm and indulgent with the grandchildren, but her strict education by nuns in an Anglican school high in the Himalayas had had a lasting effect, as had the life of a military wife, enduring a war and then raising a child and learning to cook (having been brought up with servants) under rationing. Sitting in her immaculately kept apartment, I observed that the combination VHS–DVD player she'd received as a housewarming gift was still not hooked up to the TV, four years later. I didn't want to ask, but I had to ask.

She didn't even have to think about it. Next Sunday, lunch. My wife and I showed up to the sound of sizzling in the kitchen: the woman who seemed mostly to subsist on Ensure was cooking bangers and mash. She had dressed up. After lunch, she chose a chair and we began recording. I'd get to ask questions after the story was over. When she'd had enough, she'd say "Matthew, turn it off."

We went for lunch every week – and she cooked every week, traditional English fare. We didn't always record, but usually we did. The process was about a lot more than collecting stories for posterity – it was about getting to know my grandmother in a richer way. It changed the dynamic, allowing us to open up and share more details than we were accustomed to in the somewhat ritualized ways grandkids visit with grandparents. Those last years with Nana were some of the best.

In my work life I was spending time in the archives of another interesting woman (who had also lived in London), Hilda Doolittle or H.D., a writer who at the time was seriously understudied. H.D.'s story has enough flashy elements – séances, spies, wars, Sigmund Freud, artists, critics, experimental cinema, millionaires, polyamory – to make a fantastic miniseries, but I was focussed on her unique spirituality and the way she used it to bind together and constantly revise her personal mythology in her poems, fiction, memoir, notes, letters, journals, and even marginalia. In her very last days H.D. was making new revisions to her personal story or myth that cast new light on events from decades earlier, uniting past and present in a living, breathing story that fed a remarkable collection of literary production.

In conversations with Bill I realized that his project with CIRN was an open-ended study in the very kinds of activities that had made such a difference in my life with my grandmother. I knew the story sessions helped our relationship, and all my senses told me it helped with her resilience as well: her mind seemed to sharpen, she seemed to come alive in cooking meals, her mood was lifted as she revealed, a glint in her eye, things I might not have guessed about her – even her symptoms seemed milder as we engaged with her stories. And here, at my university, was a group studying this very phenomenon.

Interdisciplinary narrative studies seemed far indeed from modernist literary studies, and I am still catching up on the literature, but I found that in approaching the works and interview transcripts with the same eye I took to H.D.'s archive, I found incredible literary richness in these stories, this "data." I had done collaborative work before, though always with fellow modernist scholars. But gathered round the table with this diverse group, I found the conversations actually focussed more deeply on certain topics rather than spiralling out into the theoretical concerns of the individual disciplines. And some of the most riveting conversations turned out to be about the things, the objects in people's lives.

Things are vital for storytelling, whether in prose or poetry. The things we notice, the things we keep, and the things we pass on shape much of our lives. And it so happens that things are central, crucial to the poetic movement H.D. founded, imagism. In thinking about literary things and their relation to meaning-making in light of these discussions, in engaging with the transcripts and stories, and in conversation with experts in life-writing and downsizing, we realized that our pooled observations needed to be worked into a book exploring the role of things in life-writing. I feel very lucky that this team was right there, at my own university, and I feel even luckier that I was so immediately and unreservedly welcomed into a conversation that had already been going on. It has stretched me to think new, unfamiliar thoughts, but it has also taken me deeper into what I was already doing.

Jennifer Estey

When we began discussing that the focus of this book would be on "cherished objects," I remembered a small token that I received years ago. When I was fifteen, my best friend invited me to attend a Pathfinders' trip. I was not a member, but I was thrilled to be included. On the two-night trip we stayed in a cabin, went snowshoeing and sliding, and had a bonfire. Other girls my age from different schools and some counsellors were in attendance. I met so many new people, but I was nervous, and to relieve this I began telling stories. I used stories to break the ice, share aspects of my life, and, most importantly, make people laugh. I told so many stories, in fact, that on the last night of the retreat when we were all sitting around the campfire I received the "storyteller" medal. The "medal" was two to three inches in diameter and made from aluminium foil. Through a punched hole on the top of it was a long, thick piece of twisted white and blue yarn, its ends tied together so that it could be worn around my neck. On the front, pressed into the foil was the date, "Jan 18/19 2003." Below this was the one word "Storyteller."

While it has been more than fifteen years, I still have the medal – a piece of yarn attached to shaped aluminium foil – since it captures a meaningful time from my youth where lasting relationships were formed, many laughs were had, and in spite of being an outsider, I felt included. In the past, I was a storyteller; however, as I pursued my education I found the value in story-listening.

I graduated with my Bachelor of Social Work degree at STU, but my journey into the world of narrative began with my Bachelor of Arts. In 2015 I graduated with honours in sociology and minors in both English and psychology. During my undergraduate degree, I took an "Introduction to Narrative" course taught by Clive Baldwin in which I was introduced to narrative ideas and approaches. I learned about basic narrative concepts and their application. I was drawn to the interdisciplinary nature of narrative and how these methods explore human experience. By 2015 I had co-authored two articles on narrative and the self (Baldwin & Estey, 2015; Baldwin, Carty, & Estey, 2015).

As the lead research assistant for this "things that matter" project, I attended all three of the one-day workshops and conducted the pre- and post-interviews with those who consented to be part of our study. During the interviews, I felt honoured and humbled to hear the participants' stories, and later was keen to help with analysing the data so that I could use narrative methods to better understand them. I am particularly interested in autobiographical reasoning, a process of personal reflection that serves to connect the relationships between the past, present, and future stages in a person's life. Storytelling can help people remember events that have been in "storage" by making connections between their memories and bringing forgotten memories to the forefront of their minds. For instance, a story about sewing a quilt can trigger memories relating to when the quilt was made, the process of obtaining the fabric as a gift or a purchase, and details about other characters in the story. Sharing the story creates space for reflecting on the events.

Narrative is a thread that has run through much of my life. At times it has been in the forefront while at others it has drifted into the background, but it has always been present. Storytelling, I have learned, is an effective way to create new relationships, to teach and learn lessons, and to organize lived experiences. Its potential is endless to empower the storyteller, to be therapeutic you could even say, above all when there is an intent and active listener.

Denise Resmi

I am a recent graduate from STU, where I received a Bachelor of Applied Arts in criminology. My involvement with the project is recent and, at least to me, unexpected. Since I began university, gerontology had been off my radar. In October 2017 I was poring over student job postings when a particular qualification caught my eye: to paraphrase, it was "good at reading."

If there is one thing I am confident in, it is my ability to read well. From a young age, I have been an avid reader. My appetite for stories could not be satiated. Accordingly, I carried books with me almost constantly. I often fell asleep with a lit lamp and an open book on my pillow. When I move to a new town, I take great delight in visiting its library, a place where I can find sanctuary. So, my curiosity was piqued; those small words were enough for me to apply to be a research assistant with CIRN.

Initially, I was hired to assist Bill and Matte in preparing for the "Narrative Matters" conference in the Netherlands in the summer of 2018. Since then, the project has evolved and I have been grateful to continue assisting in the data analysis. A welcome side effect of working with CIRN is that I have re-evaluated my previous experiences with older adults.

About halfway towards my bachelor's degree, I took a year to work at a hospital as a security guard. The work was mundane, mostly consisting of making patrols and writing reports. One day, I was called to assist a patient back to the geriatric unit. I exited the office to find a woman in remarkable attire. She was wearing a long, dark fur coat that stood out due to how luxurious it was. The coat was befitting of a film set, but rather unusual for New Brunswick, and her small frame was swimming in it. After a long day of wear, she found it too difficult to carry it back to her room. As she handed it to me, I was surprised by its weight.

We slowly made our way through the hospital while she excitedly told me about her day and the special occasion that warranted the coat: a visit from family. Unfortunately for many patients, visits were few and far between. She was delighted to dress in her finest clothes. Our chat was cut short a few minutes later so I never learned the origins of the extravagant coat.

Despite knowing little about this patient, I believe this coat was her cherished object. It likely had a story or meaning attached to it – why else bring such an impractical piece of clothing to the hospital? It is fascinating to consider how objects travel with us through our lives. From the moment an object enters our stories, we cannot anticipate the stories it will accumulate. The variety of objects presented in this book attests to this. Often, they do not stand out like a fur coat in a hospital. Something as small and ordinary as a piece of paper, we have found, can be packed with meaning.

With this experience in mind, I have found it a privilege to read our participants' stories. I am constantly amazed by the depth of each one. I have immensely enjoyed my small role in supporting the brilliance around the table; this project has been the highlight of my time in university. It is also been my initiation, or "chapter one," into the world of narrative ideas. While I am sure more chapters are to come, I will always hold this one dear.

Erin Whitmore

The stories that women tell and write about their lives have fascinated me for many years. More than that, however, is the interest I have in understanding the function these stories serve in women's lives in their efforts to understand themselves and engage in and shape the world around them. Reading, listening to, and engaging critically with these stories about self, family, and community reveals much about how meaning-making works in relation to everything from the quotidian routines of daily life to the complex systems within which we all live and that shape individual lives in distinct ways. While completing my PhD in English literature, I became increasingly interested in how women used stories to strategically engage in the world around them and enter spaces and conversations from which they had been largely excluded. While appearing on the surface to uphold dominant narratives about gender sustained within patriarchal and colonialist regimes, the women writers I studied were simultaneously authoring shadow stories that challenged these dominant ways of organizing society by revealing the negative impact of these systems on those with less power.

Alongside my engagement with women's literature was my engagement with the stories women were telling me on the volunteer crisis and support line that I worked with during graduate school. The stories women shared about violence, abuse, racism, poverty, and isolation provided concrete evidence of a collective shadow story of pervasive harm and inequality that was – and continues to be – all too real. When I completed my PhD, my interest in understanding these shadow stories, and the ways women imagined how these stories might be used to transform structures and systems that reproduce and sustain inequality, took me outside of the university and literary studies into the field of social work. Over the past ten years, I have worked in the area of violence against women and gender-based violence, first at a community-based sexual assault centre, then as a researcher and policy analyst on gender equality issues with a provincial government, then as a researcher with the National Inquiry into Missing and Murdered Indigenous Women and Girls, and currently as director of a national non-profit organization focussed on addressing and preventing violence against women and gender-based violence. At the centre of these experiences – and the place I return to again and again to ground myself and my work – are the stories that women tell and write about their everyday lives. I remain convinced that these stories offer the clues and expertise necessary to creating a more just world.

A central theme that I've witnessed emerge from the many stories I've heard women tell about their lives – including the story told by "Harriet" that I discuss in Chapter 8 – is that of their relationship to their hopes, dreams, and possibilities. More often than not, women's stories about possibility in the contexts and settings that I've heard them told are about the loss or absence of the possibilities they once imagined for themselves, their families, and their communities. To be sure, thinking about "things that matter" in the context of stories of women's lives that have been shaped by violence, trauma, harm, inequality, and loss is fraught: for anyone living in a violent home, struggling with poverty, or lacking housing, the notion of collecting "things" centres more explicitly on those things necessary to basic survival rather than a sentimental or nostalgic holding onto excessive possessions. When one is forcibly removed from one's home by a colonial government and sent to a residential school, or when one is forced to flee one's home in order to escape violence and abuse, it is stories about the absence rather than the presence of things that hold perhaps the most profound site of understanding and meaning.

Working with the CIRN team on this project has allowed me to explore the significance of stories about the presence, absence, and transience of things as gateways into much larger stories about ageing, gender, trauma, family, war, and marriage, to name just a few of the broader social issues explored in this collection. In particular, it has provided me an opportunity to weave together disparate threads about the role and function of women's stories, and to extend my thinking about the importance of these stories into women's later life where they continue to offer poignant teachings and function as powerful motivators for change. Supporting women at all stages of life in telling the story of possibility – lost or found – is a vital part of honouring, grieving, and celebrating various facets of women's experiences that remains largely ignored, particularly for older women who are themselves often forgotten or ignored. As the many women who have shared their stories with me have taught me, rather than stories of personal failure, women's stories of lost hopes or possibilities and the "things" associated with them are powerful sites through which systemic inequality is exposed and women's resistance to that inequality is recognized and articulated. The story told by Harriet is no exception.

Marcea Ingersoll

My routes to this writing have been circuitous, moving outwards and then in looping returns. Originally from New Brunswick, I left in the 1990s for what was supposed to be a one-year sojourn; however, life has a way of leading you down pathways you never imagined. So the story of a one-year deferral of my graduate work became a series of narrative encounters across continents and provinces, until I returned to my studies nearly fifteen years later. Between the bookends of leaving after my undergraduate degree at STU and returning to Canada to take up graduate work at Queen's University in Kingston, the pages of my story became filled by my days as an international school teacher. I learned my craft, teaching and learning alongside wonderful colleagues and students from a host of different nationalities. In this multicultural mix far removed from the rural New Brunswick classrooms where I became a student, I began to form a teaching identity that is the foundation from which I now write about education.

Growing up on an island in the Bay of Fundy was my first real course in narrative. As a child I spent many hours listening to the stories woven across the five living generations of family members. My graduate work at Queen's introduced me to stories as not merely an influential force in people's lives but a valid form of scholarship. My doctoral work focussed on Canadian teacher identity along the journey of international teaching, framed within the phases of leaving home, teaching internationally, and coming home. I could never have imagined, when I began my PhD, that I would write my life into the framework I crafted in my research.

After two decades away from my homeplace, New Brunswick called me home again and in a narrative loop I returned to STU – this time as an assistant professor. The power of story along our life's journey permeates my thinking, teaching, and research.

Being a part of CIRN has drawn me into a circle of colleagues with an attuned understanding of narrative along the life course. This project in particular has taken me back to the stories of my childhood, reminding me of moments spent with my parents, grandparents, great-grandparents, and great-great grandmother. Working with CIRN has opened an opportunity to engage with the stories of seniors, and to consider how intergenerational narratives as "things" and about "things" are part of our individual, familial, and social legacy.

Anthazia Kadir

I have spent most of my life searching for meaning about the world around me. This quest to find answers about life and the universe has led me thus far to devote most of my adult life to the field of education and writing. Over my twenty-plus years as an educator I have had several roles, from student teacher to language department head to mentor and instructor for teachers in training.

My journey as an educator started in 1996 in my native country, Guyana. My formative years in teachers' college afforded me opportunities to meet some interesting educators: interesting because they were dedicated and committed more to the art of teaching than to its technical dimensions. It was in my second year at the Cyril Potter College of Education that I found myself at a crossroads, having to decide what subject would be my major. I thought I had it all figured out. I wanted, almost religiously, to major in English language studies. However, grace threw me into a drama class, and I was scared. I thought I would never make it out alive, but I did, graduating in 1997 as the best teacher within my batch. My ability to find my best self during one of the most questioning periods of my training was due mostly to the fact that I fell heir to the nurturing guidance of one of the Caribbean's most acclaimed playwrights, Ronald Hollingsworth. I was timid and shy, prone to stage fright, but Mr. Hollingsworth saw something in me that I could not at the time name. Our collaboration has led to many theatre and story-writing projects.

After completing teachers' college, I taught English language arts and drama at the high school level for ten years. While in Guyana I also worked in teacher education. Additionally, I worked as a journalist and travel writer. I migrated to Toronto in 2007 and entered York University to read for an Honours BA, majoring in English with a minor in philosophy.

During my years at York I worked as an academic advisor, facilitated creative writing workshops for seniors, and in 2009 published my first novel, *What a Woman Wants* (Kadir, 2009). In 2010 I was approached by Afzal Shaq, a writer and broadcaster in Pakistan. Mr. Shaq had read some of my poetry through the Internet and reached out to me in an email. We developed a connection through a mutual desire for a more peaceful world. As we continued to exchange emails, suddenly he asked me to be part of one of his dreams to translate his life story from Phasto/Urdu into English. That translation, *Daughter of Pharaoh*, came out in 2011, the very year Mr. Shaq passed away (Kadir & Shaq, 2011).

After six years in Ontario my travels took me to Saskatchewan, where I taught English language arts and creative writing to high school students within an Indigenous context. I was also part of the Saskatchewan Writers' Guild and facilitated life-writing workshops for a variety of participants. Currently, I am completing an MEd in curriculum studies at the University of New Brunswick focussing on culturally responsive approaches within curriculum design and classroom implementation. I also continue to work in education and facilitate creative writing workshops for seniors, immigrants, and educators.

At the onset of a third decade in education and writing, coupled with my journey to complete my master's degree, I realize through research, reading, writing, and leading workshops over many geographic landscapes that there seem to be more questions than answers about the calling that has chosen me, more questions about life, about progressive education and educational reform. Moreover, while I struggle to comprehend issues with my career as an educator, my role as a life-writing facilitator has increased my acceptance of the fact that life is always in flux.

The arts have allowed me to tell stories, stories about ourselves to ourselves. In the process of sharing and telling stories comes healing, I find, that strengthens my resilience to face life's challenges and, through mindful practices, to develop the capacity to reflect with joy amidst the frailties of life.

Brandi Estey-Burtt

A resident of rural New Brunswick, I recently completed my PhD in English literature at Dalhousie University in Halifax, Nova Scotia. A large part of my motivation for doing graduate work has been my fascination with how people tell stories about their everyday lives. Most of the narratives I focus on involve religion, and they consider how spirituality and the sacred infuse many people's sense of ethics, as well as their appreciation for what author Marilynne Robinson (2004) describes as the "incandescence" of daily life (p. 44).

As I discovered while doing MA degrees in both fields, religious studies and literary studies attend to how people knit meaning together into narratives that shape their identity; our stories are imbued with our values, our perceptions of ourselves, and our relationships with others. I study texts that embrace human frailty while also meditating on the pain of vulnerability, and the closer I got to completing my doctorate on contemporary literature, the more I realized that stories bear a heavy burden. As tellers, readers, and listeners, it is our responsibility to treat the stories that circulate around us and through us with care and respect.

Since moving back to the small community in New Brunswick in which I grew up, I have become interested in how people meld their sense of the sacred with their love for the environment, for their rural communities, and for sustainable modes of living. I have been part of several local projects that ask what kinds of stories community members tell about the resilience of their rural areas in the face of contemporary challenges such as lack of employment, environmental degradation, shortage of health care services, and an ageing population. The thread that binds these stories together is a persistent gratitude to the community at large for acting like a family and providing important social and personal supports during difficult times. Such stories of family and care weave the individual into a shared narrative of communal identity and resilience.

This "things that matter" project offers a wonderful opportunity to explore how people invest deep emotions and meaning into particular objects. Growing up, I would love the times when my sister, my mom, and I would make cupcakes together in the kitchen. Not long ago, my mom was cleaning out her cupboards and asked me if I wanted any of her dishes or utensils. I immediately thought of the bowl in which we mixed the icing for those cupcakes. That bowl has become a symbol for me of family relationships and how activities like preparing food join people together. It marks an important touchstone in my personal narrative and reminds me that stories nourish people on a very fundamental level. I can see similar dynamics at work in many of the stories we describe in this book. The individuals profiled throughout – older adults who are reflecting on past events and relationships in their lives – have generously shared with us their time and their stories. Through this activity, they have helped us better understand the complexities of ageing, illuminating in particular how objects can motivate us to reflect on the experience of growing old.

Deborah (Deb) Carr

My shift from clerical work to a writing career happened in mid-life, when the comfort of the federal government job that I'd held for seventeen years slowly sunk into disenchantment. I felt purposeless. I didn't know who or what I wanted to be, but knew I could no longer remain in place. Without any idea what direction I might pursue, I made a clean break and left my job. An open landscape lay ahead with no horizon in sight. Sometime during my subsequent wanderings, a friend reminded me of my habit of crafting work occurrences into humorous stories. "You're a writer," she said. "You just don't realize it yet."

Sometimes we need another's perspective to reveal the strength of our own story. Through a serendipitous – or perhaps inevitable – series of events, I fell into freelance work with a regional newspaper. My assignments involved interviewing entrepreneurs, woodlot owners, craftspeople about their work. Intuitively, I searched for the desire in each, and dug below the surface of our conversations to ferret out their hidden motivations and obstacles. Sifting through reams of interview notes afterwards, I loved searching for patterns with which to shape the emerging story. While not an accepted journalistic practice, I secretly wrote for the interviewee, rather than the reader. I wanted them to see themselves through my eyes, to understand the strength of their own story.

I found myself particularly drawn to individuals who had discovered one beautiful thing that gave them joy, and pursued it, becoming a master at their craft: the Acadian baker who put his children through university with plain white bread baked in a wood-fired oven that he designed himself; the electronics technologist-by-day who worked long hours into the night carving exquisite violin bows from exotic wood; the woodsman/mobile farrier who lumbered with a beloved team of Belgian horses, just as his grandfather had taught him. These were lives well lived.

Eventually I sought magazine work, giving me more freedom to tell the stories I wanted to share. I became so enthralled with back stories that I undertook to write the biography of an eighty-year-old Polish-Canadian naturalist, Mary Majka. We met for interviews weekly over the span of several years. At times, I worried about bringing up the buried pain and loss of her past. Other times, I despaired that I would ever understand her many paradoxes and complexities. It wasn't until I began to piece together the chronology and look for themes that I started to appreciate the many threads that weave through our lives, and how it's often the smallest of experiences that contribute the most profound clues to our inner desires. I learned to pay attention not only to what was said but to how it was said and, sometimes more importantly, what was left unsaid.

After the book *Sanctuary: The Story of Naturalist Mary Majka* (Carr, 2010) was published, I asked how she felt about the overall experience. "It was not pleasant to recall. In the moment I was regretting this. Once I started to talk about it to you, I was reliving those things; I dreamed about those things. I knew that I had buried these things and forgotten about them. You were searching my soul, trying to get much deeper than I expected or wanted to go. But now, I wouldn't have wanted it any other way. The memories were revived and it was a good thing. I don't have any regrets" (personal communication).

The enduring and cleansing power of story was becoming clearer to me. Writing became my own spiritual practice, a way to determine who and where I am; where I might go next. I began delivering writing workshops to help others excavate those obscure yet important memories, working with them to discover the significance and to shape memory into story.

In 2012 I was invited by Medical Ambassadors of Haiti to teach rural villagers life-writing skills over a period of three weeks. The experience showed me the tremendous potential that understanding our stories has to strengthen feelings of self-worth and resilience. Both my experiences in Haiti and then later with the St. Thomas University project have been gifts that enriched my own appreciation for the work I do. Bill, Matte, and their team continue to involve me in the many research streams resulting from this initiative. The discoveries they've graciously shared with me have reinforced and enhanced my own love of stories and my desire to help others find value and meaning in their lived experiences, while clarifying my own.

Shelley Swift

I am a relocation and transition specialist, often referred to as a senior move manager, and, as such, I work essentially with seniors who are in the process of downsizing, as they work towards moving to new, usually smaller, homes.

My cumulative personal and professional experiences over several years led me to this work, at a time when individuals and families are seeking more assistance and support with this often daunting and potentially overwhelming task. For some, of course, it is easy for various reasons, and the decisions flow naturally. For many, however, the sorting and disposition of belongings collected over a lifetime, which is only one aspect of the process, requires a great deal of time, energy, and perseverance. Indeed, it is often the most challenging one, and one where I find my participation most personal and rewarding. I have learned a great deal about the tangible items that people accumulate, care for, and value throughout their lives, and the wide range of things they have come to treasure, whether it be books, china, art, historical papers and artefacts, or family heirlooms passed down through the generations. And I have learned about their wide-ranging reasons for doing so. I have learned, too, that the importance placed by the owner is not necessarily commensurate with the monetary value of the item, but often reflects a sentimental attachment that holds even deeper meaning.

As a result, it is comforting for those choosing between what to keep, and what not to, to be able to discuss the provenance and meaning of their cherished things, and to revisit memories that they invoke. Decisions made in this way tend to provide more satisfying results for those who enjoy that luxury and a more seamless and happy transition to a simpler lifestyle. That is why I treasure my grandmother's doughnut cutter – an object that I say more about in Chapter 15.

Clive Baldwin

On the top shelf of a bookcase in my office there is a quite unassuming cardboard box. It is pretty enough but, other than that, unremarkable. No self-respecting burglar would bother about it. In the box is an assortment of "things" – several books, including Herman Hesse's *Wandering* and Bishop and Spring's *Formative Undercurrents of Compulsory Knowledge: Some Comparative Historical Observations on Learning and Schools* – acronym FUCKSCHOOL! – a pine cone or two, a watch, some photos, a few programs for events, and a variety of bits and bobs that to the outsider would appear as a random assortment of detritus. Indeed, there is nothing obvious that would link these things together save that they are in the same box, and the box belongs to me.

I occasionally use items from this box in my social work classes. I bring in a plastic bag of "stuff," stuff from my box and other randomly selected items, place it on a table in front of the class, and say "deal with it." After some initial confusion, the students start to look at the stuff; sometimes they will pick up items and try to make sense of what they see before them (this, of course, is a metaphor for social work). They usually struggle, and they search for clues as to what they might deduce about the person whose stuff this is. Some items they imbue with more importance than others; some items are dismissed as insignificant. After a while they come to some agreement regarding what, at least minimally, they might be able to say about the owner of these things. Of course, they are usually far off the mark, other than being able to identify the stuff as mine. It is, again of course, unfair to expect anything else – how are they to know the significance of any particular item? The interesting thing, however, is that in all the times I have given students this exercise, they have never asked me what any of it means, even when they have identified the stuff as mine. Had they done so, they might not have thrown the pine cones to the side, dismissing them as irrelevant when, in fact, I collected these the first time I visited the grave of the one person who, at the time, I could not imagine the world without.

My memory box is just that, my memory box. It does not have to make sense to anybody else, and the items in it do not have to be linked in any way, save that they are holders of people, places, and times that I revisit when I think of where I have come from, where I am now, and (the absence of the Apocalypse permitting) where I might go. And, of course, there are memories that, however significant, cannot be held in a box: the mansion I built in my heart for her before she died.

All of this may appear, and perhaps even feels, a tad self-indulgent, but I shall come to the point in the hope of redeeming the text so far. I do not come from a story-telling family. Indeed, though I joke about it, it is true that I know the lineage of my border collie (to her great-great grandparents) more than I know that of my own family (my grandparents). I came to narrative much later, thanks to my doctoral supervisor and the Jesuits. First, my doctoral supervisor, Dr. Tim Booth, taught me how to construct a life story out of what appeared to be the merest of fragments: I remember him telling me once that, after two and a half hours of recorded interviews with a research participant, the longest answer he had received was "a rabbit an' all, and a ferret." Second, I learnt to reflect, or at least reflect properly, deeply, from the Jesuits. I learnt the importance of the little stuff – how God is to be found in the mundane as much as, if not more than, in the spectacular. I learnt also that when people tell me the story of their lives I am standing on holy ground, and I must remember to remove my hobnail boots.

I have learnt the importance of telling stories through listening to those of people whose stories do not often get told, or who have not been able to, or allowed to, tell their stories: mothers wrongly accused of child abuse, family carers of people living with dementia, transabled people, and individuals who identify as other-than-human. Listening to their stories requires accepting and working with fragments, paying close attention to the seemingly irrelevant, and, above all, asking what it all means. No doubt, in learning how others make sense of themselves through the stories they tell, I hope to find ways of doing so for myself.

Appendix 2: Interview Questions

Before Workshops

1. You have signed up for this series of workshops. Can you tell me what you hope to get out of them?
2. What sort of life story things have you done in the past, if any?
   Examples: writing in a journal, story writing, scrapbooking, family genealogy
   Yes: What do you feel were the benefits of these methods? How did they help – or hinder – you in telling your life story?
   No: What has prompted you to think about exploring your life story now?
3. What role has story telling generally played within your family, both in the past and in the present?
4. Tell me one or two stories about your life that you would like to share. Bill and Clive, the organizers behind this research project, would like to listen to these later, so could you tell your stories for them?
   Example: a key turning point in your life
5. What was your experience of coming to the first workshop and what, if anything, did you get out of it?
6. Do you have any other comments you would like to make?

After Workshops

1. When we arranged this interview, I asked you to write one story that you told me the first time we met. Can you tell me which story you have chosen to write?
   a. What was it like to write that story?
   b. Telling and writing stories can be two distinct processes. Can you comment on the differences between writing and telling your

story? (*Prompt*: How has writing affected your interpretation of the story? Experiences, feelings towards it, new insights?)

2. Can you talk about the overall impact that participating in the workshops had on you, if any?
   a. Were there exercises in the workshops you found especially helpful or meaningful? Why do you think that is?
   b. Have you continued to work with the exercises?
      i. If so, which ones and why?
      ii. If not, are there any particular reasons why not?
   c. Can you talk about how your process of writing, such as drafting, editing, revising, and so on, affects your interpretation of the story?
3. What was it like for you to share your stories with others, either with the group as a whole, or at the table?
   a. What was it like to have other people share their stories with you?
   b. What for you is the importance of sharing stories (if indeed sharing stories is important to you), and why is that?
4. Can you tell me about your experience of the workshops in terms of where you see your story going? (*Prompt*: Next chapters)
5. In what way, if at all, have the workshops influenced your sense of what constitutes a good story? (*Prompt*: What does constitute a good story?)
6. What life lessons would you like to pass on to others? If you had to choose one story to pass on, what would that story be?
7. What motivates you to write?
8. If you were to tell your story as a whole, how would you structure it? (*Prompt*: Thematically, chronologically, lessons to be learned, key relationships)
   a. There is increasing interest nowadays in the metaphor of life as a story; do you have any thoughts as to how that might apply to your life? (*Prompt*: Some people, for instance, say things like, "My life is book" or "I have a story to tell.")
   b. What themes, if any, are part of your story?
   c. Did the workshops contribute to how you would structure your story? If so, how?
9. If you were asked to write your life story, where would you begin? (*Prompt*: A lot of people don't know where to begin, tell me about that.)
10. How, if at all, does writing help generate different perspectives on your life?
11. Are there stories that you wouldn't tell?
    a. What is it about these stories that makes them untellable? (*Prompt*: I'm not asking you to tell me those stories, just what it is

about those stories that makes them unrelatable, e.g., too embarrassing, painful, boring, etc.?)

12. Some people report times when they came to a crossroads and had to choose which way to go. Can you think of a time when this was so for you? Can you tell me about a path not taken? (*Prompt*: During the initial interview you described at least one turning point; how would life have been different had you taken a different path?)
    a. Some writers provide the reader with more than one ending. What possible endings might you have in your mind for your story?
13. If you could reinvent yourself, what stories would you tell? (*Prompt*: It doesn't have to be based in reality; it could be anything.)
14. How, if at all, have the workshops impacted the role of storytelling in your life?
15. Do you have any comments on the process of participating in this research, including these interviews?

General prompt: I sense there is a story linked to this story; can you share that with me? Would you mind telling me more about that?

References

Abbott, H. (2002). *The Cambridge introduction to narrative.* New York: Cambridge University Press.

Adichie, C.N. (2009). *The danger of a single story* [Video]. TED conference. https://www.ted.com/talks/chimamanda_ngozi_adichie_the_danger_of_a_single_story/c.

Ahmed, S. (2006). *Queer phenomenology: Orientations, objects, others.* Durham: Duke University Press.

Ahmed, S. (2017). *Living a feminist life.* Durham: Duke University Press.

AIDS Memorial Quilt. (n.d.). Retrieved December 2, 2019, from https://www.aidsmemorial.org/quilt-history.

Albom, M. (1997). *Tuesdays with Morrie: An old man, a young man, and life's greatest lesson.* New York: Doubleday.

Albright, D. (1994). Literary and psychological models of the self. In U. Neisser & R. Fivush (Eds.), *The remembering self: Construction and accuracy in the self-narrative* (pp. 19–40). New York: Cambridge University Press.

Alheit, P. (1995). Biographical learning: Theoretical outline, challenges, and contradictions of a new approach in adult education. In P. Alheit, A. Bron-Wojciechowska, E. Brugger, & P. Dominice (Eds.), *The biographical approach in European adult education,* (pp. 57–74). Vienna: Verband Wiener Voksbildung.

Allen, D., & Springsted, E. (1994). *Spirit, nature, and community: Issues in the thought of Simone Weil.* Albany: SUNY Press.

Anderson, C., & MacCurdy, M. (Eds.) (2000). *Writing and healing: Toward an informed practice.* Urbana: National Council of Teachers of English.

Anderson, E. (2020) *Material spirituality in modernist women's writing.* London: Bloomsbury Academic.

Andrews, M. (2014). *Narrative imagination and everyday life.* New York: Oxford University Press.

Appaduari, A. (Ed.). (1988). *The social life of things: Commodities in cultural perspective.* Cambridge: Cambridge University Press.

Astor-Aguilera, M.A., & Harvey, G. (Eds.). (2018). *Rethinking relations and animism: Personhood and materiality*. London: Routledge.

Atkinson, R. (1995). *The gift of stories: Practical and spiritual applications of autobiography, life stories, and personal mythmaking*. Westport: Bergin & Garvey.

Atkinson, R. (2006). Life stories, autobiography, and personal narrative. *LLI Review*, 1, 88–89.

Atwood, M. (1996). *Alias Grace*. Toronto: Doubleday.

Auslander, L. (2005). Beyond words. *American Historical Review*, 110, 1015–1045. https://doi.org/10.1086/ahr.110.4.1015

Baddeley, J., & Singer, J. (2007). Charting the life story's path: Narrative identity across the life span. In J. Clandinin (Ed.), *Narrative inquiry: Mapping a methodology* (pp. 177–202). Thousand Oaks: Sage.

Bakhurst, D. (2001). Memory, identity, and the future of cultural psychology. In D. Bakhurst & S. Shanker (Eds.), *Jerome Bruner: Language, culture, and self* (pp. 184–198). Thousand Oaks: Sage.

Baldick, C. (2008). *The Oxford dictionary of literary terms*. Oxford: Oxford University Press.

Baldwin, C. (2010). Narrative, supportive care, and dementia: A preliminary exploration. In J. Hughes, M. Lloyd-Williams, & G. Sachs (Eds.), *Supportive care for the person with dementia.* (pp. 245–252). Oxford: Oxford University Press.

Baldwin, C., Carty, B., & Estey, J. (2015). Aging, spirituality, and narrative: Loss and repair. *Narrative Works*, 5(2), 1–24. https://journals.lib.unb.ca/index.php/NW/article/view/25012

Baldwin, C., & Estey, J. (2015). The self and spirituality: Overcoming narrative loss in aging. *Journal of Aging and Spirituality in Social Work*, 34(2), 205–222. https://doi.org/10.1080/15426432.2014.999978

Bamberg, M. (2006). Stories: Big or small – Why do we care? *Narrative Inquiry*, 16(1), 139–147. https://doi.org/10.1075/ni.16.1.18bam

Barusch, A. (2008). *Love stories of later life: A narrative approach to understanding romance*. New York: Oxford University Press.

Bateson, M. (2007). Narrative, adaptation, and change. *Interchange*, 38(3), 213–222. https://doi.org/10.1007/s10780-007-9030-3

Bauer, J., & McAdams, D. (2004). Personal growth in adults' stories of life transitions. *Journal of Personality*, 72(3), 573–602. Medline:15102039. https://doi.org/10.1111/j.0022-3506.2004.00273.x

Bauer, J., & Park, S. (2010). Growth is not just for the young: Growth narratives, eudaimonic resilience, and the aging self. In P. Frye & C. Keyes (Eds.), *New frontiers in resilient aging: Life-strengths and well-being in late life* (pp. 60–89). New York: Cambridge University Press.

Baumeister, R.F., & Vohs, K.D. (2002). The pursuit of meaningfulness in life. In C. Snyder & S. Lopez (Eds.), *Handbook of positive psychology* (pp. 608–628). New York: Oxford University Press.

Beardslee, W. (1990). Stories in the postmodern world: Orienting and disorienting. In D. Griffin (Ed.), *Sacred interconnections: Postmodern spirituality, political economy, and art* (pp. 163–175). Albany: SUNY Press.

Belk, R.W. (1988). Possessions and the extended self. *Journal of Consumer Research*, 15(2), 139–168. https://doi.org/10.1086/209154

Bell, T., & Spikins, P. (2018). The object of my affection: Attachment security and material culture, *Time and Mind*, 11(1), 23–39. https://doi.org/10.1080/1751696X.2018.1433355

Berman, H. (1994). *Interpreting the aging self: Personal journals of later life.* New York: Springer.

Berry, T. (1987). Creative energy. *Cross Currents*, 37(2–3), 179–186.

Betterton, S. (2015). *The history of quilts and patchwork worldwide with photographic reproductions.* Rene Press.

Bettleheim, B. (1989). *The uses of enchantment: The meaning and importance of fairy tales.* New York: Vintage.

Bhattacharyya, P., & Pradhan, R.K. (2019). Exploring cherishing: A qualitative approach. *The Qualitative Report*, 24(7), 1511–1536. https://doi.org/10.46743/2160-3715/2019.3257

Bianchi, E. (1991). A spirituality of aging. In L. Cahill & D. Meith (Eds.), *Aging* (pp. 58–64). London: SCM Press.

Birren, J., & Deutchman, D. (1991). *Guiding autobiography groups for older adults: Exploring the fabric of life.* Baltimore: Johns Hopkins University Press.

Birren, J., Kenyon, G., Ruth, J.-E., Schroots, J., & Svensson, T. (Eds.). (1996). *Aging and biography: Explorations in adult development.* New York: Springer.

Birren, J., & Svensson, C. (2006). Guided autobiography: Writing and telling the stories of lives. *LLI Review*, 1(1), 1–10.

Bivona, M., Kahlbaugh, P., & Budnick, C. (2020). Writing wisdom, reviewing identity: Positive outcomes of participating in a memoir course for older adults. *International Journal of Life Review and Reminiscence*, 7(1), 9–21.

Blair, K. (March 30, 2019). Why do women prefer gay men as friends? A lack of anxiety related to gay men's sexual intent increases women's comfort. *Psychology Today*. https://www.psychologytoday.com/ca/blog/inclusive-insight/201903/why-do-women-prefer-gay-men-friends

Blix, B., Hamran, T., & Normann, H. (2015). Roads not taken: A narrative positioning analysis of older adult's stories about missed opportunities. *Journal of Aging Studies*, 35, 169–177. https://doi.org/10.1016/j.jaging.2015.08.009

Bluck, S. (2017). Remember and review or forget and let go? Views from a functional approach to autobiographical memory. *International Journal of Life Review and Reminiscence*, 4(1), 3–7.

Bluck, S., & Liao, H.-W. (2013). I was therefore I am: Creating self-continuity through remembering our personal past. *International Journal of Life Review and Reminiscence*, 1(1), 7–12.

Bochner, A., & Ellis, C. (2016). *Evocative autoethnography: Writing lives and telling stories.* New York: Routledge.

Bohlmeijer, E., Kramer, J., Smit, F., Onrust, S., & Marwijk, H. (2009). The effects of integrative reminiscence on depressive symptomatology and mastery of older adults. *Journal of Community Mental Health, 45,* 467–484. Medline:19777348. https://doi.org/10.1007/s10597-009-9246-z

Bohlmeijer, E., & Westerhof, G. (2013). Life review as a way to enhance personal growth in midlife: A case study. *International Journal of Life Review and Reminiscence,* 1(1), 13–18.

Bohlmeijer, E., Westerhof, G., & Lamers, S. (2014). The development and validation of the Narrative Foreclosure Scale. *Aging and Mental Health,* 18(7), 879–888. Medline:24678959. https://doi.org/10.1080/13607863.2014.896865.

Bohlmeijer, E., Westerhof, G., Randall, W., Tromp, T., & Kenyon, G. (2011). Narrative foreclosure: Preliminary considerations toward a new sensitizing concept. *Journal of Aging Studies,* 25(4), 364–370. https://doi.org/10.1016/j.jaging.2011.01.003

Bohn, A. (2011). Normative ideas of life and autobiographical reasoning in life narratives. In T. Habermas (Ed.), *The development of autobiographical reasoning in adolescence and beyond: New directions for child and adolescent development,* no. 131 (pp. 19–30). San Francisco: Jossey-Bass.

Bolton, G. (2006). Writing from objects. In G. Bolton, V. Field, & K. Thompson (Eds.), *Writing works: A resource handbook for therapeutic writing workshops and activities* (pp. 74–96). London: Jessica Kingsley.

Bolton, G., Field, V., & Thompson, K. (Eds.). (2006). *Writing works: A resource handbook for therapeutic writing workshops and activities.* London: Jessica Kingsley.

Bourdieu, P. (1987). *Distinction: A social critique of the judgement of taste.* Cambridge, MA: Harvard University Press.

Bowen, S., Brenton, J., & Elliott, S. (2019). *Pressure cooker: Why home cooking won't solve our problems and what we can do about it.* New York: Oxford University Press.

Bridges, W. (1980). *Transitions: Making sense of life's changes.* Toronto: Addison-Wesley.

Brockmeier, J. (2002). Possible lives. *Narrative Inquiry,* 12(2), 455–466. https://doi.org/10.1075/ni.12.2.18bro

Brown, B. (1999). The secret life of things (Virginia Woolf and the matter of modernism). *Modernism/Modernity,* 6(2), 1–28. https://doi.org/10.1353/mod.1999.0013

Brown, B. (2001). Thing theory. *Critical Inquiry,* 28(1), 1–22.

Brown, C. (2012). Anti-oppression through a postmodern lens: Dismantling the master's conceptual tools in discursive social work practice. *Critical Social Work,* 13(1), 34–65. https://doi.org/10.22329/csw.v13i1.5848

Brown, K. (2020). Punitive reform and the cultural life of punishment: Moving from the ASBO to its successors. *Punishment & Society: International Journal of Penology*, 22(1), 90–107. https://doi.org/10.1177/1462474519831347

Bruner, J. (1986). *Actual minds, possible worlds.* Cambridge, MA: Harvard University Press.

Bruner, J. (1987). Life as narrative. *Social Research*, 71(3), 691–711. https://doi.org/10.1353/sor.2004.0045

Bruner, J. (1999). Narratives of aging. *Journal of Aging Studies*, 13(1), 7–9. https://doi.org/10.1016/S0890-4065(99)80002-4

Bruner, J. (2001). Self-making and world-making. In J. Brockmeier & D. Carbaugh (Eds.), *Narrative and identity: Studies in autobiography, self and culture* (pp. 25–38). Amsterdam: John Benjamins.

Bruner, J., & Kalmar, D. (1998). Narrative and metanarrative in the construction of the self. In M. Ferrari & R. Sternberg (Eds.), *Self-awareness: Its nature and development*(pp. 308–331). New York: Guilford.

Bruner, J., & Weisser, S. (1991). The invention of self: Autobiography and its forms. In D.R. Olson & N. Torrance (Eds.), *Literacy and Orality* (pp. 129–148). New York: Cambridge University Press.

Burstow, B. (2003). Toward a radical understanding of trauma and trauma work. *Violence Against Women*, 9(11), 1293–1317. https://doi.org/10.1177/1077801203255555

Butala, S. (2005). The memoirist's quandary. *McGill Journal of Education*, 40(1), 43–54.

Butler, R. (1963). The life review: An interpretation of reminiscence in the aged. *Psychiatry*, 26, 65–76. https://doi.org/10.1080/00332747.1963.11023339

Byatt, A.S. (2008, June 21). Twisted yarns. *The Guardian.* https://www.theguardian.com/books/2008/jun/21/saturdayreviewsfeatres.guardianreview9

Calasanti, T., Slevin, K., & King, N. (2006). Ageism and feminism: From "et cetera" to centre. *National Women's Studies Association Journal*, 18(1), 13–30. https://doi.org/10.1353/nwsa.2006.0004

Calion, M. (1986). Some elements in a sociology of translation: Domestication of the scallops and fishermen of St Brieuc Bay. In J. Law (Ed.), *Power, action and belief* (pp. 196–233). London: Routledge & Kegan Paul.

Cameron, J. (1995). *The artist's way morning pages journal: A companion volume to the artist's way.* New York: Penguin.

Campbell, J. (1949). *The hero with a thousand faces.* New York: Pantheon.

Campbell, J., & Moyers, B. (1988). *The power of myth.* New York: Doubleday.

Cappeliez, P. (2017). The worth of personal memories: Reviewing, letting go, or ... obliterating? *International Journal of Life Review and Reminiscence*, 4(1), 1–2.

Caputo, J. (1997). *Deconstruction in a nutshell.* New York: Fordham University Press.

Carney, G. (2018). Towards a gender politics of aging. *Journal of Women & Aging*, 30(3), 242–258. https://doi.org/10.1080/08952841.2017.1301163

Carr, D. (2010). *Sanctuary: The story of naturalist Mary Majka*. Fredericton: Goose Lane.

Carson, R. (1962). *Silent spring*. Greenwich, CT: Fawcett Crest.

Carstensen, L., Isaacowitz, D., & Charles, S. (1999). Taking time seriously: A theory of socioemotional selectivity. *American Psychologist*, 54, 165–181. https://doi.org/10.1037//0003-066x.54.3.165

Carstensen, L., & Mikels, J. (2005). At the intersection of emotion and cognition: Aging and the positivity effect. *Current Directions in Psychological Science*, 14, 117–121. https://doi.org/10.1111/j.0963-7214.2005.00348.x

Casey, E. (1987). *Remembering: A phenomenological study*. Bloomington: Indiana University Press.

Chandler, S., & Ray, R. (2002). New meanings for old tales: A discourse-based study of reminiscence and development in later life. In J. Webster & B. Haight (Eds.), *Critical advances in reminiscence work: From theory to application* (pp. 76–94). New York: Springer.

Chapman, S. (2005). Theorizing about aging well: Constructing a narrative. *Canadian Journal on Aging*, 24(1), 9–18. https://doi.org/10.1353/cja.2005.0004

Charon, R. (2006). *Narrative medicine: Honoring the stories of illness*. New York: Oxford University Press.

Chavese, R., Molina, M., Lizama, C., Sosa, C., & Torres, C. (2020). To know and not to know: Dialogic social inquiry. In S. McNamee, M. Gergen, C. Camargo-Borges, & E. Rasera (Eds.), *The Sage handbook of social constructionist practice* (pp. 77–85). Thousand Oaks: Sage.

Chavis, G. (2011). *Poetry and story therapy: The healing power of creative expression*. London: Jessica Kingsley.

Cheek, C., & Piercy, K. (2004). Quilting as age identity expression in traditional women. *International Journal of Aging and Human Development*, 59(4), 321–337. https://doi.org/10.2190/T1R0-D8TW-ML6Y-VYYL

Cheek, C., & Yaure, R. (2017). Quilting as a generative activity: Studying those who make quilts for wounded service members. *Journal of Women & Aging*, 29(1), 39–50. https://doi.org/10.1080/08952841.2015.1021652

Chopra, D. (2014). *The future of God: A practical approach to spirituality for our times*. New York: Harmony.

Chudacoff, H. (2000). *The age of the bachelor: Creating an American subculture*. Princeton: Princeton University Press.

Clandinin, J. (Ed.). (2007). *Handbook of narrative inquiry: Mapping a methodology*. Thousand Oaks: Sage.

Coates, T. (2015). *Between the world and me*. New York: Spiegel & Grau.

Cohen, G. (2005). *The mature mind: The positive power of the aging brain*. Boston: Basic.

Cohen, L. (1992). Anthem [Song]. On *The future.* Parkwood: Columbia.

Cole, T. (2002). *Life stories: Aging and the human spirit* [Video]. National Film Network.

Coleman, P. (1999). Creating a life story: The task of reconciliation. *The Gerontologist,* 39(2), 133–139. https://doi.org/10.1093/geront/39.2.133

Coleman, T., & Wiles, J. (2020). Being with objects of meaning: Cherished possessions and opportunities to maintain aging in place. *The Gerontologist,* 60(1), 41–49. https://doi.org/10.1093/geront/gny142

Connor, K., & Davidson, J. (2003). Development of a new resilience scale: The Connor-Davidson Resilience Scale (CD-RISC). *Depression and Anxiety,* 18, 71–82. https://doi.org/10.1002/da.10113

Costa, P., & McRae, R. (1985). *The NEO personality inventory.* Odessa, FL: Psychological Assessment Resources.

Craig, C., & Huber, J. (2007). Relational reverberations: Shaping and reshaping narrative inquiries in the midst of storied lives and contexts. In J. Clandinin (Ed.), *Handbook of narrative inquiry: Mapping a methodology* (pp. 251–279). Thousand Oaks: Sage.

Csikszentimihalyi, M., & Beattie, O. (1979). Life themes: A theoretical and empirical exploration of their origins and efforts. *Journal of Humanistic Psychology,* 19(1), 45–63. https://doi.org/10.1177/002216787901900105

Csikszentmihalyi, M., & Rathunde, K. (1990). The psychology of wisdom: An evolutionary interpretation. In R. Sternberg (Ed.), *Wisdom: Its nature, origins, and development* (pp. 25–51). New York: Cambridge University Press.

Csikszentmihalyi, M., & Rochberg-Halton, E. (1981). *The meaning of things: Domestic symbols and the self.* Cambridge: Cambridge University Press.

Curtis, B., & Eldredge, J. (1997). *The sacred romance: Drawing closer to the heart of God.* New York: Thomas Nelson.

Dant, T. (2001). Fruitbox/toolbox: Biography and objects. *Auto/Biography,* 9(1–2), 11–20.

Danto, A. (1985). *Narration and knowledge.* New York: Columbia University Press.

Davis, J., & Franks, T. (1950). *How far is heaven?* [Song].

de Medeiros, K. (2007). Beyond the memoir: Telling life stories using multiple literary forms. *Journal of Aging, Humanities, and The Arts,* 1, 159–167. https://doi.org/10.1080/19325610701638052

de Medeiros, K. (2011). Telling stories: How do expressions of self differ in a writing group versus a reminiscence group? In G. Kenyon, E. Bohlmeijer, & W. Randall (Eds.), *Storying later life: Issues, investigations, and interventions in narrative gerontology* (pp. 159–176). New York: Oxford University Press.

de Medeiros, K. (2013). *Narrative gerontology in research and practice.* New York: Springer.

de Medeiros, K., Kennedy, Q., Cole, T., Lindley, R., & O'Hara, R. (2007). The impact of autobiographic writing on memory performance in older adults: A preliminary investigation. *American Journal of Geriatric Psychiatry*, 15(3), 257–261. Medline:17322137. https://doi.org/10.1097/01.JGP.0000240985.10411.3e

de Medeiros, K., & Lagay, F. (2000). "Share your lifestory" workshop manual [Unpublished manuscript].

de Medeiros, K., Mosby, A., Hanley, K., Pedraza, M., & Brandt, J. (2011). A randomized clinical trial of a writing workshop and intervention to improve autobiographical memory and well-being in older adults. *International Journal of Geriatric Psychiatry*, 26, 803–811. Medline:21744383. https://doi.org/10.1002/gps.2605

de Medeiros, K., & Rubinstein, R. (2015). "Shadow stories" in oral interviews: Narrative care through careful listening. *Journal of Aging Studies*, 34, 162–168. Medline:26162737. https://doi.org/10.1016/j.jaging.2015.02.009

Denzin, N. (1989). *Interpretive interactionism* (Vol. 16, Applied Social Research Methods Series). Thousand Oaks: Sage.

Denzin, N. (1996). *Interpretive ethnography: Ethnographic practices for the 21st century*. Thousand Oaks: Sage.

DeSalvo, L. (1999). *Writing as a way of healing: How telling our stories transforms our lives*. Boston: Beacon.

Dominicé, P. (2000). *Learning from our lives: Using educational biographies with adults*. San Francisco: Jossey-Bass.

Dubovská, E., Chrz, V., Tavel, P., Poláčková-Šolcová, I., & Růžička, J. (2016). Narrative construction of resilience: Stories of older Czech adults. *Ageing and Society*, 37(9), 1–25. https://doi.org/10.1017/S0144686X16000581

Dyl, J., & Wapner, S. (1996). Age and gender differences in the nature, meaning, and function of cherished possessions for children and adolescents. *Journal of Experimental Child Psychology*, 62(3), 340–377. https://doi.org/10.1006/jecp.1996.0034

Eakin, P.J. (1999). *How our lives become stories: Making selves*. Ithaca: Cornell University Press.

Edwards, V. (Ed.) (2018). *Remembered: A collection of stories from the "Writing Our Lives" class of 2017*. Fredericton, NB.

Eliot, T.S. (2005). Tradition and the individual talent. In L. Rainey (Ed.), *Modernism: An anthology*. (pp. 152–156). London: Blackwell.

Ellis, C., & Berger, L. (2002). Their story/my story/our story: Including the researcher's experience in interview research. In J. Gubrium & J. Holstein (Ed.), *Postmodern interviewing* (pp. 849–875). Thousand Oaks: Sage.

Erikson, E. (1963). *Childhood and society*. New York: W.W. Norton.

Erikson, E. (1968). *Identity: Youth and crisis*. New York: W.W. Norton.

Erikson, E., Erikson, J., & Kivnick, H. (1986). *Vital involvement in old age*. New York: W.W. Norton.

Ettinger, L.F., & Hoffman, E. (1990). Quilt making in art education: Toward a participatory curriculum metaphor. *Art Education*, 43(4), 40–47. https://doi.org/10.2307/3193214

Ferguson, N. (Ed.). (1997). *Virtual history: Alternatives and counterfactuals.* London: Papermac.

Ferraro, R., Escolas, J., & Bettman, J. (2011). Our possessions, our selves: Domains of self-worth and the possession-self link. *Journal of Consumer Psychology*, 21(2), 169–177. https://doi.org/10.1016/J.JCPS.2010.08.007

Fireman, G., McVay, T., & Flanagan, O. (Eds.). (2003). *Narrative and consciousness: Literature, psychology, and the brain.* New York: Oxford University Press.

Fish, S. (1980). *Is there a text in this class? The authority of interpretive communities.* Cambridge, MA: Harvard University Press.

Fivush, R. (1994). Constructing narrative, emotion, and gender in parent-child conversations about the past. In U. Neisser & R. Fivush (Eds.), *The remembering self: Construction and accuracy of the life narrative* (pp. 136–157). New York: Cambridge University Press.

Fivush, R., Haden, C., & Reese, E. (1995). Remembering, recounting, and reminiscing: The development of autobiographical memory in social context. In D. Rubin (Ed.), *Remembering our past: Studies in autobiographical memory* (pp. 341–359). New York: Cambridge University Press.

Fowler, J. (1981). *Stages of faith: The psychology of human development and the quest for meaning.* San Francisco: Harper & Row.

Frank, A. (2010). *Letting stories breathe: A socio-narratology.* Chicago: University of Chicago Press.

Frank, A. (2013). *The wounded storyteller* (2nd ed.). Chicago: University of Chicago Press.

Franklin, J. (2007). *Telling true stories: A non-fiction writers' guide from the Nieman Foundation at Harvard University.* New York: Plume.

Franklin, P. (2000). Object choice: Marcel Duchamp's fountain and the art of queer art history. *Oxford Art Journal*, 23(1), 23–50. https://doi.org/10.1093/oaj/23.1.23

Freeman, M. (1993). *Rewriting the self: History, memory, narrative.* New York: Routledge.

Freeman, M. (2000). When the story's over: Narrative foreclosure and the possibility of self-renewal. In M. Andrews, S. Slater, C. Squire, & A. Treacher (Eds.), *Lines of narrative: Psychosocial perspectives* (pp. 81–91). London: Routledge.

Freeman, M. (2010). *Hindsight: The promise and peril of looking backward.* New York: Oxford University Press.

Fry, P., & Debats, D. (2011). Sources of human life-strengths, resilience, and health. In P. Fry & C. Keyes (Eds.), *New frontiers in resilient aging: Life-strengths and well-being in late life* (pp. 15–59). New York: Cambridge University Press.

Frye, N. (1990). *Words with power: Being a second study of "The Bible and Literature."* New York: Harcourt Brace Jovanovich.

Fulford, R. (1999). *The triumph of narrative: Storytelling in the age of mass culture.* Toronto: Anansi.

Fuller, D. (2004). *Writing the everyday: Women's textual communities in Atlantic Canada.* Montreal: McGill-Queen's University Press.

Furlong, D., Randall, W., Baldwin, C., McKenzie-Mohr, S., & McKim, E. (2015, October 23). The importance of the stories of others: Narrative embeddedness as a feature of resilience [Paper presentation]. Canadian Association on Gerontology, Calgary, AB.

Gardner, H., & Winner, H. (1978). The development of metaphoric competence: Implications for humanistic disciplines. *Critical Inquiry*, 5(1), 123–141. https://doi.org/10.1086/447976

Gawande, A. (2014). *Being mortal: Medicine and what matters in the end.* New York: Metropolitan Books.

Gibson, K.R., & Ingold, T. (1994). *Tools, language, and cognition in human evolution.* Cambridge: Cambridge University Press.

Gold, J. (2002). *The story species: Our life-literature connection.* Toronto: Fitzhenry & Whiteside.

Goldberg, N. (1986). *Writing down the bones: Freeing the writer within.* Boston: Shambala.

Gordon, C.A. (1871). Remarks on the Prussian Siege of Paris in some of its relations to hygiene and surgery. *British Medical Journal*, 2(559), 313. Medline:20746349. https://doi.org/10.1136/bmj.2.559.313

Green, O., & Ayalon, L. (2019). "Home is where my couch is": The role of possessions in the process of moving and adjusting to continuing care retirement communities. *Qualitative Health Research*, 29(4), 577–589. Medline:29947582. https://doi.org/10.1177/1049732318780350

Grigoriou, T. (2004). *Friendship between gay men and heterosexual women: An interpretative phenomenological analysis.* Families & Social Capital ESRC Research Group. London: South Bank University.

Gullette, M. (2004). *Aged by culture.* Chicago: University of Chicago Press.

Habermas, T. (2010). Autobiographical reasoning: Arguing and narrating from a biographical perspective. *New Directions for Child and Adolescent Development*, 131, 1–17. Medline:21387528. https://doi.org/10.1002/cd.285

Habermas, T. (2019). *Emotion and narrative: Perspectives in autobiographical storytelling.* Cambridge: Cambridge University Press.

Haight, B. (2007). The life review: Historical approaches. In J. Kunz & F. Soltys (Eds.), *Transformational reminiscence: Life story work* (pp. 67–81). New York: Springer.

Hammarskjöld, D. (1964). *Markings.* (L. Sjöberg & W. Auden, Trans.). New York: Ballantine.

Hampl, P. (1999). *I could tell you stories: Sojourns in the land of memory.* New York: W.W. Norton.

Hannan, L., Carney, G., Devine, P., & Hodge, H. (2019). A view from old age: Women's lives as narrated through objects. *Life Writing*, 16(1), 51–67. https://doi.org/10.1080/14484528.2019.1521259

Harman, G. (2009). *Prince of networks: Bruno Latour and metaphysics.* Melbourne: Re.press.

Hartman-Stein, P. (2011). Creative writing groups: A promising avenue for enhancing working memory and emotional well-being. In P. Hartman-Stein & A. La Rue (Eds.), *Enhancing cognitive fitness in adults: A guide to the use and development of community-based programmes* (pp. 199–212). New York: Springer.

Hatlen, B. (1995). The imagist poetics of H.D.'s "Sea Garden." *Paideuma*, 24(2–3), 107–130.

Hecht, A., & O'Brien Tyrell, M. (2007). Life stories as heirlooms: The personal history industry. In J. Kunz & F. Soltys (Eds.), *Transformational reminiscence: Life story work* (pp. 85–106). New York: Springer.

Heilbrun, C. (1988). *Writing a woman's life.* New York: Ballantine.

Herman, D. (2008). Storyworld. In D. Herman, M. Jahn, & M.-L. Ryan (Eds.), *Routledge encyclopedia of narrative theory* (p. 569). London: Routledge.

Hermans, H. (2001). The dialogical self: Toward a theory of personal and cultural positioning. *Culture and Psychology*, 7, 243–281. https://doi.org/10.1177/1354067X0173001

Hesse, H. (1961). *Journey to the east.* New York: Farrar, Straus, & Giroux.

Hewes, G. (1995). A history of speculation on the relation between tools and language. In K. Gibson & T. Ingold (Eds.), *Tools, language, and cognition in human evolution* (pp. 20–30). Cambridge: Cambridge University Press.

Hills, R. (1977). *Writing in general and short story in particular.* Boston: Bantam.

Hillstrom, K. (2012). *The September 11 Terrorist Attacks.* Detroit: Omnigraphics.

Hoinacki, L. (1996). *El Camino: Walking to Santiago de Compostela.* University Park: Pennsylvania State University Press.

Holstein, J., & Gubrium, J. (2000). *The self we live by: Narrative identity in a postmodern world.* New York: Oxford University Press.

Hooker, K., & Kaus, C.R. (1992). Possible selves and health behaviors in later life. *Journal of Aging and Health*, 4(3), 390–411. https://doi.org/10.1177/089826439200400304

Hooyman, N., Browne, C., Ray, R., & Richardson, V. (2002). Feminist gerontology and the life course. *Gerontology & Geriatrics Education*, 22(4), 3–26. https://doi.org/10.1300/J021v22n04_02

Hoppmann, C., Gerstorf, D., Smith, J., & Klumb, P. (2007). Linking possible selves and behavior: Do domain-specific hopes and fears translate into daily activities in very old age? *Journal of Gerontology: Psychological Sciences*, 62B(2), P104–P111. https://doi.org/10.1093/geronb/62.2.P104

Hoppmann, C., & Smith, J. (2007). Life-history related differences in possible selves in very old age. *International Journal of Aging and Human Development*,

64(2), 109–127. Medline:17451041. https://doi.org/10.2190/GL71-PW45-Q481-5LN7

Howarth, L. (2020). Narrative, objects, and the construction of the self: How we might remember when we have forgotten. *International Journal of Information, Diversity, & Inclusion*, 4(1), https://jps.library.utoronto.ca/index.php/ijidi/article/view/32841/25591

Humphreys, H. (2000). *Afterimage.* Toronto: HarperCollins Canada.

Humphries, C., & Smith, A.C.T. (2014). Talking objects: Towards a post-social research framework for exploring object narratives. *Organization*, 21(4), 477–494. https://doi.org/10.1177/1350508414527253

Hunter, C. (2019). *Threads of life: A history of the world through the eye of a needle.* London: Sceptre.

Hunter, E., & Rowles, G. (2005). Leaving a legacy: Toward a typology. *Journal of Aging Studies*, 19(3), 327–347. https://doi.org/10.1016/j.jaging.2004.08.002

Hydén, L.-C., Lindemann, H., & Brockmeier, J. (Eds.). (2014). *Beyond loss: Dementia, identity, and personhood.* New York: Oxford University Press.

Hyvärinen, M., Hydén, L.-C., Saarenheimo, M., & Tamboukou, M. (Eds.). (2010). *Beyond narrative coherence.* Philadelphia: John Benjamins.

Ingersoll, M., & Whitty, P. (2021). Critical narrative nostalgia: Places, spaces, and privilege. In E. Lyle & S. Mahani (Eds.), *Sister scholars: Untangling issues of identity as women in academe* (pp. 41–48). New York: DIO Press.

Ingold, T. (2011). *Being alive: Essays on movement, knowledge and description.* London: Routledge.

Johnson, M., & Walker, J. (Eds.). (2016). *Spiritual dimensions of ageing.* Cambridge: Cambridge University Press.

Josselson, R. (2007). The ethical attitude in narrative research: Principles and practicalities. In J. Clandinin (Ed.), *Handbook of narrative inquiry: Mapping a methodology* (pp. 537–566). Thousand Oaks: Sage.

Joyce, J. (1968). *Ulysses.* Middlesex: Penguin.

Jung, C. (1976). The stages of life. In J. Campbell (Ed.), *The portable Jung* (pp. 3–22). London: Penguin.

Kadir, A. (2009). *What a woman wants.* Bloomington: Xlibris.

Kadir, A., & Shaq, A. (2011). *Daughter of Pharoah.*

Kadir, A., & Skov-Nielsen, E. (Eds.). (2018). *Arrivals and departures: The stories we tell.* Foraging Chapbook no.1. Fredericton: The Fiddlehead.

Kaminsky, M. (1992). Story of the shoe box: On the meaning and practice of transmitting stories. In T. Cole (Ed.), *Handbook of the humanities and aging* (pp. 307–327). New York: Springer.

Kelly, J. (2012, 23 May). ASBO – The end of an era. *BBC Online.* www.bbc.co.uk/news/magazine-18164426.

Kenyon, G. (2011). On suffering, loss, and the journey to life: Tai Chi as narrative care. In G. Kenyon, E. Bohlmeijer, & W. Randall (Eds.), *Storying later life: Issues, investigations, and interventions in narrative gerontology* (pp. 237–251). New York: Oxford University Press.

Kenyon, G., Bohlmeijer, E., & Randall, W. (Eds.) (2011). *Storying later life: Issues, investigations, and interventions in narrative gerontology*. New York: Oxford University Press.

Kenyon, G., Clark, P., & de Vries, B. (Eds.). (2001). *Narrative gerontology: Theory, research, and practice*. New York: Springer.

Kenyon, G., & Randall, W. (1997). *Restorying our lives: Personal growth through autobiographical reflection*. Westport: Praeger.

Kenyon, G., & Randall, W. (2001). Narrative gerontology: An overview. In G. Kenyon, P. Clark, & B. de Vries (Eds), *Narrative gerontology: Theory, research, and practice* (pp. 3–18). New York: Springer.

Kenyon, G., & Randall, W. (2015). Introduction: Special issue on "narrative care." *Journal of Aging Studies*, 34, 143–145.

King, L., & Hicks, J. (2007). Whatever happened to "what might have been"? Regrets, happiness, and maturity. *American Psychologist*, 63(7), 625–636. Medline:17924747. https://doi.org/10.1037/0003-066X.62.7.625

King, L., & Mitchell, L. (2015). Lost possible selves and personality development. In K. Cherry (Ed.), *Traumatic stress and long-term recovery* (pp. 309–325). New York: Springer.

King, L., & Raspin, C. (2004). Lost and found possible selves, subjective well-being, and ego development in divorced women. *Journal of Personality*, 72(3), 603–632. Medline:15102040. https://doi.org/10.1111/j.0022-3506.2004.00274.x

King, T. (2003). *The truth about stories: A native narrative*. Toronto: Anansi.

Kohlberg, L. (1984). *The psychology of moral development: The nature and validity of moral stages*. San Francisco: Harper & Row.

Kopp, S. (1976). *If you meet the Buddha on the road, kill him!* Toronto: Bantam.

Koschwanez, H., Kerse, N., Darragh, M., Jarrett, P., Booth, R., & Broadbent, E. (2013). Expressive writing and wound healing in older adults: A randomized controlled trial. *Psychosomatic Medicine*, 75, 581–590. Medline:23804013. https://doi.org/10.1097/PSY.0b013e31829b7b2e

Kotre, J. (1984). *Outliving the self: Generativity and the interpretation of lives*. Baltimore: Johns Hopkins University Press.

Kotre, J. (1999). *Make it count: How to generate a legacy that gives meaning to your life*. New York: Free Press.

Krasner, J. (2005). Accumulated lives: Metaphor, materiality, and the homes of the elder. *Literature and Medicine*, 24(2), 209–230. https://doi.org/10.1353/lm.2006.0008

Kroger, J., and Adair, V. (2008). Symbolic meanings of valued personal objects in identity transitions of late adulthood. *Identity*, 8(1), 5–24. https://doi.org/10.1080/15283480701787251

Kunz, J., & Soltys, F. (Eds.). (2007). *Transformational reminiscence: Life story work.* New York: Springer.

Labouvie-Vief, G. (1990). Wisdom as integrated thought: Historical and developmental perspectives. In R. Sternberg (Ed.), *Wisdom: Its nature, origins, and development* (pp. 52–83). New York: Cambridge University Press.

Latour, B. (1988). Mixing humans and nonhumans together: The sociology of a door-closer. *Social Problems,* 35(3), 298–310.

Latour, B. (1991). Technology is society made durable. In J. Law (Ed.), *A sociology of monsters: Essays on power, technology and domination* (pp. 103–131). London: Routledge.

Latour, B. (2005). *Reassembling the social: An introduction to actor-network-theory.* Oxford: Oxford University Press.

Lawrence-Lightfoot, S. (2009). *The third chapter: Passion, risk, and adventure in the 25 years after 50.* New York: Sarah Crichton Books.

Lepore, S., & Smyth, J. (Eds.). (2002). *The writing cure: How expressive writing promotes health and emotional well-being.* Washington, DC: American Psychological Association.

Letherby, G., & Davidson, D. (2015). Embodied storytelling: Loss and bereavement, creative practices, and support. *Illness, Crisis & Loss,* 23(4), 343–360. https://doi.org/10.1177/1054137315590745

Levin, J. (2020). *Black hole survival guide.* New York: Knopf.

Linde, C. (1993). *Life stories: The quest for coherence.* New York: Oxford University Press.

Lively, P. (2013). *Ammonites and leaping fish: A life in time.* London: Fig Tree.

Loevinger, J. (1976). *Ego development: Conceptions and theories.* San Francisco: Jossey-Bass.

Lombao, D., Guardiola, M., & Mosquera, M. (2017). Teaching to make stone tools: New experimental evidence supporting a technological hypothesis for the origins of language. *Scientific Reports,* 7, 14394. https://doi.org/10.1038/s41598-017-14322-y

MacGregor, N. (2010, 19 January). Making us human: (2,000,000–9000 BC). Episode of *A history of the world in 100 objects* [Radio series]. BBC. https://www.bbc.co.uk/sounds/play/b00pwn7m

MacGregor, N. (2011). *A history of the world in 100 objects.* London: Allen Lane.

Mader, W. (1996). Emotionality and continuity in biographical contexts. In J. Birren, G. Kenyon, J-E. Ruth, J. Schroots, & T. Svensson (Eds.), *Aging and biography: Explorations in adult development* (pp. 39–60). New York: Springer.

Marks, S. (2011). The power of stories left untold: Narratives of Nazi followers. In G. Kenyon, E. Bohlmeijer, & W. Randall (Eds.), *Storying later life: Issues, investigations, and interventions in narrative gerontology* (pp. 101–110.) New York: Oxford University Press.

Markus, H. (2006). Foreword. In C. Dunkel & J. Kerpelman (Eds.), *Possible selves: Theory, research, and applications* (pp. ix–xiv). New York: Nova Science.

Markus, H., & Nurius, P. (1986). Possible selves. *American Psychologist*, 41(9). 954–969. https://doi.org/10.1037/0003-066X.41.9.954

Mather, M., & Carstensen, L.L. (2005). Aging and motivated cognition: The positivity effect in attention and memory. *Trends in Cognitive Sciences*, 9, 496–502. Medline:16154382. https://doi.org/10.1016/j.tics.2005.08.005

Maurois, A. (1986). Biography as a work of art. In S.B. Oates (Ed.), *Biography as high adventure: Life-writers speak on their art* (pp. 3–17). Amherst: University of Massachusetts Press.

McAdams, D. (1988). *Power, intimacy, and the life story: Personological inquiries into identity*. New York: Guilford.

McAdams, D. (1996). Narrating the self in adulthood. In J. Birren, G. Kenyon, J-E. Ruth, J. Schroots, & T. Svensson (Eds.), *Aging and biography: Explorations in adult development*(pp. 131–148). New York: Springer.

McAdams, D. (2001a). *The person: An integrated introduction to personality psychology*. New York: Harcourt.

McAdams, D. (2001b). The psychology of life stories. *Review of General Psychology*, 5(2), 100–122. https://doi.org/10.1037/1089-2680.5.2.100

McAdams, D. (2006). *The redemptive self: Stories Americans live by*. New York: Oxford University Press.

McAdams, D. (2008). Personal narratives and the life story. In O. John, R. Robins, & L. Pervin (Eds.), *Handbook of personality: Theory and research* (pp. 242–262). New York: Guilford.

McAdams, D., & Bowman, P. (2001). Narrating life's turning-points: Redemption and contamination. In D. McAdams, R. Josselson, & A. Lieblich (Eds.), *Turns in the road: Narrative studies of lives in transition* (pp. 3–34). Washington, DC: American Psychological Association.

McAdams, D., & Logan, R. (2004). What is generativity? In E. de St Aubin, D. McAdams, & T. Kim (Eds.), *The generative society: Caring for future generations* (pp. 15–31). Washington, DC: American Psychological Association.

McFadden, S., & Atchley, R. (Eds.). (2001). *Aging and the meaning of time*. New York: Springer.

McKendy, J. (2006). "I'm very careful about that": Narrative agency of men in prison. *Discourse & Society*, 17(4), 473–502. https://doi.org/10.1177/0957926506063128

McLean, K. (2008). The emergence of narrative identity. *Social and Personality Psychology Compass*, 2(4), 1685–1702. https://doi.org/10.1111/j.1751-9004.2008.00124.x

Meretoja, H. (2014). *The narrative turn in fiction and theory: The crisis and return of storytelling from Robbe-Grillet to Tournier*. London: Palgrave Macmillan.

Merrill, N., & Fivush, R. (2016). Intergenerational narratives and identity across development. *Developmental Review*, 40, 72–92. https://doi.org/10.1016/j.dr.2016.03.001

Michael, M. (1996). *Constructing identities: The social, nonhuman and change.* London: Sage.

Miller, D. (2008). *The comfort of things.* Cambridge: Polity.

Mishler, E.G. (1991). *Research interviewing: Context and narrative.* Cambridge, MA: Harvard University Press.

Mitchell, S. (Director). (2006). *Tell me* [Film]. Talisman Films. https://www.shandimitchell.com/tell-me

Moore, T. (1992). *Care of the soul: A guide for cultivating depth and sacredness in everyday life.* New York: HarperCollins.

Moore, T. (2000). Neither here nor there. *Parabola*, 25(1), n.p.

Morgan, T., Uomini, N., & Rendell, L. (2015). Experimental evidence for the co-evolution of hominin tool-making teaching and language. *Nature Communications*, 6, 6029. https://doi.org/10.1038/ncomms7029

Morris, C. (2011). *Remembering the AIDS Quilt.* East Lansing: Michigan State University Press.

Morson, G. (1994). *Narrative and freedom: The shadows of time.* New Haven, CT: Yale University Press.

Morton, B. (1999). *Starting out in the evening.* New York: Berkley.

Morton, S., & Guildford, J. (Eds.). (1994). *Separate spheres: The world of women in the 19th-century Maritimes.* Fredericton: Acadiensis.

Mulkerns, H., & Owen, C. (2008). Identity development in emancipated young adults following foster care. *Smith College Studies in Social Work*, 78(4), 427–449. https://doi.org/10.1080/00377310802378594

Myerhoff, B. (1992). *Remembered lives: The work of ritual, storytelling, and growing older.* Ann Arbor: University of Michigan Press.

Myss, C. (1996). *Anatomy of the spirit: The seven stages of power and healing.* New York: Three Rivers.

Neisser, U., & Libby, L. (2000). Remembering life experiences. In E. Tulving & F. Craik (Eds.), *The Oxford handbook of memory* (pp. 315–332). New York: Oxford University Press.

Nelson, H. (2001). *Damaged identities: Narrative repair.* Ithaca: Cornell University Press.

Nelson, K., & Fivush, R. (2000). Socialization of memory. In E. Tulving & F. Craik (Eds.), *The Oxford handbook of memory* (pp. 283–295). New York: Oxford University Press.

Nord, C. (2013). A day to be lived: Elderly people's possessions for everyday life in assisted living. *Journal of Aging Studies*, 27, 135–142. Medline:23561278. https://doi.org/10.1016/j.jaging.2012.12.002

Norris, J., Kuiack, S., & Pratt, M. (2004). "As long as they go back down the driveway at the end of the day": Stories of the satisfactions and challenges of grandparenthood. In M. Pratt & B. Fiese (Eds.), *Family stories and the life course: Across time and generations* (pp. 327–398). Mahwah: Erlbaum.

Ochs, E., & Capps, L. (2002). *Living narrative: Creating lives in everyday storytelling.* Cambridge, MA: Harvard University Press.

Olson, D., & Torrance, N. (Eds.). (1991). *Literacy and orality.* New York: Cambridge University Press.

O'Neill, P., Birren, J., & Svensson, C. (2011). Narrative and gender differences: How men and women interpret their lives. In G. Kenyon, E. Bohlmeijer, & W. Randall (Eds.), *Storying later life: Issues, investigations, and interventions in narrative gerontology* (pp. 143–158). New York: Oxford University Press.

Ong, A., & Bergeman, C. (2010). The socioemotional basis of resilience in later life. In P. Fry & C. Keyes (Eds.), *New frontiers in resilient aging* (pp. 230–257). New York: Cambridge University Press.

Ott, K. (2014, August 19). Spinsters, confirmed bachelors, and LGBTQ collecting. *O Say Can You See: Stories from the Museum.* https://americanhistory.si.edu/blog/2014/08/spinsters-confirmed-bachelors-and-lgbtq-collecting.html

Pals, J. (2006). Narrative identity processing of difficult life experiences: Pathways of personality development and positive self-transformation in adulthood. *Journal of Personality,* 74(4), 1079–1109. Medline:16787429. https://doi.org/10.1111/j.1467-6494.2006.00403.x

Pasupathi, M., & Mansour, E. (2006). Adult age differences in autobiographical reasoning in narratives. *Developmental Psychology,* 42(5), 798–808. https://doi.org/10.1037/0012-1649.42.5.798

Pearson, C. (1989). *The hero within: Six archetypes we live by.* San Francisco: Harper & Row.

Pennebaker, J. (1990). *Opening up: The healing power of confiding in others.* New York: Avon.

Pennebaker, J., & Seagal, J. (1999). Forming a story: The health benefits of narrative. *Journal of Clinical Psychology,* 55(10), 1243–1254. Medline:11045774. https://doi.org/10.1002/(SICI)1097-4679(199910)55:10<1243::AID-JCLP6>3.0.CO;2-N

Petrelli, D., & Whittaker, S. (2010). Family memories in the home: Contrasting physical and digital mementos. *International Journal of Personal and Ubiquitous Computing,* 14(2), https://doi.org/10.1007/s00779-009-0279-7

Phenice, L., & Griffore, R. (2013). The importance of object memories for older adults. *Educational Gerontology,* 39(10), 741–749. https://doi.org/10.1080/03601277.2013.766536

Phoenix, C., & Smith, B. (2011). Telling a (good?) counterstory of aging: Natural bodybuilding meets the narrative of decline. *Journals of Gerontology, Series B: Psychological Sciences and Social Sciences,* 66(5), 628–639. https://doi.org/10.1093/geronb/gbr077

Pinnegar, S., & Daynes, G. (2007). Locating narrative inquiry historically: Thematics in the turn to narrative. In J. Clandinin (Ed.), *Handbook of narrative inquiry: Mapping a methodology* (pp. 3–34). Thousand Oaks: Sage.

Polkinghorne, D. (1988). *Narrative knowing and the human sciences.* Albany: SUNY Press.

Polkinghorne, D. (2004). *Practice and the human sciences: The case for a judgment-based practice of care.* Albany: SUNY Press.

Polster, E. (1987). *Every person's life is worth a novel: How to cut through emotional pain and discover the fascinating core of life.* New York: W.W. Norton.

Pound, E. (1954). A retrospect. In T.S. Eliot (Ed.), *Literary essays of Ezra Pound* (pp. 3–14). London: Faber & Faber.

Price, L.L., Arnaud, E.J., & Curasi, C.F. (2000). Older consumers' disposition of special possessions. *Journal of Consumer Research,* 27(2), 179–201. https://doi.org/10.1086/314319

Prince. (1984). When doves cry [Song]. On *Purple Rain.* Paisley Park Records.

Progoff, I. (1975). *At a journal workshop: The basic text and guide for using the Intensive Journal.* New York: Dialogue House Library.

Raggatt, P. (2006). Multiplicity and conflict in the dialogical self: A life-narrative approach. In D. McAdams, R. Josselson, & A. Lieblich (Eds.). *Identity and story: Creating self in narrative* (pp. 15–35). Washington, DC: American Psychological Association.

Rainer, T. (1978). *The new diary: How to use a journal for self-guidance and expanded creativity.* Los Angeles: Jeremy P. Tarcher.

Rainer, T. (1998). *Your life as a story: Discovering the "new autobiography" and writing memoir as literature.* New York: Jeremy P. Tarcher.

Rak, J. (2018). The hidden genre: Diaries and time. *European Journal of Life Writing,* 7, 85–89. https://doi.org/10.5463/ejlw.7.262

Ramsey, J., & Bleizner, R. (2013). *Spiritual resiliency and aging: Hope, relationality, and the creative self.* Amityville: Baywood.

Randall, W. (2001). Storied worlds: Acquiring a narrative perspective on aging, identity, and everyday life. In G. Kenyon, P. Clark, & B. de Vries (Eds.), *Narrative gerontology: Theory, research, and practice* (pp. 31–62). New York: Springer.

Randall, W. (2007). From computer to compost: Rethinking our metaphors for memory. *Theory & Psychology,* 17(5), 611–633. https://doi.org/10.1177/0959354307081619

Randall, W. (2010). Storywork: Autobiographical learning in later life. In C. Clark & M. Rossiter (Eds.), *Narrative perspectives on adult education: New directions for adult learning and continuing education,* no. 126 (pp. 25–36). San Francisco: Jossey-Bass.

Randall, W. (2011). Memory, metaphor, and meaning: Reading for wisdom in the stories of our lives. In G. Kenyon, E. Bohlmeijer, & W. Randall (Eds.),

Storying later life: Issues, investigations, and interventions in narrative gerontology (pp. 20–38). New York: Oxford University Press.

Randall, W. (2013). The importance of being ironic: Narrative openness and personal resilience in later life. *The Gerontologist*, 53(1), 9–16. https://doi .org/10.1093/geront/gns048

Randall, W. (2014). *The stories we are: An essay on self-creation* (2nd ed.). Toronto: University of Toronto Press.

Randall, W. (2019). The end of the story? Narrative openness in life and death. *Narrative Works: Issues, Investigations, and Interventions*, 9(2), 152–170.

Randall, W. (2020). Strengthening our stories in the second half of life: Narrative resilience through narrative care. In S. McNamee, M. Gergen, C. Camargo-Borges, & E. Rasera (Eds.), *The Sage handbook of social constructionist practice* (pp. 444–454). Thousand Oaks: Sage.

Randall, W. (2023). The poetics of growing old: Metaphoric competence and the philosophic homework of later life. In O. Lehmann & O. Synnes, *A poetic language of ageing* (pp. 137–154). London: Bloomsbury.

Randall, W., Baldwin, C., McKenzie-Mohr, S., McKim, E., & Furlong, D. (2015). Narrative and resilience: A comparative analysis of how older adults story their lives. *Journal of Aging Studies*, 34, 155–161. Medline:26162736. https:// doi.org/10.1016/j.jaging.2015.02.010

Randall, W., & Kenyon, G. (2001). *Ordinary wisdom: Biographical aging and the journey of life.* Westport: Praeger.

Randall, W., & Kenyon, G. (2002). Reminiscence as reading our lives: Toward a wisdom environment. In J. Webster & B. Haight (Eds.), *Critical advances in reminiscence work: From theory to application* (pp. 233–253). New York: Springer.

Randall, W., & Khurshid, K. (2017). Narrative development in later life: A novel perspective. *Aging, Culture, Humanities: An Interdisciplinary Journal*, 3, 125–161. https://doi.org/10.7146/ageculturehumanities.v3i.130158

Randall, W., Lewis, B., & Achenbaum, A. (2022). *Fairy tale wisdom: Stories for the second half of life.* ElderPress.

Randall, W., & McKim, E. (2008). *Reading our lives: The poetics of growing old.* New York: Oxford University Press.

Randall, W., Prior, S., & Skarborn, M. (2006). How listeners shape what tellers tell: Patterns of interaction in lifestory interviews and their impact on reminiscence with elderly interviewees. *Journal of Aging Studies*, 20, 381–396. https://doi.org/10.1016/j.jaging.2005.11.005

Ray, R. (2000). *Beyond nostalgia: Aging and life-story writing.* Charlottesville: University Press of Virginia.

Ray, R. (2004). Toward the croning of feminist gerontology. *Journal of Aging Studies*, 18, 109–121. https://doi.org/10.1016/j.jaging.2003.09.008

Reissman, K., & Speedy, J. (2007). Narrative inquiry in the psychotherapy professions: A critical review. In J. Clandinin (Ed.), *Handbook of narrative inquiry: Mapping a methodology* (pp. 426–456). Thousand Oaks: Sage.

Reker, G., & Chamberlain, K. (Eds.). (2000). *Exploring existential meaning: Optimizing human development across the lifespan.* Thousand Oaks: Sage.

Resnick, B., Gwyther, L., & Roberto, K. (Eds.). (2011). *Resilience in aging: Concepts, research, and outcomes.* New York: Springer.

Richardson, L. (1994). Writing: A method of inquiry. In N. Denzin & Y. Lincoln (Eds.), *A handbook of qualitative research.* Thousand Oaks: Sage.

Ricoeur, P. (1981). Narrative time. In W.J.T. Mitchell (Ed.), *On narrative* (pp. 165–186). Chicago: University of Chicago Press.

Riordan, R. (2016). *The hammer of Thor.* Disney Hyperion.

Robinson, M. (2004). *Gilead.* San Francisco: HarperPerennial

Rogerson, M. (1998). Reading the patchworks in *Alias Grace. Journal of Commonwealth Literature,* 33(1), 5–22. https://doi.org/10.1177/002200949803300102

Rosenblatt, L. (1978). *The reader, the text, the poem: The transactional theory of the literary work.* Carbondale: Southern Illinois University Press.

Rosenblatt, L. (1985). Viewpoints: Transaction versus interaction – A terminological rescue operation. *Research in the Teaching of English,* 19, 96–107.

Rosenblatt, L. (1986). The aesthetic transaction. *Journal of Aesthetic Education,* 20, 122–127. https://doi.org/10.2307/3332615

Rosenblatt, L. (1994). The transactional theory of reading and writing. In H. Singer & R. Ruddell, (Eds.), *Theoretical models and processes of reading* (pp. 1057–1092). Newark: International Reading Association.

Rotter, J.B. (1966). Generalized expectancies for internal versus external control of reinforcement. *Psychological Monographs: General and Applied, 80*(1), 1–28. https://doi.org/10.1037/h0092976

Rubin, D. (1995). Introduction. In D. Rubin (Ed.), *Remembering our past: Studies in autobiographical memory* (pp. 1–15). New York: Cambridge University Press.

Rubinstein, R. (1987). The significance of personal objects to older people. *Journal of Aging Studies,* 1(3), 225–238. Medline:25195721. https://doi.org/10.1016/0890-4065(87)90015-6

Ruffing, J. (2011). *To tell the sacred tale: Spiritual direction and narrative.* Mahwah: Paulist Press.

Ruth, J.-E., & Kenyon, G. (1996). Biography in adult development and aging. In J. Birren, G. Kenyon, J.-E. Ruth, J. Schroots, & T. Svensson (Eds.), *Aging and biography: Explorations in adult development* (pp. 1–20). New York: Springer.

Ruth, J.-E., & Öberg, P. (1996). Ways of life: Old age in a life history perspective. In J. Birren, G. Kenyon, J-E. Ruth, J. Schroots, & T. Svensson (Eds.), *Aging and biography: Explorations in adult development* (pp. 167–186). New York: Springer.

Ruth, J.-E., & Vilkko, A. (1996). Emotions in the construction of autobiography. In C. Maggai & S. McFadden (Eds.), *Handbook of emotion, adult development, and aging* (pp. 167–181). San Diego: Academic Press.

Ryan, E., Elliot, G., & Meredith, S. (Eds.). (1999). *From me to you: Intergenerational connections through storytelling.* Hamilton: Centre for Gerontological Studies, McMaster University.

Ryan, E., Pearce, K., Anas, A., & Norris, J. (2004). Writing a connection: Intergenerational communication through stories. In M. Pratt & B. Fiese (Eds.), *Family stories and the life course: Across time and generations* (pp. 375–398). Mahwah: Erlbaum.

Sacks, O. (1987). *The man who mistook his wife for a hat, and other clinical tales.* New York: Summit.

Sandell, R., Lennon, R., & Smith, M. (2018). *Prejudice and pride: LGBTQ heritage and its contemporary implications.* Research Centre for Museums and Galleries, University of Leicester.

Sarbin, T. (1986). The narrative as a root metaphor for psychology. In T. Sarbin (Ed.), *Narrative psychology: The storied nature of human conduct* (pp. 3–21). New York: Praeger.

Sarbin, T. (1998). Believed-in imaginings: A narrative approach. In J. de Rivera & T. Sarbin (Eds.), *Believed-in imaginings: The narrative construction of reality* (pp. 15–30). Washington, DC: American Psychological Association.

Sarton, M. (1977). *Journal of a solitude.* New York: W.W. Norton.

Sarton, M. (1981). *The house by the sea.* New York: W.W. Norton.

Schachter-Shalomi, Z., & Miller, R. (1995). *From age-ing to sage-ing: A profound new vision of growing older.* New York: Warner.

Schacter, D. (1996). *Searching for memory: The brain, the mind, and the past.* New York: Basic Books.

Schaie, K., & Willis, S. (2000). A stage theory model of adult cognitive development revised. In R. Rubinstein, M. Moss, & M. Kleban (Eds.), *The many dimensions of aging* (pp. 175–193). New York: Springer.

Schiff, B., McKim, E., & Patron, S. (Eds.). (2017). *Life and narrative: The risks and responsibilities of storying experience.* New York: Oxford University Press.

Schofield, G., Larsson, B., & Ward, E. (2017). Risk, resilience, and identity construction in the life narratives of young people leaving residential care. *Child and Family Social Work*, 22, 782–791. https://doi.org/10.1111/cfs.12295

Schopenhauer, A. (2004). *Counsels and maxims* (T.B. Saunders, Trans.). Whitefish: Kessinger.

Scott-Maxwell, F. (1968). *The measure of my days.* London: Penguin.

Senft, C. (1995). Cultural artifact and architectural form: A museum of quilts and quilt making. *Journal of Architectural Education*, 48(3), 144–153. https://doi.org/10.2307/1425349

Sherman, E. (1991a). *Reminiscence and the self in old age.* New York: Springer.

Sherman, E. (1991b). Reminiscentia: Cherished objects as memorabilia in late life reminiscence. *International Journal of Aging and Human Development*, 33(2), 89–100. Medline:1955210. https://doi.org/10.2190/FJW1-60UF-WW1R-FP2K

Sherman, E. (1994). The structure of well-being in the life narratives of the elderly. *Journal of Aging Studies*, 8(2), 149–158. https://doi.org/10.1016/S0890-4065(05)80003-9

Sherman, E. (2010). *Contemplative aging: A way of being in later life.* Pennsauken, NJ: BookBaby.

Sherman, E., & Dacher, J. (2005). Cherished objects and the home: Their meaning and roles in late life. In G.D. Holmes and H. Chaudhury (Eds.), *Home and identity in late life: International perspectives* (pp. 63–79). New York: Springer.

Sherman, E., & Newman, E.S. (1978). The meaning of cherished personal possessions for the elderly. *International Journal of Aging and Human Development*, 8(2), 181–192. Medline:892918. https://doi.org/10.2190/m1h4-2ntb-92ga-ak32

Shields, C., & Anderson, M. (Eds.). (2001). *Dropped threads: What we aren't told.* Toronto: Vintage Canada.

Sierpina, M. (2007, Fall). Pentimento Project: Celebrating the power of lifestory writing and sharing groups. *LLI Review*, 7, 84–94.

Sinats, P., Scott, D., McFerran, S., Hittos, M., Cragg, C., LeBlanc, T., & Brooks, D. (2005). Writing ourselves into being: Writing as spiritual self-care for adolescent girls. Part One. *International Journal of Children's Spirituality*, 10(1), 17–29. https://doi.org/10.1080/13644360500039329

Singer, J. (1996). The story of your life: A process perspective on narrative and emotion in adult development. In C. Magai & S. McFadden (Eds.), *Handbook of emotion, adult development, and aging* (pp. 443–463). San Diego: Academic Press.

Singer, J., & Blagov, P. (2004). The integrative function of narrative processing: Autobiographical memory, self-defining memories, and the life story of identity. In D. Beike, J. Lampinen, & D. Behrend (Eds.), *The self and memory* (pp. 117–138). New York: Psychology Press.

Singer, J., & Bluck, S. (2001). New perspectives on autobiographical memory: The integration of narrative processing and autobiographical reasoning. *Review of General Psychology*, 5, 91–99. https://doi.org/10.1037/1089-2680.5.2.91

Singer, J., & Skerrett, K. (2014). *Positive couple therapy: Using we-stories to enhance resilience.* New York: Routledge.

Smith, B., & Montforte, J. (2020). Stories, new materialism and pluralism: Understanding, practising, and pushing the boundaries of narrative analysis. *Methods in Psychology*, 2. 1–8. https://doi.org/10.1016/j.metip.2020.100016

Smith, D. (1987). *The everyday world as problematic: A feminist sociology.* Toronto: University of Toronto Press.

Smith, J., & Freund, A. (2002). The dynamics of possible selves in old age. *Journal of Gerontology: Psychological Sciences*, 57B(6), P492–P500. Medline:12426431. https://doi.org/10.1093/geronb/57.6.p492

Snaza, N., Sonu, D., Truman, S., & Zaliwska, Z. (Eds.). (2016). *Pedagogical matters: New materialisms and curriculum studies.* New York: Peter Lang.

Solanki, A., Bateman, T., Boswell, G., & Hill, E. (2006). *Anti-social behaviour orders*. London: Youth Justice Board.

Soltys, F., & Kunz, J. (2007). Reminiscence group work. In J. Kunz & F. Soltys (Eds.), *Transformational reminiscence: Life story work* (pp. 85–107). New York: Springer.

Spector-Mersel, G. (2011). Mechanisms of selection in claiming narrative identities: A model for interpreting narratives. *Qualitative Inquiry*, 17(2), 172–185. https://doi.org/10.1177/1077800410393885

Spector-Mersel, G. (2017). Life story reflection in social work education: A practical model. *Journal of Social Work Education*, 53(2), 286–299. https://doi .org/10.1080/10437797.2016.1243498

Staudinger, U., Marsiske, M., & Baltes, P. (1995). Resilience and reserve capacity in later adulthood: Potentials and limits of development across the life span. In D. Cicchetti & D. Cohen (Eds.), *Developmental psychopathology*, Vol. 2: *Risk, disorder, and adaptation* (pp. 801–847). New York: John Wiley.

Sternberg, R.J. (1998). *Love is a story: A new theory of relationships*. New York: Oxford University Press.

Stevens, D., Camic, P., & Solway, R. (2019). Maintaining the self: Meanings of material objects after a residential transition later in life. *Educational Gerontology*, 45(3), 214–226. https://doi.org/10.1080/03601277.2019.1601832

Stone, E. (2008). *Black sheep and kissing cousins: How our family stories shape us*. New Brunswick, NJ: Transaction.

Stout, D., & Chaminade, T. (2012). Stone tools, language, and the brain in human evolution. *Philosophical Transactions of the Royal Society London B: Biological Sciences*, 367(1585), 75–87. Medline:22106428. https://doi.org /10.1098/rstb.2011.0099

Synnes, O. (2015). Narratives of nostalgia in the face of death: The importance of lighter stories of the past in palliative care. *Journal of Aging Studies*, 34, 169–176. Medline:26162738. https://doi.org/10.1016/j.jaging.2015.02.007

Synnes, O., & Frank, A. (2020). Home as cultural imaginary at the end of life. In B. Pasveer, O. Synnes, & I. Moser (Eds.), *Ways of home making in care for later life* (pp. 19–40). London: Palgrave Macmillan.

Taylor, D. (2001). *Tell me a story: The life-shaping power of our stories*. St. Paul: Bog Walk.

Taylor, S., & Brown, J. (1994). Positive illusions and well-being revisited: Separating fact from fiction. *Psychological Bulletin*, 116(1), 21–27. Medline:8078971. https://doi.org/10.1037/0033-2909.116.1.21

Thomas, T. (2014). "Once a foster child …": Identity construction in former foster children's narratives. *Qualitative Research Reports in Communication*, 15(1), 84–91. https://doi.org/10.1080/17459435.2014.955596

Thompson, K. (2011). *Therapeutic journal writing: An introduction for professionals*. London: Jessica Kingsley.

Thompson, L., & Chatterjee, H. (2014). Assessing well-being outcomes for arts and heritage activities: Development of a museum well-being measures toolkit. *Journal of Applied Arts and Health*, 5(1), 29–50. https://doi.org/10.1386/jaah.5.1.29_1

Tobin, S. (1996). Cherished possessions: The meaning of things. *Generations*, 20(3), 46–49.

Tornstam, L. (1997). Gerotranscendence: The contemplative dimension of aging. *Journal of Aging Studies*, 11(2), 143–154. https://doi.org/10.1016/S0890-4065(97)90018-9

Turner, M. (1996). *The literary mind.* New York: Oxford University Press.

Ulrich, L.T. (2001). *The age of homespun: Objects and stories in the creation of an American myth.* New York: Vintage.

Van Hoof, J., Janssen, M., Heesakkers, C., Van Kersbergen, W., Severijns, L., Willems, L., Marston, H., Janssen, B., & Nieboer, M. (2016). The importance of possessions for the development of a sense of home of nursing home residents. *Journal of Housing for the Elderly*, 30(1), 35–51. https://doi.org/10.1080/02763893.2015.1129381

Wagamese, R. (2012). *Indian horse.* Madeira Park: Douglas & McIntyre.

Wahlstrom, R.L. (2006). *The Tao of writing: Imagine. create. flow.* Avon: Adams Media.

Wakefield, D. (1990). *The story of your life: Writing a spiritual autobiography.* Boston: Beacon.

Walker, J. (2016). Spiritual development in later life. In M. Johnson & J. Walker (Eds.), *Spiritual dimensions of ageing* (pp. 249–269). Cambridge: Cambridge University Press.

Wapner, S., Demick, J., & Redondo, J.P. (1990). Cherished possessions and adaptation of older people to nursing homes. *International Journal of Aging and Human Development*, 31(3), 219–235. Medline:2272702. https://doi.org/10.2190/GJPL-ATJY-KJA3-8C99

Webster, J. (2002). Reminiscence functions in adulthood: Age, race, and family dynamics correlates. In J. Webster & B. Haight (Eds.), *Critical advances in reminiscence: From theory to application* (pp. 140–152). New York: Springer.

Webster, J. (2003). An exploratory analysis of a self-assessed wisdom scale. *Journal of Adult Development*, 10, 13–22. https://doi.org/10.1023/A:1020782619051

Webster, J. (2011). A new measure of time perspective: Initial psychometric findings for the Balanced Time Perspective Scale (BTPS). *Canadian Journal of Behavioural Science / Revue Canadienne Des Sciences Du Comportement*, 43(2), 111–118.

Webster, M. (2008). *Quilts: Their story and how to make them* [ebook #24682].

White, M., & Epston, D. (1990). *Narrative means to therapeutic ends.* New York: W.W. Norton.

Whitmore, E. (2005a, February 26). Literary environment: Women's environmental strategies in nineteenth-century Canada [Paper presentation].

13th Annual Conference on Student Research, University of New Brunswick, Fredericton, NB.

Whitmore, E. (2005b, June 21). "'Trilobite cookies' and other delicacies: Femininity, environmentalism, and literature in early Canadian Natural History Societies" [Paper presentation]. Living and Being in the Word Conference, Association for the Study of Literature and Environment, University of Oregon, Eugene, OR.

Williams, R. (2007). *Where God happens: Discovering Christ in one another* (2nd ed.). Boston: New Seeds.

Willis, P. (1977). *Learning to labour: How working class kids get working class jobs.* Farnborough: Saxon House.

Wilson, S. (2009). Quilting as narrative art: Metafictional construction in *Alias Grace.* In H. Bloom (Ed.), *Margaret Atwood: Bloom's modern critical views* (2nd edition). New York: Chelsea House.

Wingard, B., & Lester, J. (2001). *Telling our stories in ways that make us stronger.* Adelaide: Dulwich Centre.

Wink, P., & Schiff, B. (2002). To review or not to review? The role of personality and life events in life review and adaptation to older age. In J. Webster & B. Haight (Eds.), *Critical advances in reminiscence: From theory to application* (pp. 44–60). New York: Springer.

Witzling, M. (2009). Quilt language: Towards a poetics of quilting. *Women's History Review,* 18(4), 619–637. https://doi.org/10.1080/09612020903138351

Wong, P. (1995). The processes of adaptive reminiscence. In B. Haight & J. Webster (Eds.), *The art and science of reminiscing: Theory, research, methods, and applications* (pp. 23–35). Washington, DC: Taylor and Francis.

Wong, P., & Watt, L. (1991). What types of reminiscence are associated with successful aging? *Psychology and Aging,* 6(2), 272–279. Medline:1863396. https://doi.org/10.1037//0882-7974.6.2.272

Woodward, K. (2003). Against wisdom: The social politics of anger and aging. *Journal of Aging Studies,* 17(1), 55–67. https://doi.org/10.1016/S0890-4065(02)00090-7

Woolf, V. (1944). Solid objects. In *A haunted house and other stories,* collected by Leonard Woolf (82). New York: Harcourt, Brace.

Yngvesson, B. (2003). Going "home": Adoption, loss of bearings, and the mythology of roots. *Social Text,* 24(1), 7–27. https://doi.org/10.1215/01642472-21-1_74-7

Index

www.ingramcontent.com/pod-product-compliance
Lightning Source LLC
Chambersburg PA
CBHW020453030426
42337CB00011B/97
9781487524470